D1756264

Landmark Papers in Neurology

Landmark Papers in . . . series

Titles in the series

Landmark Papers in Rheumatology
Edited by Richard A. Watts and David G. I. Scott

Landmark Papers in Neurosurgery, Second Edition
Edited by Reuben D. Johnson and Alexander L. Green

Landmark Papers in Anaesthesia
Edited by Nigel R. Webster and Helen F. Galley

Landmark Papers in Nephrology
Edited by John Feehally, Christopher McIntyre, and J. Stewart Cameron

Landmark Papers in Allergy
Edited by Aziz Sheikh, Thomas Platts-Mills, and Allison Worth

Landmark Papers in General Surgery
Edited by Graham MacKay, Richard Molloy, and Patrick O'Dwyer

Landmark Papers in Cardiovascular Medicine
Edited by Aung Myat and Tony Gershlick

Landmark Papers in Neurology

Edited by

Martin R. Turner
Nuffield Department of Clinical Neurosciences,
University of Oxford, Oxford, UK

Matthew C. Kiernan
Brain and Mind Research Institute,
The University of Sydney, Camperdown, Australia

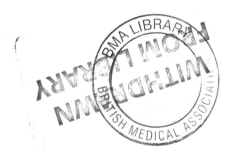

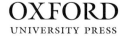

UNIVERSITY PRESS

UNIVERSITY PRESS

Great Clarendon Street, Oxford, OX2 6DP,
United Kingdom

Oxford University Press is a department of the University of Oxford.
It furthers the University's objective of excellence in research, scholarship,
and education by publishing worldwide. Oxford is a registered trade mark of
Oxford University Press in the UK and in certain other countries

Published in the United States of America by Oxford University Press
198 Madison Avenue, New York, NY 10016, United States of America

British Library Cataloguing in Publication Data
Data available

Library of Congress Control Number: 2015937783

ISBN 978–0–19–965860–2

Printed and bound by
CPI Group (UK) Ltd, Croydon, CR0 4YY

Acknowledgements

We dedicate this book to Sally and Clare, in recognition of their support throughout this 'landmarks' expedition. The pursuit of knowledge, in any academic discipline, belies an inherent conflict that does nothing to ease the day-to-day challenges imposed by children and their busy lifestyles. The tolerance of our wives is enormously appreciated, though not assumed.

We thank our children (Abigail and Barnaby; Tighe, Roisin, Saoirse, and Jarlath) for their entertainment; our parents (David and Pamela; Joan and Colm) for their wisdom and belief; and our siblings (Sarah; Carol and Margaret) for their essential contributions to the tapestry of life.

The value of this book hinged on the participation of true experts in their fields. Book chapter writing is a very hard sell to busy academics, and we are grateful for the enthusiasm our authors showed for this concept.

Contents

Contributors

James R. Burrell
Neuroscience Research Australia,
and University of New South Wales,
Randwick, Australia

Alan Carson
Robert Fergusson Unit,
Royal Edinburgh Hospital,
Edinburgh, UK

Patrick F. Chinnery
Mitochondrial Research Group,
Institute for Ageing and Health,
Newcastle University,
Newcastle, UK

Alasdair Coles
Department of Clinical Neurosciences,
University Neurology Unit,
Cambridge Biomedical Campus,
Cambridge, UK

Alastair Compston
Department of Clinical Neurosciences,
University Neurology Unit,
Cambridge Biomedical Campus,
Cambridge, UK

David R. Cornblath
Department of Neurology,
Johns Hopkins University School
of Medicine,
Baltimore, USA

Andrew Eisen
Neurology UBC,
Vancouver, Canada

Jennifer Fugate
Division of Critical Care Neurology,
Mayo Clinic,
Rochester, USA

Jan van Gijn
Department of Neurology and
Neurosurgery,
University Medical Centre,
Utrecht, The Netherlands

Peter J. Goadsby
Headache Group,
NIHR-Wellcome Trust Clinical
Research Facility,
King's College London
London, UK

Gráinne S. Gorman
Mitochondrial Research Group,
Institute for Ageing and Health,
Newcastle University,
Newcastle, UK

John R. Hodges
Neuroscience Research Australia and
University of New South Wales,
Randwick, Australia

Gregory L. Holmes
Department of Neurological Sciences
University of Vermont College of
Medicine,
Burlington, USA

Richard A.C. Hughes
Cochrane Neuromuscular Disease Group,
MRC Centre for Neuromuscular Disease,
National Hospital for Neurology and
Neurosurgery,
Queen Square,
London, UK

Matthew C. Kiernan
Brain and Mind Research Institute,
The University of Sydney,
Camperdown, Australia

Satoshi Kuwabara
Department of Neurology,
Graduate School of Medicine,
Chiba University,
Chiba, Japan

A. J. Lees
Reta Lila Weston Institute of
Neurological Studies,
University College London,
London, UK

Jon Stone
Department of Clinical Neurosciences,
Western General Hospital,
Edinburgh, UK

Elsdon Storey
Department of Neuroscience,
Monash University,
Alfred Hospital,
Melbourne, Australia

Michael Swash
Departments of Neurology and
Neuroscience,
Royal London Hospital,
Queen Mary University of London,
London, UK,
Institute of Neuroscience, University
of Lisbon,
Lisbon, Portugal

Kevin Talbot
Nuffield Department of Clinical
Neurosciences,
University of Oxford,
Oxford, UK

Martin R. Turner
Nuffield Department of Clinical
Neurosciences,
University of Oxford,
Oxford, UK

Angela Vincent
Nuffield Department of Clinical
Neurosciences,
John Radcliffe Hospital,
Oxford, UK

Charles Warlow
Department of Clinical Neurosciences,
Western General Hospital,
Edinburgh, UK

Eelco Wijdicks
Division of Critical Care Neurology,
Mayo Clinic,
Rochester, USA

Chapter 1

Technical advances in neuroscience

Martin R. Turner, Matthew C. Kiernan,
and Kevin Talbot

1.0 **Introduction**

Advances in neuroscience knowledge, mapped out in each chapter of this book, were the product of clinico-anatomical methods pioneered by Charcot, Gowers, and Osler, combined with great technological developments over past centuries. The study of the brain and mind emerged from what were essentially elitist gentlemen's clubs. Surgeons, with those variably designated physicians, anatomists, and pathologists, all contributed to what would take many decades to coalesce as the modern concept of neuroscience. Books were then the preserve of a relatively few privileged scholars. Ideas were proffered and debated in printed correspondence, far from the modern digital delivery at the press of a button from all continents of the globe.

The science fiction writer and scholar, Isaac Asimov (1920–1992), eluded to the fact that it has often been serendipitous observations from the application of technology that has characterized major scientific advances: 'The most exciting phrase to hear in science, the one that heralds new discoveries, is not "Eureka!" (I found it!) but "That's funny . . ."' [1]. Predictions of the technological future have often been spectacularly misjudged, either through over-inflated visions of fledgling concepts, or entirely unimagined ones. Key technologies that allowed the testing of neuronal functions undoubtedly catalysed the intellectual leaps in the understanding of the nervous system in health and disease. The core technologies that have driven the very rapid developments in neuroscience have emerged from a period of less than a century and can be divided into those associated with neuroimaging, neurotransmission, and molecular biology.

Neuroimaging spans the sub-cellular and systems levels of neuroscience, beginning with electron microscopy and then, 50 years later, magnetic resonance imaging and increasingly sophisticated mathematical modelling of brain function. These developments have been interleaved with the improved understanding of neurotransmission, starting with the seminal observations made from giant squid axon recordings, which were translated into clinically useable tools through the application of electric current, and later with magnetic stimulation. It is during the last 50 years that a molecular framework for these concepts emerged, with the cloning of genes that began in Duchenne muscular dystrophy, paving the way for the wider human genome project. The visualization of the downstream cellular consequences of genetic dysfunction was then transformed by the discovery of green fluorescent protein, and the production of disease-specific neurons through reprogramming of stem cells heralds new possibilities for the modelling of neurological disease.

1.1 **Electron microscopy of the nervous system**

Main paper: Knoll M, Ruska EZ. Das elektronenmikroskop. *Physik* 1832; 78:318–39.

Background

The oldest known sketch of the nervous system has been attributed to the polymath Ibn al-Haytham (965–*c*.1040) and is said to be based on the teachings of the Roman physician, Galen of Pergamum, nine centuries prior [2]. From the earliest detailed gross anatomy of the brain observed by English physician Thomas Willis (1621–1675) and documented by his colleague and preeminent architect, Christopher Wren (1632–1723) [3], to the exquisite drawings of neuronal circuitry by Spanish neuroscientist and Nobel Laureate, Santiago Ramón y Cajal (1852–1934), the images that continue to dominate and define neuroscience seem to oscillate between the large and very small. This ongoing struggle to reconcile the 'cell' and the 'system' in neuroscience has clear parallels in the particle and astronomical branches of modern physics. Perhaps it should come as no surprise that it is technological leaps in physics that have had the most profound impact on the development of neuroscience.

The Dutch draper and lens maker, Antonie Philips van Leeuwenhoek (1632–1723), is credited with the first observation of single-celled organisms, for which he used the Latin term *animalcules* ('little animals'). He constructed over 500 microscopes, several with a magnification of over 250 times, but was notoriously unwilling to share his lens-making secrets. The Royal Society of London published his letter in 1673 detailing his observations of lice, among other things. Thus began a regular correspondence of ideas seemingly far from the modern constraints of peer review, although the Society soon dispatched observers in response to increasing scepticism voiced by other scientists about Leeuwenhoek's findings.

The cell is a fundamental unit in biology, and it was the English polymath, Robert Hooke (1635–1703), who first coined the term in relation to the appearance of 'compartments' in magnified cork tissue, documented in his 1665 book *Micrographia*. Hooke had worked with both Thomas Willis and Robert Boyle during his time in Oxford. He was an architect and, as well as performing the majority of the surveys after the Great Fire of London, Hooke curated many experiments at the Royal Society.

> By the means of Telescopes, there is nothing so far distant but may be represented to our view; and by the help of Microscopes, there is nothing so small as to escape our inquiry; hence there is a new visible World discovered to the understanding. By this means the Heavens are open'd and a vast number of new Stars and new Motions, and new Productions appear in them, to which all the ancient Astronomers were utterly strangers. By this the Earth itself, which lyes so neer to us, under our feet, shews quite a new thing to us, and in every little particle of its matter, we now behold almost as great a variety of Creatures, as we were able before to reckon up in the whole Universe itself. [4]

The eventual visualization of the contents of Hooke's cells provided the foundations for the modern understanding of cell biology, though the existence of such sub-cellular structures was questioned and, if present at all, were thought likely to be too dynamic and transient to visualize. The resolution of optical microscopes is inherently limited by the wavelength of the illuminating light, and so a leap in technology was needed.

Methods

In 1924, French physicist, Louis (seventh duc) de Broglie (1892–1987), published a dissertation, *Recherches sur la théorie des quanta* (Research on Quantum Theory), hypothesizing that all matter, notably electrons, possessed a wave property similar to light. He went on to receive the Nobel Prize for Physics for his wider theory in 1929 [5]. Electrons have wavelengths thousands of times shorter than those of light, and it was a German electrical engineer, Ernst August Friedrich Ruska (1906–1988), only in his twenties at the time, who suggested that focusing electrons on an object would yield far greater resolution than conventional light microscopes.

Results

With his colleague, Max Knoll (1897–1969), Ruska's prototype electron microscope (EM) was constructed in 1929, and consisted of a cathode-ray tube with a coil to focus the electron beam and form the image of an object on a fluorescent screen. By 1931, the application of two electromagnetic lenses had achieved 16-fold magnification (Fig. 1.1).

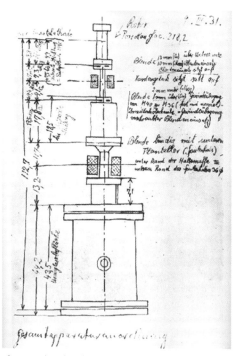 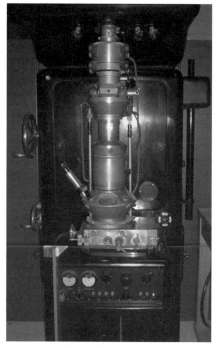

Fig. 1.1 Sketches by Ernst Ruska (left) and his prototype electron microscope c.1933 (right).

Fig. 1.1(left) reproduced from *Ann. Phys.*, 404(6), Knoll, M. and Ruska, E., Beitrag zur geometrischen Elektronenoptik. II., p. 641–661, Copyright (1932), with permission from John Wiley and Sons.

Fig. 1.1(right) reproduced from Electron Microscope Deutsches Museum, First Electron Microscope with Resolving Power Higher than that of a Light Microscope, taken from <https://www.flickr.com/photos/93452909@N00/176059674>, reprinted with permission under the Creative Commons License 2.0.

In addition to the technical hurdles, many thought that the vacuum required for the instrument and the intensity of the electron beam would threaten the preservation of the very structures under study. Two companies, Siemens & Halske in Berlin and Carl Zeiss in Jena, took on the challenge. Ruska joined Siemens as a research engineer in 1937 and two years later, the first commercial electron microscope was produced. Ernst's brother, Helmut (a physician), was greatly enthused and, together with physicist Bodo von Borries, went on to apply electron microscopy to visualize viruses for the first time [6]. Later developments included the scanning electron microscope for more detailed surface images, magnifications of the order of 500,000 times, and images with nanometer resolution.

Conclusions and critique

A fuller appreciation, if not also direct visualization of the microscopic world, has arguably increased human survival more than any other scientific knowledge. In neuroscience, an understanding of physical neuronal interactions and axonal microstructure has been pivotal as a framework to comprehend the non-directly observable underlying biochemical pathways (Fig. 1.2). There are inherent limitations with electron microscopy however. Specimens have to be observed in a vacuum and the tissues fixed prior. If non-conductive, then the surface at least must be sprayed, typically with gold alloy.

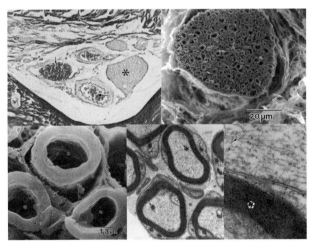

Fig. 1.2 Light microscopy (top left) shows the nerve (*) with surrounding blood vessels (arrows). Progressive magnification using scanning electron microscopy of the nerve in cross-section (top right and bottom left) with nerve fibres (*) and collagen (arrow). Individual mitochondria can be seen (bottom middle (arrows)), inside myelinated nerves, with endoneurial collagen fibres (*) and the Schwann cell lamina (**) at 4440x magnification. At 42,000x magnification (bottom right), the laminae of the myelin (*) and individual neurofilaments (arrow) can be seen.

Reproduced with permission from Prof. Dr. Ii-sei Watanabe, Institute of Biomedical Sciences, University of São Paulo.

Ruska performed research at Siemens until 1955. For his electron microscope, he received the Nobel Prize for Physics in 1986 (shared with Heinrich Rohrer and Gerd Binnig for their design of the scanning tunnelling microscope, which allows surface imaging at the atomic level). Ruska commented at the end of his Nobel lecture:

> We should not, therefore, blame those scientists today who did not believe in electron microscopy at its beginning. It is a miracle that by now the difficulties have been solved to an extent that so many scientific disciplines today can reap its benefits. [7]

He also observed that his discovery was not the end of the story:

> The light microscope opened the 1st gate to the microcosm. The electron microscope opened the 2nd gate. What will we find opening the 3rd gate? [8]

1.2 **Towards a molecular understanding of neurotransmission**

Main paper: Hodgkin AL, Huxley AFJ. A quantitative description of membrane current and its application to conduction and excitation in nerve. *Physiol* 1952; 117; 500–44.

Background

Neuroscience is at an exciting crossroads—one where the mind and the computer meet. Cutting-edge technology is allowing computers to read our minds and our minds to control computers. Even more ambitious aims lie ahead—it is conceivable that brain-implanted microchips will eradicate the need for computers as we know them, and that damaged body parts may be replaced by neuroprostheses. Much of the original knowledge regarding the workings of the human nervous system was derived from *in vitro* and *in vivo* approaches in cellular and animal models. However, the advent of technological advances has led to new concepts in the understanding of human nerve activation, signal transmission, and brain information processing, with the translation of the original techniques into a clinical setting. The fundamental concept that governs the entirety of neuroscience relates to neurotransmission. Central to describing neurotransmission is an understanding of the 'action potential'. Neural transmission involving myelinated axons of the human nervous system occurs by means of salutatory conduction (Fig. 1.3), with action potentials advancing between successive nodes of Ranvier:

> Like a kangaroo travelling at speed, the action potential advances at near-uniform velocity, but it is powered by discrete kicks of inward membrane current at nodes of Ranvier. [9]

The chief role of human axons remains that of impulse transmission and information processing, which in turn depends on the electrical cable structure, voltage-dependent ion channels of the axonal membrane, and neurotransmitters. While Louis-Antoine Ranvier (1835–1922) established the existence of nodes in myelinated axons more than a hundred years ago, it has only been over recent decades that an understanding of the molecular structure of the axonal membrane and its constituent ion channels has developed.

Methods

From 1948 to 1952, Alan Hodgkin (1914–1998) and Andrew Huxley (1917–2012) reprised their work on the giant squid axon, based in Plymouth. The pair had originally started their research in 1938, using Hodgkin's university laboratories based in Cambridge, which he then subsequently transported in his car and trailer to Plymouth. Plymouth had been chosen as a source of giant squid axons. Previous work had been undertaken across a range of species—Carcinus (crab), Sepia (cuttlefish), frogs, and lobsters—but Hodgkin realised that Loligo (squid) provided a big enough mass of tissue into which an electrode could be inserted.

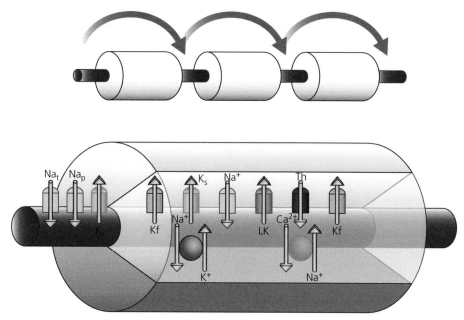

Fig. 1.3 (Upper panel) Saltatory conduction, with the action potential (arrow) jumping from one node of Ranvier to the next. (Lower panel) Molecular dissection of the axon: different channels are distributed unevenly along the axonal membrane. Sodium (Na+) channels are found in high concentrations at the node, as are slow potassium (K+) channels. Fast potassium channels (Kf) are almost exclusively paranodal. Inward rectifier channels (Ih), permeable to both K+ and Na+ ions, act to limit axonal hyperpolarization, whereas the Na+/K+ pump (circles) serves to reverse ionic fluxes that may be generated through activity.

Their early work was forced to be abandoned by the outbreak of the Second World War, although their skill sets were keenly taken up by the Royal Air Force, specifically for radar development:

> . . . by June 1940 the war had gone so disastrously and the
>
> need for centimetric radar was so pressing that I was forced
>
> to bury my interest in neurophysiology for nearly five years.[10]

On return to research after the war, and re-invigoration of their experimental set up in Plymouth, Hodgkin and Huxley encountered their next problem—no squid:

> First there have been no squid. . . Last Thursday I went out
>
> on the trawler. . . it got rough and I got very sick. . . we had
>
> much to learn about the best season and place to catch squid.[10]

With refinements in their fishing and experimental techniques, improved equipment, and prolonged periods of experimentation using a range of buffering solutions, Hodgkin and Huxley obtained all the voltage-clamp data that they needed to define their theory of nerve conduction and excitation. They were also supported by a network of collaborators, most notably, Bernard Katz (1911–2003) from mid-July 1949. Subsequent mathematical modelling techniques were crucial, with Huxley solving differential equations to develop and construct the original models of a computed action potential. However, it took the pair a further two years to analyse and write up their results from their experimental data obtained in Plymouth.

Results

Hodgkin and Huxley synthesized years of research and experimentation dating back to 1938 to create their 1952 classic citation [11]. They divided their manuscript into three parts: first, discussing results of their early studies; secondly, deriving a mathematical form of their experimental results; and, finally, establishing that the findings in entirety could account for the processes of nerve conduction and excitation. Specifically, they determined the total inward movement of sodium ions and the total outward movement of potassium ions associated with the passage of a nerve impulse. In their simple and typically understated way, the final sentence of their 1952 *Journal of Physiology* opus reads:

> It is concluded that the responses of an isolated giant axon of Loligo to electrical stimuli are due to reversible alterations in sodium and potassium permeability arising from changes in membrane potential.[11]

Conclusions and critique

On the basis of this landmark manuscript, Hodgkin and Huxley shared the Nobel Prize for Medicine in 1963 and both were subsequently to receive knighthoods. The understanding of impulse conduction spawned developments across all fields of neuroscience. The basic techniques developed for their original studies were made more universally accessible through development of patch clamping by Erwin Neher (1944–) and Bert Sakmann (1942–) in 1976, who in turn also shared the Nobel Prize in 1991. The patch clamping technique enabled a small area of membrane to be voltage-clamped to provide information about the current flow through individual ion channels. With a better understanding of ion channel physiology and function, there arose important therapeutic implications, as pharmacological manipulation of these channels and pumps provided new therapeutic strategies for neurological disorders. Specifically, these specialized techniques promoted drug discovery through incremental approaches of individual ion currents (e.g. anti-epileptic and pain medications exerting therapeutic effect via axonal sodium channels).

The discovery that virulent nerve poisons block the sodium channel has led, in turn, to understanding the mechanisms of conduction block. Tangentially, a review of bioterrorism suggested that biowarfare agents may critically include paralysing neurotoxins such as tetrodotoxin and saxitoxin [12]. These two naturally occurring neurotoxins cause

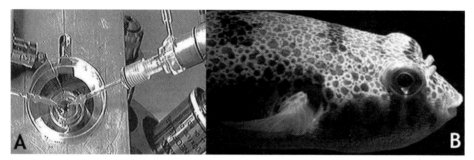

Fig. 1.4 Patch-clamp studies involving the investigation of Na+ channel function in dorsal root ganglia in the spinal cord. (A) Tetrodotoxin (TTX) may be accidentally ingested by consuming puffer fish (B)]. TTX is present in high concentrations in the liver, ovaries, intestines, and skin of these fish. Fugu (puffer fish fillets) is a delicacy in Japan and, although processing of fugu is licensed, puffer fish poisoning accounts for more deaths than any other type of food poisoning in Japan.

Reproduced from *The Lancet*, 4, Isbister GK, Kiernan MC, Neurotoxic marine poisoning, p. 219–228, Copyright (2005), with permission from Elsevier.

severe paralysis of prompt onset: both are derived from fish or shellfish—tetrodotoxin (from puffer fish), saxitoxin (from micro algae in bivalve shellfish)—and are effective after oral ingestion. These toxins bind to sodium channels, blocking propagation of nerve action potentials and, if consumed orally, cause paralysis within minutes to hours [13] (Fig. 1.4).

BMA

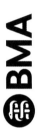

BMA Library

|.....||.|.|.||||||..||..||.|.|.||

Freepost RTKJ-RKSZ-JGHG
British Medical Association
PO Box 291
LONDON
WC1H 9TG

FREE RETURN POSTAGE FOR STUDENTS & FY DOCTORS!

Use this label for the **FREE** return of books to the BMA Library

1.3 **Diagnostic translations: the advent of clinical neurophysiology**

Main paper: Gilliatt RW, Sears TA. Sensory nerve action potentials in patients with peripheral lesions. *Journal of Neurology, Neurosurgery & Psychiatry* 1958; 21:109–18.

Background

For a neurologist, clinical neurophysiology represents the electrical equivalent of the stethoscope and, as such, an extension of the clinical examination. Clinical neurophysiological methods such as electroencephalography (EEG) and somatosensory and motor-evoked potentials have been adapted to investigate brain function, providing insight into the phenomenal plasticity of the brain. The most exciting aspect of these advances is that, when combined with powerful medical imaging, these techniques are starting to enable an understanding of the innermost workings of the brain and its role in determining our behaviour. At a more basic and fundamental level, clinical neurophysiology plays a critical role in the diagnosis, classification, and prognosis of neurological disease. In the peripheral nervous system, sensory and motor nerve conduction studies (NCS), in combination with electromyography, have remained the method of choice for the clinician investigating nerve function in patients.

Methods

Dr T.A. Sears graduated in 1952 and took up a position as a physiologist in the EEG Department at Queen Square. In the mid-1950s, Dr Roger Gilliatt (1922–1991), then a Senior Registrar at the Middlesex Hospital, attended the Queen Square clinic twice per week to learn and help with electromyograph (EMG) recordings. The pair combined their expertise to attempt to record sensory nerve responses in patients with peripheral nerve lesions. In their initial approaches, digital nerves of the fingers were stimulated with single electrical shocks and the action potential recorded over the median and ulnar nerves.

Results

Sears and Gilliatt determined that small sensory action potentials could be invariably recorded in normal subjects, such that the absence of a response could be regarded as a reliable sign of 'disturbed function'. Their early recording of nerve signals required 'averaging' and their photographic method drew on the fact that any stimulus time-locked signals would summate as 'latent images' in the emulsion to form a clear and discrete image, whereas random electrical or biological 'noise' would not. Specialized instrumentation was developed, coupled with good skin preparations and low-resistance electrodes, paramount for success to record 5–20 microvolts signals, being of even lower amplitude and dispersed in disease states.

Having established the technique, Gilliatt and Sears went on to study 41 neurological patients with a range of conditions, to establish that neuropathy was associated with small amplitude compound nerve potentials, that were delayed in latency. All carpal tunnel syndrome patients with severe sensory loss had abnormalities of their nerve potentials and the authors concluded that, as a diagnostic procedure, their method provided objective information about sensory nerve function and required minimal patient cooperation, other than asking the patient to lie in a relaxed state.

Conclusions and critique

Sears later recalled some scepticism from clinicians who seemed averse to electrophysiologically based laboratory findings [14]. With time, it became evident that slowed and blocked conduction with subsequent recovery was the hallmark of demyelination. However, it also soon became apparent that recovery processes such as remyelination, or axonal regeneration and remyelination, could lead to dissociation between clinical and laboratory findings—a major advance in understanding.

Based on this knowledge, these early techniques were adapted into further clinical neurophysiological methods such as somatosensory and motor-evoked potentials, to investigate specific cortical areas and to provide information regarding the mechanisms of cortical dysfunction and, later, neuroplasticity. Evoked potentials became the traditional neurophysiological technique employed by clinicians to aid localization of neurological abnormalities across the central and peripheral nervous system (e.g. central demyelination such as multiple sclerosis; Fig. 1.5). As a further example of adaptation of conventional technologies for more novel purposes, recent studies that incorporated evoked response technology have demonstrated alterations in sensorimotor representation in professional pianists following tactile stimulation, suggesting a stronger plasticity for cortical reorganization in this group [15].

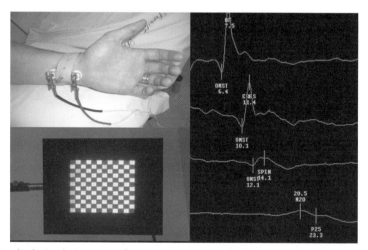

Fig. 1.5 Standard stimulating set-up for somatosensory evoked responses; and resultant evoked recording (right panel). Electrical stimulation of the ulnar nerve at the wrist (top left panel) evokes far-field potentials as the evoked signal passes through the axilla (AX; 'underarm'), Erb's point (brachial plexus), spinal cord (SPIN), and the cortex (N20 up-deviated wave recorded at 20 ms and positive wave P25 deviating downwards (right panel)). Conduction delays between segments can be used to localize the level of neurological disease (e.g. spinal cord versus cortical level). Visual chequer-board (lower left panel) is used to generate visual evoked recordings.

1.4 **Magnetic resonance imaging of the brain**

Main paper: Damadian R. Tumor detection by nuclear magnetic resonance. *Science* 1971; 171(3976):1151–3.

Background

German physicist, Wilhelm Conrad Röntgen (1845–1923), is credited with the discovery of X-rays in 1895, for which he received the Nobel Prize for Physics in 1901 (he did not give a lecture). He created the first X-ray image of a human body part, namely the bones of his wife Bertha's hand, with the radiopaque bulge of her wedding ring also clearly visible. On seeing the image she is said to have exclaimed 'I have seen my death!'. When, at the turn of the century, an Italian radiologist, Alessandro Vallebona (1899–1987), proposed a method to represent a single slice of the body, so began the rapid development of non-invasive human body imaging or 'tomography'.

In 1949, an electrical engineer, (later Sir) Godfrey Hounsfield (1919–2004), began work at EMI working on weapons' guidance and radar. He developed a computer for his idea of synthesizing data from X-rays applied at various angles around an object. The theoretical development needed for reconstruction of the image in slices was provided by South African physicist, Allan McLeod Cormack (1924–1998), and thus emerged computed (axial) tomography, the C(A)T scan, for which they shared the 1979 Nobel Prize for Physiology or Medicine [16, 17].

Methods

The concept of nuclear magnetic resonance began in 1946 with the Swiss physicist, Felix Bloch (1905–1983), and colleagues' 'Nuclear induction experiment' [18] and, independently, by American physicist, Edward Mills Purcell (1912–1997), and colleagues' 'Resonance absorption by nuclear magnetic moments in a solid' [19]. These experiments observed the variation in relaxation times of the nuclear magnetic moment of protons, for which Bloch and Purcell shared the Nobel Prize for Physics in 1952 [20, 21].

A quarter of a century later, American physician, Raymond Vahan Damadian (b. 1936), reported that tumours within several different tissues in rats, including the brain, could be distinguished by the 'motional freedom of the tissue water molecules' [22], and he obtained a patent for his whole-body human cancer-detecting apparatus (Fig. 1.6). Two years later, American chemist, Paul Lauterbur (1929–2007), coined the term 'zeugmatography' (from the Greek for 'joining') in relation to a novel concept that removed the image resolution limitation of the wavelength of the radiation field. Instead, he proposed observing the induced local interactions of two fields, one interacting with the object, and the other limiting the interaction to a small region (gradient field) [23].

British physicist, (later Sir) Peter Mansfield (b. 1933), then took up the baton. A true 'rocket scientist'—having first worked, aged 18, in the Rocket Propulsion Department of the UK Ministry of Supply—his PhD thesis (awarded in 1962) was entitled 'Proton magnetic resonance relaxation in solids by transient methods'. The leap into a clinical

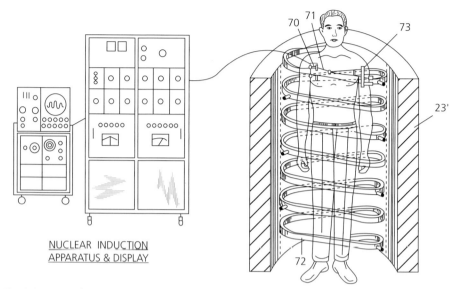

Fig. 1.6 Raymond Damadian's 'apparatus and method for detecting cancer in tissue'.
Reproduced from the US Patent and Trademark Office. Patent number 3789832 filed 17 March 1972, issued Feb 5, 1974.

application for magnetic resonance imaging (MRI) that he pioneered required the development of faster, 'pulsed' sequences and novel image reconstruction methods [24]. He and Lauterbur shared the Nobel Prize for Physiology or Medicine in 1990 [25, 26], but the absence of Damadian remains contentious [27].

Results

Specific application of MRI to the brain soon followed [28, 29], and faster sequences (e.g. echo-planar imaging (EPI)) and computer processing speeds, combined with cheaper and more compact data storage, allowed scanning times to drop dramatically. Research into the pathogenesis and therapeutic response in stroke, multiple sclerosis, and, more recently, neurodegenerative disorders, has come to rely heavily on MRI. However, it is the more recent advanced applications of MRI such as diffusion-weighted, and its later refinement, diffusion tensor imaging (DTI), that have taken MRI into the realm of *in vivo* histopathology, allowing the deeper integrity of white matter tracts to be probed in health and disease [30]. Being sensitive to the movement of water in tissues, not just the water content, DTI exploits the relatively restricted, directional 'anisotropic' movement of protons (largely water) within healthy, intact nerve fibre tracts, compared to the more 'isotropic' movement able to occur in damaged tissue. Information about the principle direction of water movement allows the tracking of large fibres between brain regions [31], in a technique known as tractography (Fig. 1.7).

A further important development in MRI has been the ability to study brain function non-invasively. The established link between neuronal activity and blood flow can be

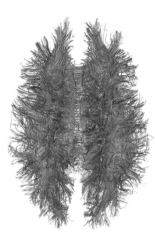

Fig. 1.7 Brain white matter fibre tracts discernable using diffusion tensor MRI and tractography.
Adapted from *PLoS One*, 3(12), X. Gigandet, P. Hagmann, M. Kurant, L. Cammoun, R. Meuli and J. P. Thiran, Estimating the confidence level of white matter connections obtained with MRI tractography, p. e4006, Copyright (2008), with permission under the Creative Commons License 2.0.

measured indirectly, using MRI, by exploiting a difference in the paramagnetic properties of oxygenated and deoxygenated blood (termed 'blood oxygenation level-dependent' or 'BOLD' imaging). Since the first report over two decades ago [32], this technique continues to lead insights into brain function [33].

Conclusions and critique

As well as the evolution of a non-invasive imaging tool without the hazards of ionizing radiation, the specific impact of MRI on the understanding of central nervous system structure and function, in addition to its routine place in the modern practice of clinical neurology, cannot be over-estimated. No one could have imagined, half a century ago, that the human brain could be seen in such detail non-invasively. What is becoming apparent, with time, is the gradual evolution of MRI away from the histological image seen by the naked eye (the radiologist's view), to constructs based upon new ways of analysing the digital information encoded within thousands of voxels of ever-decreasing size and the higher concept of the brain as a network (the neuroscientist's view). In a 2005 paper, Sporns and colleagues encapsulated this emerging concept:

> To understand the functioning of a network, one must know its elements and their interconnections. The purpose of this article is to discuss research strategies aimed at a comprehensive structural description of the network of elements and connections forming the human brain. We propose to call this dataset the human 'connectome,' and we argue that it is fundamentally important in cognitive neuroscience and neuropsychology. The connectome will significantly increase our understanding of how functional brain states emerge from their underlying structural substrate, and will provide new mechanistic insights into how brain function is affected if this structural substrate is disrupted. [34]

The Human Connectome Project (<http://www.humanconnectomeproject.org>) now proposes to map the MRI connectomes of 1200 healthy adults, plus twin pairs and their siblings from 300 families. It is hoped that this will reveal the relative contributions of genes and environment in shaping brain circuitry, pinpoint relevant genetic variation, and shed light on the organization of brain networks.

1.5 **Transcranial magnetic stimulation: unlocking brain circuitry**

Main paper: Barker AT, Jalinous R, Freeston IL. Non-invasive magnetic stimulation of the human motor cortex. *The Lancet* 1985;1(8437):1106–07.

Background

Transcranial magnetic stimulation (TMS) is a non-invasive method to excite neurons in the brain that has evolved as a clinical technique to successfully delineate mechanisms of neurodegeneration in movement disorders (e.g. Parkinson's disease) and other neurodegenerative diseases such as motor neurone disease [35]. In simple terms, TMS represents a mechanism to decode brain circuitry and the involvement of neurotransmitters at different levels of conscious thought and vegetative function. For example, TMS has the capability to completely paralyse the brainstem and, thereby, stop effective breathing and heart function, the latter through effects mediated by the vagal nerve. Understanding circuitry in turn suggests novel therapeutic avenues, in addition to serving as a useful monitoring device for therapies.

Methods

Dr Patrick Merton (1920–2000) and colleagues established that electrical stimulation of the brain was possible, but that the technique was painful and technically challenging [36]. As a result, Barker and colleagues set to work to establish a non-invasive process involving TMS. They established a system that could stimulate the brain every 3 seconds using a flat coil. Magnetic stimulators were developed that consisted of a capacitor that stored charge which, when discharged, initiated a flow of current through the coil to generate a magnetic field.

Results

Barker and colleagues observed that when the magnetic coil was placed over the scalp and discharged, movements of the opposite hand or leg could be obtained 'without any distress or pain'. They could also stimulate peripheral nerves without pain. By means of explanation, their TMS technique induced an electric field in nearby conductors (later determined to be cortical neurons), thereby resulting in current flow and neural stimulation. Given that the neural anatomy in the brain is complex, the point of excitation occurs at bends, branch points, or at the transition from cell body to axon. As such, the orientation of neurons, relative to the induced electric field, determines which neurons become activated (Fig. 1.8).

A pulse discharged by means of TMS causes a population of neurons in the neocortex to depolarize and discharge an action potential. If used in the *primary motor cortex*, such a process will produce a motor-evoked potential (MEP). If used over the *occipital cortex*, 'phosphenes' (flashes of light) may be detected. In most other areas of the cortex, the participant does not consciously experience any effect, but his or her behaviour may be slightly altered (e.g. slower reaction time during a cognitive task).

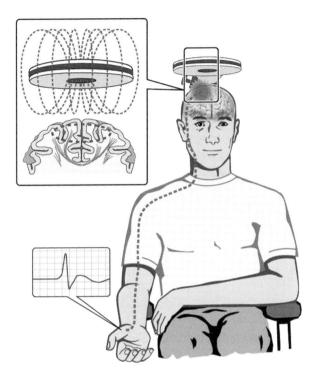

Fig. 1.8 Transcranial magnetic stimulation excites a network of neurons in the underlying motor cortex with motor-evoked potentials recorded from a contralateral limb.

Conclusions and critique

Barker and colleagues realized that their system would be particularly useful for interrogation of the motor system by activating the corticospinal tract. Subsequently, TMS has been successfully utilized as a method to investigate the circuitry and connectivity of the brain. Motor threshold (MT), or the ease with which the corticomotoneurons become excited, was subsequently determined to be mediated by excitability of cortical and thalamo-cortical axons via voltage-dependent Na^+ channels [37]. Inhibition of voltage-dependent Na^+ channels with epilepsy medications such as carbamazepine, phenytoin, and lamotrigine, increases MT.

With further development, TMS has achieved wider potential applications involving diagnosis and treatment, particularly with repetitive TMS (rTMS). Long-lasting changes in neuronal activity may be obtained using rTMS, which has a potential therapeutic role in conditions such as stroke (to promote neuroplasticity) and major depression. The TMS technique has delineated greater resolution in cerebral functional localization and establishment of causal relationships between the stimulated area and behaviour [38]. TMS represents a novel method for modulating the neuronal activity underlying sensory processing, motor planning, language, and consciousness, and may even be of use in differentiating organic from psychogenic paralysis [39].

1.6 **The first neurological disease gene identified by positional cloning**

Main paper: Koenig M, Hoffman EP, Bertelson CJ, Monaco AP, Feener C, Kunkel LM. Complete cloning of the Duchenne muscular dystrophy (DMD) cDNA and preliminary genomic organization of the DMD gene in normal and affected individuals. *Cell* 1987; 50:509–17.

Background

As with the Human Genome Project, a word of explanation is required to justify the inclusion of generic technological advances, relevant to the whole of medicine, as landmarks in the history of neurology. The central nervous system is unique in its complexity and in the extent to which recent evolution has selected for specialization of cellular function. The number of genes, or more accurately, gene variants, selectively expressed in the nervous system far exceeds that for any other organ system. Consequently, there are more single gene disorders in neurology than in any other specialty, and advances in genetics can be expected to have a transformative effect on neurological practice. From the 1970s, classical 'forward genetic' approaches had taken disorders in which the biochemical defect was known (e.g. haemoglobinopathies) and used deoxyribonucleic acid (DNA) or protein sequencing to demonstrate mutations in the obvious candidate genes and protein products. The discovery that DNA variants could be used to create genetic linkage maps by following segregation within individual pedigrees, tracking a disease phenotype against markers in known locations, ushered in the era of positional cloning [40]. In this situation, a gene could be cloned without any prior assumption about the biochemical pathway involved.

The X chromosome presented one of the earliest targets for positional cloning strategies, since 95% of the genome could immediately be excluded by the pattern of inheritance. The Duchenne muscular dystrophy (DMD) locus was identified by British geneticist, Kay Davies, who cloned fragments of the X chromosome flanking the DMD gene on Xp21 [41], setting the scene for the eventual discovery, some 7 years later, of what remains the largest mammalian locus encoding a single protein.

Methods

Having established the approximate location of the DMD gene on Xp21, a number of research groups proceeded to clone the whole region from X chromosome- specific libraries. The very large region where the DMD gene is located is vulnerable to deletion events, which explains why 30% of cases are *de novo*. This allowed researchers to screen patients with probes from the candidate region and identify areas that were missing, compared to controls. These deletions were used to produce a restriction map (based on the pattern and location of restriction enzyme sites) with flanking regions bounding the gene. Sequence comparison across different species allowed the definition of regions of conservation likely to represent coding DNA [42]. Using probes from this region, the complete coding sequence, of what was to be named the dystrophin gene, was assembled from fragments of a muscle-specific complementary DNA library.

Results

Extending over more than 14 kb of coding DNA and several hundred kb of genomic sequence, the DMD gene remains of the largest genes to be identified (Fig. 1.9). Both the size and intron–exon structure of the gene give clues to the high rate of *de novo* deletion mutations found in boys with DMD. The immediate impact of the identification of the primary structure of the DMD gene was an improvement in the speed and accuracy of pre-natal diagnosis in families already affected by the birth of a boy with DMD. However, the major outcome of the cloning and sequencing of this gene was that it gave rise to an era of improved understanding of the biology of the disease. Prediction of the primary protein sequence soon led to the production of anti-dystrophin antibodies, the demonstration that this was absent from the muscle membrane of DMD patients and the unequivocal proof that Duchenne and Becker muscular dystrophy are allelic disorders.

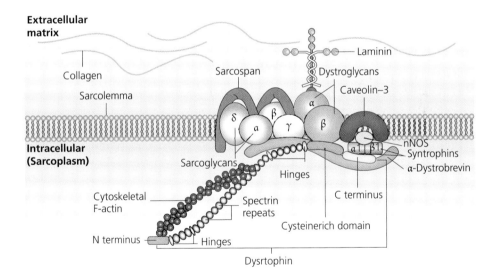

Fig. 1.9 Prior to the cloning of the gene for dystrophin, the existence of the complex of proteins linking the extracellular matrix to the actin cytoskeleton was unknown. Positional cloning was the starting point for exploring the biology of muscular dystrophy at the molecular level.

Reproduced from *Nature Reviews Molecular Cell Biology*, 7(10), Davies and Nowak, Molecular mechanisms of muscular dystrophies: old and new players, p. 762–773, Copyright (2006), with permission from Macmillan.

Conclusions and critique

The identification of neurological disease genes through positional cloning has led to start-ling expansion of our biological horizons. Who could have anticipated the emergence of triplet repeat disorders (in Huntington's disease and the cerebellar ataxias, among others) or the selective vulnerability of neurons to mutations in ubiquitously expressed proteins (e.g. SOD1 in amyotrophic lateral sclerosis (ALS))? The identification of the dystrophin coding sequence in a series of papers in 1986–88 was to be followed, in the early 1990s, by the identification of genes for Friedreich's ataxia, Huntington's disease, familial ALS, and a range of other neurological disorders. It opened an era where the neurobiological investigation of central nervous system (CNS) disease was underpinned by a mechanistic approach to disease modelling based on a clear understanding of the molecular lesion. However, it is a sobering thought that, almost 25 years after the discovery of the gene for DMD, the therapy of muscular dystrophy is still based on symptomatic treatments. The use of precisely targeted molecular biological therapy, which was initially heralded as being but a few years away after the cloning of the dystrophin gene, has been a long time in coming. The first trials of antisense oligonucleotide for 'exon skipping', aimed at restor-ing the dystrophin transcript to a functional structure, are only now taking place, and the technical issues of systemic delivery, precise molecular targeting, and efficiency *in vivo* have yet to be fully overcome.

1.7 **Reconstruction and analysis of neuroimages**

Main paper: Friston KJ, Frith CD, Liddle PF, Frackowiak RS. Comparing functional (PET) images: the assessment of significant change. *J Cereb Blood Flow Metab* 1991; 11:690–9.

Background

As much as the technological advances in neuroimaging have relied on physics, it is parallel developments in mathematics that have permitted their application. Austrian mathematician, Johann Karl August Radon (1887–1956), showed mathematically, that a function could be reconstructed from an infinite set of its projections, and his 1917 'Radon transform' became a foundation for tomography, with benefit to both electron microscopy and CT. The analysis method of French mathematician, Jean Baptiste Joseph Fourier (1768–1830), is in turn central to MRI, transforming the multiple sine waves of individual frequencies and amplitudes in the MRI signal to the frequency domain for spatial analysis.

The brain, even macroscopically, is a highly individualized anatomical structure, as well as subject to movement and change in shape due to breathing and the cardiac cycle during scanning. Image registration is the essential process of transforming a brain image dataset in the coordinates of one system to allow comparisons to be made. A French neurosurgeon, Jean Talairach (1911–2007), developed a coordinate system to describe brain structure locations based upon *post mortem* sections of a 60-year-old female brain, and this became the basis for a classical anatomical atlas for research as well as stereotactic brain surgery [43]. It paved the way for brain atlases derived from larger subject numbers, such as that of the Montreal Neurological Institute (MNI), that remain an essential part of modern neuroimaging analysis.

Methods

Karl Friston (b. 1959) and colleagues published a method for detecting areas of significant difference in brain scans acquired using positron emission tomography (PET), the method of functional brain imaging at the time. Rather than measuring differential tissue X-ray absorption (as in CT) or relaxation of proton spin (as in MRI), PET detects the radioactive decay of short-lived isotopes injected into the bloodstream. These isotopes release positively charged electrons known as positrons. When a positron collides with its matter counterpart, a negatively charged electron, there is release of energy in the form of two 511 kiloelectron volt (keV) gamma rays at 180 degrees to one another. This event forms the basis for the spatial and temporal image resolution in PET which relies on the concept of annihilation coincidence detection. Detectors consist of radio-dense material, such as bismuth germanate, which emit light when struck by high-energy gamma radiation, and photomultipliers which augment this signal. A series of rings of detectors surround the tissue of interest. Where two scintillations are recorded at 180 degrees to each other by opposing detectors on the ring within a nanosecond time frame, this event is recorded as a 'true coincidence event'.

Statistical maps were an alternative to the so-called 'region of interest' analysis which relies on *a priori* assumptions about localization. Friston and colleagues described these maps:

'as representing images of change significance, as opposed to change magnitude, allowing brain regions to be compared qualitatively in terms of relative significance. Alternatively, they have the potential to localize change at a given level of significance.'

The technique of statistical parametric mapping is now standard in functional MRI and gave its initials to a suite of image analysis tools known as 'SPM', published for international use by the Wellcome Department of Imaging Neuroscience, University College London (<http://www.fil.ion.ucl.ac.uk/spm/>). Other popular image analysis suites include Oxford University's Centre for Functional Magnetic Resonance of the Brain (FMRIB) Software Library's 'FSL' [44], and Harvard University's 'FreeSurfer' (<http://surfer.nmr.mgh.harvard.edu/>). More recent developments have included the application of Bayesian logic to image analysis, which has found particular use in studying regional connectivity in the brain [45].

Results

There are nearly 350,000 listings returned from a PubMed search using the search term 'functional MRI', equivalent to more than 300 a week since the first paper. All of these experiments depended on sophisticated mathematical methods to align scans to a standard space, as well as to model brain function and assess significant change from several thousand voxels of brain tissue between experimental contrasts, that were in turn created by careful gating of the MRI sequence and the data acquisition as subjects performed a specific task during their scan.

What is the most interesting part of the brain?' was the question posed by Behrens and colleagues [46]. They conducted a regression analysis of journal impact factor against patterns of regional brain activity from nearly 7500 published functional contrast datasets over nearly 25 years, and against experimental keywords. This revealed the frontal lobe regions of the brain and the keyword 'fear' to have had the most research impact in brain imaging to date (Fig. 1.10).

Finally, centuries-old mathematical methods are now being applied to the study of structural brain data derived from DTI. Graph theory is based on the solution, by eighteenth-century Swiss mathematician Leonhard Euler, to the 'Seven Bridges of Königsberg' problem [47]. The brain may be represented as a system of hubs (nodes or vertices), linked by tracts (edges or lines) defined using well-established tractographic techniques based on DTI data. Small-world network models of the brain envisage efficient transfer of information via an optimal number of local and long-distance connections [48]. While there is no consensus, as yet, on how to divide up the brain into its constituent hubs, this type of approach offers new potential for the mapping and understanding of network changes in neurodegenerative disorders (Fig. 1.11).

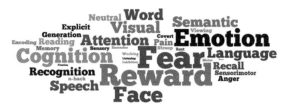

Fig. 1.10 World cloud shows the positive correlation between experimental keyword and impact factor.

Reproduced from *Trends Cogn Sci*, 17, T.E. Behrens, P. Fox, A. Laird and S. M. Smith, What is the most interesting part of the brain?, p. 2–4, Copyright (2013), with permission from Elsevier.

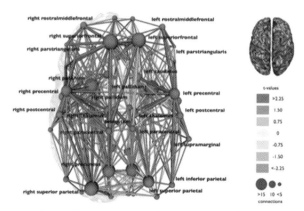

Fig. 1.11 A representation of the brain network based on graph theory showing the affected structural connections in a group of amyotrophic lateral sclerosis patients, compared with healthy controls. The size of the nodes is determined by their number of structural connections, darker if affected, according to the diffusion tensor images derived using advanced MRI.

Reproduced from *Hum. Brain Mapp.*, 35, Verstraete, E., Veldink, J.H., van den Berg, L.H., and van den Heuvel, M.P., Structural brain network imaging shows expanding disconnection of the motor system in amyotrophic lateral sclerosis, p. 1351–1361, Copyright (1932), with permission from John Wiley and Sons.

Conclusions and critique

The process of image analysis in the research setting has become gradually more automated, but is still a long way from being possible at the press of a button. Even the process of removing the skull and other tissues surrounding the brain in a consistent way, before analysis, requires complex software. Human input is still needed for quality assurance at all stages and, importantly, in the setting and interpretation of statistical thresholds. The Ig® Nobel Prizes (<http://www.improbable.com/ig/>) are to 'honor achievements that make people laugh, and then think.' The 2012 Neuroscience Ig® Nobel Prize was awarded for 'demonstrating that brain researchers, by using complicated instruments and simple statistics, can see meaningful brain activity anywhere— even in a dead salmon.' [49]. This award encapsulates a lingering suspicion among some neuroscientists about the validity of conclusions derived from functional neuroimaging. In reality, the dangers of multiple comparisons in statistics are well understood across all research disciplines, and neuroimaging is no exception.

Conclusions derived from advanced MRI techniques are typically based on comparisons across groups of subjects, and the major challenge for eventual clinical translation will be the assessment of change at the level of the individual subject. A more precise understanding of the relationship between the BOLD signal and neurovascular coupling remains one of the holy grails of functional MRI. Nonetheless, the technique stands as the leading tool for the study of the human brain at the systems level and MRI, more broadly, has come a long way from its original applications, and continues to evolve.

1.8 Visualization of neurons by live imaging with green fluorescent protein

Main paper: Chalfie M, Tu Y, Euskirchen G, Ward WW, Prasher DC. Green fluorescent protein as a marker for gene expression. *Science* 1994; 11:263(5148):802–5.

Background

Japanese organic chemist and marine biologist, Osamu Shimomura, American scientist, Martin Chalfie, and Chinese-American biochemist, Roger Tsien, shared the 100th Nobel Prize for Chemistry in 2008 for the discovery and development of the jellyfish green fluorescent protein (GFP), more correctly named *aequorin*. The group of fluorescent proteins derived from GFP are now the most important tool in contemporary neuroscience. Chalfie's work, though critical for the exploitation of GFP in neuroscience, could not have been achieved without the prior discoveries of Shimomura, who isolated the protein from the jellyfish, after painstakingly collecting many thousands of samples (50,000 were required to produce 1 mg of GFP), and showed that it became luminescent in the presence of calcium.

Methods

Chalfie was interested in mechanosensation in the nematode worm *C. elegans*. In the 1980s, he realized that GFP offered the opportunity to visualize proteins in the transparent worm. Importantly, he also appreciated that its small size and natural origins made it very likely that it would be biologically inert and not interfere with endogenous cellular processes when used to tag proteins. He obtained a cDNA encoding the aequorin molecule, which he transgenically inserted, first into *E. coli*, then into the worm genome.

Results

Chalfie was able to demonstrate that GFP could fluoresce independently of any other proteins, overturning the prevailing view that in order for fluorescence to occur in the intact animal, other enzymes, possibly unique to jellyfish, would be required. By cloning the GFP cDNA in-frame with a defined endogenous promotor, he was able to show expression in specific mechanosensitive neurons in response to external stimuli.

Conclusions and critique

The complex excitation spectrum and poor folding properties led to difficulties in exploiting wild-type GFP as an imaging tool in mammalian systems. The work of Roger Tsien, driven by the desire to image calcium flux in neurons, was critical in developing a whole series of GFP variants, ranging from green to yellow, cyan, and red, both by random mutagenesis and directly engineered structural modification. This resulted in proteins more suited to use in live imaging and, thus, completes the story of the evolution of GFP from a biological curiosity to a tool that has transformed modern neuroscience. While this might seem, at first sight, to be somewhat removed from the practice of clinical neurology, GFP has transformed the one-dimensional and static world described by Cajal into a dynamic one in which individual gene expression and the morphology and connectivity of individual neurons can be directly visualized in the whole animal, in real time. The spin offs from this discovery continue to astound. In 2007, the 'brainbow mouse', created using a combination of four types of fluorescent protein expressed stochastically, showed the complex architecture of brain regions by staining individual adjacent neurons with subtley different hues [50]. Most recently, a technique called CLARITY (Fig. 1.12) has revealed the three-dimensional architecture of the whole brain at a level of detail which, once the huge computational challenges have been solved, raises the prospect of understanding the high-level architecture of neuronal connectivity in health and disease.

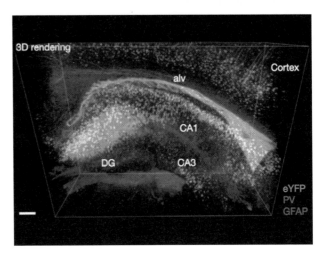

Fig. 1.12 Using a combination of fluorescent proteins and a technique for making tissue transparent, the complex architecture of neuronal and glial connections is revealed in the mouse hippocampus.

Reproduced from *Nature*, 497, Chung et al., Structural and molecular interrogation of intact biological systems, p. 332–7, Copyright (2013), with permission from Macmillan.

1.9 **The Human Genome Project**

Main paper: International Human Genome Sequencing Consortium. Initial sequencing and analysis of the human genome. *Nature* 2001; 409:860–921.

Background

The political grandstanding from American President, Bill Clinton, and British Prime Minister, Tony Blair, which accompanied the publication of this paper in *Nature* should not allow cynics to detract from the enormous significance of this work, which is one of the most important single episodes in the history of science. The ramifications will be felt for many decades to come and, like all great advances in technology, there are consequences that were not easy to perceive at the time. As with gene cloning, the significance for neuroscience and clinical neurology are proportionately greater than for any other area of medicine because of the genetic complexity of the CNS and the rapid recent evolution of the brain, allowing functional adaptation of *Homo sapiens* with the acquisition of manual dexterity and language through cortical specialization, convolution, and lateralization.

Methods

How was it achieved? The methodology of high throughput automated sequencing depended on three main scientific developments:

1 'shotgun' cloning of small fragments of DNA

2 automated fluorescent sequencers (Fig. 1.13), using an adaptation of the basic methods developed by British biochemist, Frederick Sanger, for which he won the Nobel Prize for Chemistry in 1980

3 bioinformatic techniques for reading, assembling, and annotating the resulting huge volume of sequence.

Results

This paper represented an early draft of the human genome, but laid the foundations for what was to be an extraordinary series of revelations, defying many previous assumptions about the nature of genes. Strikingly, the human genome contains fewer individual protein-coding genes than expected. The figure given in this paper of 30,000–40,000 is revealingly vague and, in fact, completely wrong. The current estimate is about 22,000—only a few thousand more than much simpler organisms such as worms and flies. Organismal complexity, therefore, turns out to be a consequence not of increasing gene number but a combination of (a) the way that genes are processed through alternate splicing and variable transcription start sites and (b) the emergence of specific functional domains, which greatly enhances the variety of protein–protein interactions. One immediate output from this work was the identification of 1.4 million single nucleotide polymorphisms, which

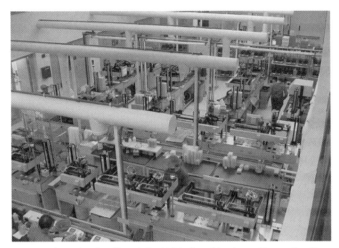

Fig. 1.13 The automated production line at the Whitehead Institute Center for Genome Research. The system consists of custom-designed factory-style conveyor belt robots that perform all functions, from purifying DNA from bacterial cultures, through setting up and purifying sequencing reactions.

Reproduced from *Nature*, 409, by ES Lander et al., Initial sequencing and analysis of the human genome, p. 860–921, Copyright (2001), with permission from Macmillan.

facilitated the emergence of genome-wide association studies and the whole field of complex genetics.

Conclusions and critique

The authors (and there were many, for this was biology's 'big science' moment akin to the kind of mega-experiments previously the domain of physics) took a rather wistful and philosophical tone in their concluding comments. With a wry nod to the famous final sentence by James Watson (USA) and Francis Crick (UK) in their paper describing the double helix, they stated: 'Finally, it is has not escaped our notice that the more we learn about the human genome, the more there is to explore.'

In the last decade, sequencing technology has become cheaper and more rapid, and the true significance of the role of genomics in neurobiology is emerging. In addition to the realization that some of the source of human variation is in the way genes are processed, it is now clear that the 97% of non-coding DNA we were taught to think of as 'junk' probably holds important clues to susceptibility to disease. Up to 10% consists of sequence under high evolutionary selection pressure (the 'dark matter'). As with undersea exploration, the deeper we get, the stranger is the world we find. Single-cell genomic sequencing is now a technical reality. Astonishingly, the genome of individual neurons in the brain appears to show a remarkable degree of variation, with up to 40% of neurons displaying deletions and duplications leading to copy number variation in individual genes [51].

How this relates to the expression of neurological disease will be an important new field of study.

In terms of gene discovery, the complete annotation of the human genome has led to rapid identification of candidate genes in whole exome projects (e.g. ion channels). Although the true era of personalized medicine depends on a much better way of distinguishing truly pathogenic from neutral variants, individual whole genome sequencing is now an economic reality.

1.10 **The production of disease-specific neurons by reprogramming of induced pluripotent stem cells**

Main paper: Ebert AD, Yu J, Rose Jr. FF, et al. Induced pluripotent stem cells from a spinal muscular atrophy patient. *Nature* 2009; 457:277–80.

Background

The inaccessibility of the nervous system and the destructive functional consequences of removal of peripheral and central nervous tissue have denied neurologists the kind of approaches available to specialists with access to bone marrow, skin, and other replaceable tissue. The 2012 Nobel Prize for Medicine was awarded to the Japanese physician, Shinya Yamanaka, for using a discrete cocktail of four transcription factors (Oct4, Sox2, Klf4, and c-Myc) to reprogram skin fibroblasts into induced pluripotent stem cells (iPSCs), effectively equivalent to embryonic stem (ES) cells, and, therefore, capable of forming the three major germlines (mesoderm, ectoderm, and endoderm) [52]. The groundwork necessary to turn ES cells into a variety of neural tissues had already been done using cells harvested directly from embryos, initially dopaminergic neurons [53] and, then, spinal motor neurons [54], based on decades of experimental work defining the molecular triggers to cell fate in the developing nervous system. There are a number of candidates for the first paper to describe the production of neurons from the skin fibroblasts of a patient with a neurological disease, but there remain only a few convincing examples of disease-relevant phenotypes in these models.

Methods

Using the Yamanaka protocol, iPS cells were generated from the skin fibroblasts of an infant with Type I spinal muscular atrophy (SMA), a fatal lower motor neuron disorder. In a now well-established protocol for producing motor neurons, iPSCs were grown in the presence of retinoic acid, SHH, cyclic AMP, ascorbic acid, glial cell line-derived neurotrophic factor, and brain-derived neurotrophic factor.

Results

After 6 weeks in culture, iPSC-derived motor neurons from the SMA patient were reduced in number and size, and showed a defective axonal morphology. Drugs known to increase the level of the defective survival motor neuron (SMN) protein in SMA showed the expected effect on motor neurons, validating this model as a potential tool for drug screening.

Conclusions and critique

The advent of iPSC-derived neuronal culture has been hailed as ushering in a new era of modelling 'disease in a dish' (Fig. 1.14). In addition to the obvious objection that neurological diseases affect systems rather than cells, a number of more technical issues must be solved before this becomes a reality. The production of primary neurons from iPSCs is

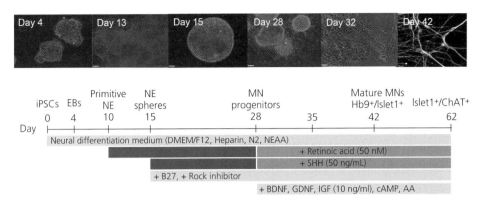

Fig. 1.14 Motor neurons in culture derived from iPS cells.

Reproduced with permission from Dr Ruxandra Mutihac, University of Oxford.

time-consuming (approximately 3 months from skin biopsy), extremely expensive, and subject to a high level of inter-experimental variation. Therefore, it is crucial to establish that changes seen in cells in culture reflect the disease itself and not differences induced by reprogramming. The ideal control cell line is one in which the genetic defect has been corrected after differentiation (which is therefore 'isogenic'). Several years of experimental refinement will be required for this method to be sufficiently high throughput to satisfy the needs of the pharmaceutical industry for screening many thousands of compounds simultaneously.

Key unanswered questions

Real-time functional neuroimaging to combine the temporal sensitivity of magnetoencephalography with the spatial resolution of magnetic resonance imaging. Such technology has the potential to illuminate the network basis of the human nervous system. If feasible, changes in connectivity and activity may be detectable years prior to the onset of symptoms and, thereby, enable primary prevention of neurodegenerative disorders.

The ability to remotely stimulate single neuronal cells and axons, and record at a molecular level. In essence, a non-invasive patch clamp would revolutionize the treatment of neurological disease. Separately, bio-assays (rather than simply bland pharmacological concentration assays) could be developed to monitor the physiological and, thereby, functional consequences of treatment interventions. It may also promote focused induction of neuronal plasticity in key areas of the brain found to have signs of pre-symptomatic neurodegeneration.

A post-genomic era of genetics. It is now clear that the protein coding sequence of genes provides only a partial explanation of how brains are built, are subsequently maintained, and, ultimately, go wrong. A complete understanding of the variation in non-coding DNA, non-coding ribonucleic acid (RNA), and epigenetic regulation would radically improve our ability to identify therapies and tailor these to the individual with neurological disease.

The ability to model nervous system function using *in vitro* three-dimensional neuronal networks. Developments in the concept of a 'disease in a dish' already involve the routine co-culture of neurones and their glial support cells to better reproduce human physiology. Three-dimensional neural networks will require novel frameworks, possibly through the use of inert single-molecule thick materials such as graphene, or from experiments conducted in zero gravity as space-based research becomes more routine.

The ability to deliver therapeutic agents to highly specific CNS cell types. Genetic therapy is now a reality in some disorders, and inactivated viruses have been used as vectors to the intracellular domain. As the nature of therapeutic interventions in this realm becomes more refined, it will be necessary to ensure highly targeted delivery of agents to small populations of cells, possibly at multiple times during various stages of CNS development.

References

1 **Applewhite AWR, Evans T, Frothingham A.** *And I Quote.* Thomas Dunne Books. New York; 2003.

2 **Schoonover C.** *Portraits of the Mind.* New York: Abrams; 2010.

3 **Talbot K.** *Great Medical Discoveries: The Anatomy of the Brain.* Oxford University, Bodleian Libraries; 18 November 2013; available at <https://www.youtube.com/watch?v=BBkBVM9x1N4>.

4 **Hooke R.** *Micrographia: or Some Physiological Descriptions of Minute Bodies Made by Magnifying Glasses with Observations and Inquiries Thereupon.* London: J. Martyn & J. Allestry, Printers to the Royal Society; 1665.

5 **de Broglie L.** *Nobel Lecture: The Wave Nature of the Electron.* The Nobel Foundation; 1929.

6 **Kruger DH., Schneck P., Gelderblom HR.** Helmut Ruska and the visualisation of viruses. *Lancet* 2000; **355**(9216):1713–7.

7 **Ruska E.** *Nobel Lecture: The Development of the Electron Microscope and of Early Electron Microscopy.* 8 December 1986; available at: http://www.nobelprize.org/nobel_prizes/physics/laureates/1986/ruska-lecture.pdf.

8 **Ruska E.** *The 2nd Gate to Microcosm: Ernst Ruska and the Electron Microscope.* 1998.

9 **Krishnan AV, Kiernan MC.** Uremic neuropathy: clinical features and new pathophysiological insights. *Muscle Nerve* 2007; **35**:273–90.

10 **Hodgkin A.** *Chance and Design: Reminiscences of Science in Peace and War.* Cambridge University Press; 1992.

11 **Hodgkin, Huxley.** *J Physiology* 1952.

12 **Donaghy M.** Neurologists and the threat of bioterrorism. *Journal of the Neurological Sciences* 2006; **249**:55–62.

13 **Isbister GK, Kiernan MC.** Neurotoxic marine poisoning. *Lancet Neurology* 2005; **4**:219–28.

14 **Sears T.** Sensory nerve action potentials in patients with peripheral lesions. *J Neurol Neurosurg Psychiatry* 2012; **83**:1137–8.

15 **Ragert P, Schmidt A, Altenmuller E, et al.** Superior tactile performance and learning in professional pianists: evidence for meta-plasticity in musicians. *Eur J Neuros* 2004; **19**:473–8.

16 **Cormack AM.** *Nobel Lecture: Early Two-Dimensional Reconstruction and Recent Topics Stemming from it.* The Nobel Foundation; 1979.

17 **Hounsfield GN.** *Nobel Lecture: Computed Medical Imaging.* The Nobel Foundation; 1979.

18 **Bloch F, Hansen WW, Packard M.** The nuclear induction experiment. *Phys Rev* 1946; **70**:474–85.

19 **Purcell EM, Torrey HC, Pound RV.** Resonance absorption by nuclear magnetic moments in a solid. *Phys Rev* 1946; **69**(1–2):37–8.

20 **Bloch F.** *Nobel Lecture: The Principle of Nuclear Induction.* The Nobel Foundation; 1952.

21 **Purcell EM.** *Nobel Lecture: Research in Nuclear Magnetism.* The Nobel Foundation; 1952.

22 **Damadian R.** Tumor detection by nuclear magnetic resonance. *Science* 1971;**171**(3976):1151–3.

23 **Lauterbur PC.** Image formation by induced local interactions: examples employing nuclear magnetic resonance. *Nature* 1973; **242**:190–1.

24 **Mansfield P, Maudsley AA.** Medical imaging by NMR. *Br J Radiol* 1977; **50**(591):188–94.

25 **Lauterbur PC.** *Nobel Lecture: All Science is Interdisciplinary—from Magnetic Moments to Molecules to Men.* The Nobel Foundation; 2003.

26 **Mansfield P.** *Nobel Lecture: Snap-Shot MRI.* The Nobel Foundation; 2003.

27 **Dreizen P.** The Nobel prize for MRI: a wonderful discovery and a sad controversy. *Lancet* 2004; **363**(9402):78.

28 **Holland GN, Moore WS, Hawkes RC.** Nuclear magnetic resonance tomography of the brain. *J Comput Assist Tomogr* 1980; **4**(1):1–3.

29 **Doyle FH, Gore JC, Pennock JM, et al.** Imaging of the brain by nuclear magnetic resonance. *Lancet* 1981; **2**(8237):53–7.

30 **Moseley ME, Cohen Y, Kucharczyk J, et al.** Diffusion-weighted MR imaging of anisotropic water diffusion in cat central nervous system. *Radiology* 1990; **176**(2):439–45.

31 **Douek P, Turner R, Pekar J, Patronas N, Le Bihan D.** MR color mapping of myelin fiber orientation. *J Comput Assist Tomogr* 1991; **15**(6):923–9.

32 **Belliveau JW, Kennedy Jr. DN, McKinstry RC, et al.** Functional mapping of the human visual cortex by magnetic resonance imaging. *Science* 1991; **254**(5032):716–9.

33 **Bandettini PA.** Twenty years of functional MRI: the science and the stories. *Neuroimage* 2012; **62**(2):575–88.

34 **Sporns O, Tononi G, Kotter R.** The human connectome: a structural description of the human brain. *PLoS Comput Biol* 2005; **1**(4):e42.

35 **Rossini PM, Rossi S.** Transcranial magnetic stimulation: diagnostic, therapeutic, and research potential. *Neurology* 2007; **68**:484–8.

36 **Merton PA, Hill DK, Morton HB, Marsden CD.** Scope of a technique for electrical stimulation of human brain, spinal cord, and muscle. *Lancet* 1982; **2**:597–600.

37 **Vucic S, Ziemann U, Eisen A, Hallett M, Kiernan MC.** Transcranial magnetic stimulation and amyotrophic lateral sclerosis: pathophysiological insights. *J Neurol Neurosurg Psychiatry* 2013; **84**:1161–70.

38 **Walsh V, Cowey A.** Transcranial magnetic stimulation and cognitive neuroscience. *Nature Reviews Neuroscience* 2000; **1**:73–9.

39 **Cantello R.** Applications of transcranial magnetic stimulation in movement disorders. *J Clin Neurophysiol* 2002; **19**:272–93.

40 **Botstein D, White RL, Skolnick M, Davis RW.** Construction of a genetic linkage map in man using restriction fragment length polymorphisms. *Am J Hum Genet* 1980; **32**: 314–31.

41 **Davies KE, Pearson PL, Harper PS, et al.** Linkage analysis of two cloned DNA sequences flanking the Duchenne muscular dystrophy locus on the short arm of the human X- chromosome. *Nucleic Acids Res* 1983; **11**:2303–12.

42 **Monaco AP, Bertelson CJ, Colletti-Feener C, Kunkel LM.** Isolation of candidate cDNAs for portions of the Duchenne muscular dystrophy gene. *Nature* 1986; **323**:646–50.

43 **Talairach J, Tournoux P.** *A Coplanar Stereotactic Atlas of the Human Brain.* Stuttgart: Thieme Verlag; 1988.

44 **Jenkinson M, Beckmann CF, Behrens TE, Woolrich MW, Smith SM.** FSL. *Neuroimage* 2012; **62**(2):782–90.

45 **Woolrich MW, Jbabdi S, Patenaude B, et al.** Bayesian analysis of neuroimaging data in FSL. *Neuroimage* 2009; **45**(1 Suppl):S173–86.

46 **Behrens TE, Fox P, Laird A, Smith SM.** What is the most interesting part of the brain? *Trends Cogn Sci* 2013;**17**(1):2–4.

47 **Jones DT, Seeley WW.** Neurodegeneration, Konigsberg, and the New York City subway: dementia researchers on edge(s). *Neurology* 2013; **81**(2):104–6.

48 **Pievani M, de Haan W, Wu T, Seeley WW, Frisoni GB.** Functional network disruption in the degenerative dementias. *Lancet Neurol* 2011; **10**(9):829–43.

49 **Bennett CM, Baird AA, Miller MB, Wolford GL.** Neural correlates of interspecies perspective taking in the post-mortem Atlantic salmon: an argument for multiple comparisons correction. 15th Annual Meeting of the Organization for Human Brain Mapping, San Francisco, USA. 2009.

50 **Livet J, Weissman TA, Kang H, et al.** Transgenic strategies for combinatorial expression of fluorescent proteins in the nervous system. *Nature* 2007; **450**(7166): 56–62.

51 **McConnell M, Lindberg MR, Brennand K, et al.** Mosaic copy number variation in human neurons. *Science* 2013; **342**:632–7.

52 **Takahashi K, Tanabe M Ohnuki M et al.** Induction of pluripotent stem cells from adult human fibroblasts by defined factors. *Cell* 2007; **131**:861–72.

53 **Kawasaki H, Mizuseki K, Nishikawa S, et al.** Induction of midbrain dopaminergic neurons from ES cells by stromal cell-derived inducing activity. *Neuron* 2000; **28**:31–40.

54 **Lee H, Shamy GA, Elkabetz Y, et al.** Directed differentiation and transplantation of human embryonic stem cell-derived motoneurons. *Stem Cells* 2007; **25**:1931–9.

Chapter 2

Coma

Jennifer Fugate and Eelco Wijdicks

2.0 **Introduction**

Becoming comatose had, of course, been a state known to physicians since antiquity and many had simply considered it to mark the end. When care improved—particularly supportive care such as mechanical ventilation—patients could be better examined and often in a less pressured situation. Over several decades, a much better understanding of mechanisms of coma, patterns of brain tissue shift, and its clinical correlates has developed. Physicians now may think they have a good handle on how to approach the comatose patient, but it was not always so. Different categories of coma—persistent vegetative state (PVS), minimally conscious state, and brain death—have been described, and often to better summarize the severity of brain injury and improvement potential (or lack thereof). Establishing the cause of coma accelerated with the widespread availability of computerized tomography (CT) scanning in the late 1970s, and this led to much better care (predominantly neurosurgical) and better outcome studies. Such studies were often seen as a way to determine an appropriate level of care. In this chapter, we have selected a collection of articles that will help the reader understand how we arrived at this level of sophistication. It will quickly become clear that it is a result of precise observations of a small group of interested physicians.

2.1 **Refining the neurological examination in coma**

Main paper: Fisher CM. The neurological examination of the comatose patient. *Acta Neurol Scand* 1969; 45(Suppl 36):1–56.

Background

In the first half of the twentieth century, an accurate neurological assessment of a comatose patient was a particularly deficient aspect of clinical neurology. There were surprisingly little data available in the medical literature or in textbooks about the examination of comatose patients. It was not until the 1960s, with the publication of several noteworthy papers, that methods of the examination and the details of approaching a diagnosis of patients in coma were described [1, 2]. In 1962, neurologist Fred Plum (1924–2010) published his observations of clinically deteriorating patients and outlined two brain herniation syndromes [2]. One year later, an anaesthesiologist, Eckenhoff, published one of the first papers that focused on the clinical care (rather than the diagnosis) of the comatose patient [3]. It was in this setting that C. Miller Fisher (1913–2012) published a classic and extraordinarily detailed paper, 'The neurological examination of the comatose patient' [1].

Methods

In the 1950s, while performing clinical studies of stroke, Fisher and his colleagues 'found it impossible to portray accurately the clinical picture in the comatose patient'. Spurred on in part by the dearth of discussion, in the literature, on the neurological examination findings in coma, Fisher described his methods of examining comatose patients and reported them in this comprehensive 56-page paper.

Results

Fisher emphasized the importance of initially just watching patients in their environments—with careful, close inspection—prior to 'doing'. The general examination of skin colour and texture, fingernails, mucous membranes, respiration patterns, autonomic stability, vital sign measurements, and general posture of the patients could be important pieces of the overall clinical picture: 'A comfortable-looking patient curled up with legs crossed will prove to be in light coma at the worst.'

Several observations of notable neurological findings in comatose patients were described here for the first time (Fig. 2.1). Fisher emphasized that ocular signs are 'the most important of the entire examination' in a comatose patient. After seeing 10 cases with clinical–pathological correlation, Fisher described ocular bobbing (an 'intermittent down and up' conjugate movement of the eyes), which he correlated with pontine pathology. He identified and reported the now well-recognized 1½ syndrome, which he actually described from observing a comatose patient's spontaneously roving eye movements. Other ocular signs were described for the first time, including 'wrong-way eyes', pontine miosis, ocular agitation, doll's eyes, eye closure and blinking in coma, and reflex blepharospasm. Fisher pointed out that the eyelid tone and length of time the eyes remain open after they are opened by the examiner are both findings that give an indication on the depth of the

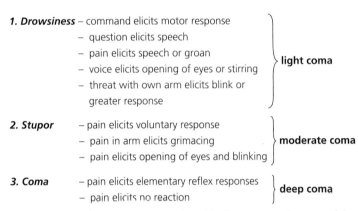

Table 1. Drowsy—Comatose States.
(Eyes persistently closed and often unblinking).

Fig. 2.1 Fisher's description of comatose states. The table shows many elements of the later Glasgow Coma Scale.

Reproduced from *Acta Neurologica Scandinavica*, 45, Fisher C.M., The Neurological Examination of the Comatose Patient, p. 5–56, Copyright (1969), with permission from John Wiley and Sons.

coma. There were also new observations about the motor examination. Bilateral decerebrate posturing resulting from acute lesions involving the supratentorial motor system was described in humans, when previously it had only been described with brainstem lesions. Unilateral decerebrate posturing due to an acute hemispheric lesion (in the hemiplegic limb, hours after an acute stroke, for example) was also newly described. Other novel observations that he reported within this paper included pseudo sixth nerve palsy and the concepts of bilateral hemispheric coma.

Conclusions and critique

The details of the neurological examination of a comatose patient were explained and reviewed. Fisher described numerous novel clinical observations in this historical paper, many of which remain useful in today's practice.

Fisher, a superbly skilled neurologist, wrote this paper based on his immense clinical experience over the years. Such a purely clinical description in this age of advancing technologies (which some may think is to the detriment of examination and observation skills) is a rarity today. There are no specific methods described in the paper, nor is there any indication as to exactly how many patients with each finding he described; yet many of his observations have stood the test of time. However, retrospectively, some of the statements in the paper may be questionable. One such example is his idea that epileptic brain tissue must be viable to sustain seizure activity and that once seizures are controlled, the brain tissue will return to normal or near normal. The majority of his observations are now well-known and classic examination findings.

It is of no surprise that other clinicians would find Fisher's observations interesting and valuable to their practice, especially in a time when there was such a lack of discourse about examining and caring for comatose patients. Interestingly, in his memoirs published decades later, Fisher professed that 'it was in the field of coma that one of the few unpleasant incidents' of his career occurred [4]. He indicated that he had discussed some of the principles of this paper with another neurologist at an academic meeting and that this person published a paper on the topic without acknowledging information from Fisher's previously relayed experience. Without providing further details about this apparently disturbing experience, he 'decided to let the matter rest' [4]. Regardless of what truly happened between Fisher and this (still unidentified) neurologist, the clinical observations that he provided in this landmark paper offered a solid foundation for generations of future neurologists when approaching, describing, and examining a comatose patient. The paper has not been widely read and may have been overshadowed by Plum and Posner's monograph on the diagnosis of stupor and coma [5] (Fig. 2.2). However, as Fisher used to say about publishing in 'less than stellar' journals, 'if it is a good paper they will find it' (personal communication).

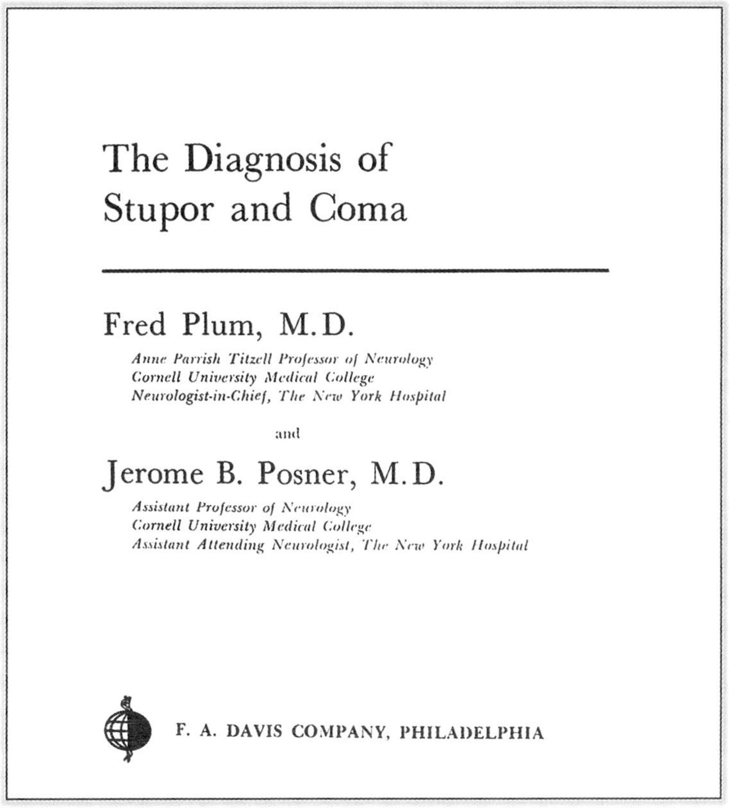

The Diagnosis of Stupor and Coma

Fred Plum, M.D.

Anne Parrish Titzell Professor of Neurology
Cornell University Medical College
Neurologist-in-Chief, The New York Hospital

and

Jerome B. Posner, M.D.

Assistant Professor of Neurology
Cornell University Medical College
Assistant Attending Neurologist, The New York Hospital

F. A. DAVIS COMPANY, PHILADELPHIA

Fig. 2.2 Plum and Posner's monograph on stupor and coma.
Reproduced from Wijdicks Eelco, The Comatose Patient, Second edition, Copyright (2014), with permission from Oxford University Press USA

2.2 **Herniation syndromes and rostrocaudal deterioration**

Main paper: McNealy DE, Plum F. Brainstem dysfunction with supratentorial mass lesions. *Arch Neurol* 1962; 7:10–32.

Background

In the early twentieth century, most clinical descriptions of precipitous neurological deterioration were nondescript. Coma was described using several elements of the neurological examination in combination with other physical findings. To depict a deteriorating patient, many textbooks described changes in pulse, respiratory rate and depth, odour of breath, pupils, and temperature [6]. In the early 1960s, physicians began to recognize acute neurological deteriorations by understanding that certain clinical signs indicated brainstem damage caused by tissue displacement through the tentorium or foramen magnum. Some of these acute clinical signs, such as a fixed pupil, irregular respiratory pattern, or acute hypertension, became identified as an impetus for neurosurgical intervention [7–11]. Earlier publications described many neurological symptoms that were not categorized into distinct stages or patterns [12, 13], and the precise course of how patients deteriorated was not widely known at the time. It would take the simple idea of just examining patients after presentation.

Methods

Neurologist, Plum, and his resident, McNealy, performed detailed neurological examinations on 52 patients with supratentorial mass lesions and secondary brainstem dysfunction [2]. They described two clinical patterns of the progression of secondary brainstem injury in great detail and termed these the uncal syndrome and the central syndrome. Not only did they clearly describe these orderly progressions of clinical signs, but they also proposed thorough anatomical and pathophysiological explanations for many of their examination findings.

Results

The 52 patients had supratentorial mass lesions, which included traumatic contusions or haemorrhages, massive ischaemic strokes, intracerebral haemorrhages, or neoplasms. A 'central syndrome', the first of the two main sequences of secondary brainstem dysfunction described, was seen in 27 patients. The central syndrome was reported to progress anatomically in predictable stages, rostrally to caudally. The diencephalic stage was characterized by impaired consciousness, Cheyne-Stokes respiration pattern, small pupils (1–3 mm), hyperactive vestibulo-ocular reflexes, and bilateral motor changes, with the development of paratonia or decorticate rigidity. This was followed by the midbrain–upper pons stage, characterized by sustained hyperventilation, slightly enlarged pupils to mid-position (3–5 mm), weaker vestibulo-ocular reflexes, and bilateral decerebrate posturing. The clinical signs continued to progress caudally to a lower pontine–upper medullary stage in which hyperventilation quietened and vestibulo-ocular reflexes and motor responses were lost. Finally, the medullary stage consisted of slow, irregular respirations, hypotension, and at end stage, apnea. During hypoxia, the pupils would widely dilate, and without respiratory support, the blood pressure would plummet.

The 'uncal syndrome', caused by lateral brainstem compression, was seen in seven patients. The early third nerve stage showed a unilateral dilated pupil (6–9 mm) with no light response. The authors explained this by third nerve compression by the posterior cerebral artery being pushed downwards by the ipsilateral herniating temporal lobe. In contrast to the central syndrome, the level of consciousness could be normal in this circumstance, and respirations were normal. The late third nerve–midbrain stage was characterized by progression into coma and decerebrate posturing. Proceeding rostrally, the midbrain–upper pons stage consisted of bilateral fixed mid-position pupils, impairment of vestibulo-ocular reflexes, and bilateral decerebrate posturing. From here on, the progression was indistinguishable from the central syndrome, with progressive loss of function by the mid to lower pons and, finally, the medulla oblongata. According to the authors, three factors could explain the rostrocaudal direction and facilitation of the downward displacement: 1) arterial compression followed by infarction and oedema; 2) venous compression followed by increased intracranial pressure (ICP); and 3) obstructive hydrocephalus at the aqueduct, further increasing ICP.

Most patients had only one of the syndromes, but five had clinical features of both. Patients who had intraventricular haemorrhage appeared to have different courses characterized by sudden coma or a succession of clinical signs that was interrupted by rapid medullary failure (irregular respiration and haemodynamic collapse).

Conclusions and critique

For the first time, orderly patterns of secondary neurological deterioration due to secondary brainstem injury were identified. Two specific patterns—the central and uncal syndromes—were described, and from these observations, a reportedly predictable succession of clinical signs (known as *rostrocaudal deterioration*) was characterized.

The clinical correlates to brain tissue shift that were described in this paper were fundamental to the basic understanding of mechanisms of coma, and these patterns were easily accepted by practicing neurologists when evaluating comatose patients. In the discussion of the paper, one of the purported uses for recognizing rostrocaudal deterioration was to aid in categorizing the diagnosis of a deteriorating comatose patient. In other words, a physician seeing a patient with progressive rostrocaudal deterioration could be almost certain that the patient was comatose because of brainstem dysfunction secondary to a supratentorial lesion, rather than from a primary brainstem lesion, metabolic encephalopathy, or psychogenic state. This particular application has become somewhat less relevant in current practice, as advances in neuroimaging—and particularly magnetic resonance imaging (MRI)—have aided our ability to diagnose and understand the cause of coma in many patients. The non-consecutive series of patients was small, with the focus on relatively slow deteriorations secondary to supratentorial lesions. Thus, the authors' findings cannot be extrapolated to all comatose patients, particularly patients with acute and rapid courses.

Some of the mechanisms that were proposed by the authors to produce the clinical signs of brain herniation have been challenged. For example, the authors explained the early fixed dilated pupil in the uncal syndrome to be due to downward movement of the posterior cerebral artery compressing the third nerve, whereas alternative explanations have been proposed, including third nerve compression between the edge of the clivus and the tentorial ridge or acute angulation of the third nerve over the clivus due to brainstem displacement [14, 15]. The specific mechanism producing a fixed unilateral pupil still remains unclear today, and more than one explanation may exist [16]. In addition, the clinical importance of herniation has been questioned. Autopsy reports of patients who were comatose prior to death from a supratentorial mass indicated that there was no pathological evidence of herniation [17]. A study in the 1980s showed that level of consciousness corresponded to horizontal displacement of the brain rather than transtentorial herniation [18]. Furthermore, experience has taught us that clinical deterioration does not always follow these characteristic patterns, and there is still a need for better understanding of mechanisms of coma in acute circumstances. Even a basic question such as how osmotic diuretics and hyperventilation resolve a fixed and dilated pupil after initiation of treatment in some patients has not been answered. Another basic question concerns when irreversibility ('the point of no return') occurs. How much should be 'lost' before we know for certain an intervention is futile? This is only established in patients with massive structural lesions with loss of all brainstem reflexes who are apneic.

2.3 **The origin of the Glasgow Coma Scale**

Main paper: Teasdale G, Jennett B. Assessment of coma and impaired consciousness. A practical scale. *Lancet* 1974; 2:81–84.

Background

In the early to mid-twentieth century, clinicians often described patients with impaired consciousness with mostly subjective, non-standardized terms such as 'somnolent', 'lethargic', 'drowsy', 'unresponsive', 'semicoma', or 'stuporous'. Textbooks in the early 1900s would also be no more specific in descriptions of the clinical features of coma. Some would describe the 'endogenous and exogenous toxic coma' and some would mention specific localization but without much elaboration [19]. In the 1970s, Jennett participated in an international study that collected data on comatose patients who had suffered head injury. Researchers began to realize that defining what constituted 'severe' head injury was inexact and could be very difficult [20]. This underlined the need for more objective coma scales. Several coma scales had already been developed, but none were consistently or systematically used. In 1974, Graham Teasdale and Bryan J. Jennett, pioneers in the field of neurosurgery, described the now well-known Glasgow Coma Scale (GCS), primarily as a research tool to objectify the depth of coma so that changes in consciousness could be accurately and reliably tracked [21].

Methods

After introducing the need for a clinical scale and briefly reviewing the existing systems, the authors detailed the new coma scale in a descriptive fashion.

Results

Notably, the GCS outlined in this paper was devoid of the numbering system so familiar today. The authors described each response of the scale in detail, beginning with the motor response, which ranged from following commands to no motor response. The authors provided specific instructions about how to perform each component of the motor examination (e.g. 'pressure is applied to the fingernail bed with a pencil') in order to standardize the examination. The flexion response to nailbed stimulation was not separated into normal versus abnormal flexion, and thus the scale consisted of 14 total points, rather than the 15 well-known today. The authors indicated the importance of recording the best motor response when there was a discrepancy, as the purpose of the scale was to indicate the patient's level of consciousness, not to localize the brain injury. The verbal response included the following categories: orientation, confused conversation, inappropriate speech, incomprehensible speech, and no verbal response. When outlining the various eye-opening responses, the authors warned against using eye movements to judge whether patients could interact with the environment because of the difficulty of interpreting these movements. They indicated that when testing for eye opening, the stimulus should be applied to the limbs because facial stimuli such as supraorbital or temporomandibular joint pressure may cause grimacing and closure of the eyelids.

The reliability of the GCS was then tested among 'several doctors and nurses'. Disagreements were reported to be rare, but there were no data or statistics provided. When the observers were asked only whether patients were conscious or unconscious, one in five clinicians disagreed with the majority opinion.

Conclusions and critique

The GCS—a coma scale incorporating motor, verbal, and eye-opening responses—was described in this paper and led to the standardization of the assessment of comatose patients.

Although this surprisingly brief paper was descriptive, rather than a formal study, it made a tremendous impact because it called attention to and proposed a solution to the limitations of existing systems. What is even more remarkable is that the scale could predict deterioration in a time without readily available CT scans. The GCS became a widely used clinical scale and was incorporated into many trauma and critical care classification systems and outcome prediction models. The practice of totalling the GCS to a sum score has unfortunately become widespread, but Jennett and Teasdale had always emphasized that a patient's level of consciousness should be described using all three separate responses [22].

Over the years, understandable criticisms of the GCS have emerged. Perhaps in part because the three components are unequally weighted (six points for motor, four for eyes, and five for verbal) and because points are still given for absent responses, some have difficulty remembering the scale, leading to unreliable and inaccurate scores. This is particularly a problem among relatively inexperienced clinicians [23]. In one study, when physicians were asked to name the scale components, they accurately identified only three of the six motor responses, three of the four eye responses, and two of the five verbal responses [24]. In addition, the verbal component, which comprises one-third of the scale, cannot be assessed in intubated patients, which is an exceedingly common problem. Sum scores are now ubiquitous and some physicians may use a GCS of 3 for any unresponsive patient (we occasionally have seen a GCS of 1 noted in reports). The GCS also does not provide any information about brainstem function—perhaps the most critical component of the evaluation of a comatose patient. Despite these drawbacks, the GCS can be quickly formulated, and can be a useful communication aide.

Newer coma scales have surfaced since the description of the GCS [25–29] and, currently, the FOUR (Full Outline of UnResponsiveness) score seems to have staying power. This scale is an attempt to summarize the bare essentials in a coma examination and incorporates motor response, eye opening and eye movements, brainstem reflexes, and respiratory pattern. The FOUR score has been validated in multiple studies in multiple intensive care units (ICUs) throughout the world [30–33]. It was found to be a better predictor of ICU mortality than the GCS in a recent study evaluating > 1,500 critically ill patients [34]. Physicians can see the usefulness of the FOUR score and there is a likelihood it will become widely accepted—forgetting the GCS will be less likely.

2.4 **Herniation dogma disputed**

Main paper: Ropper AH. Lateral displacement of the brain and level of consciousness in patients with an acute hemispheral mass. *N Engl J Med* 1986; 314:953–58.

Background

The uncal and central herniation syndromes described by McNealy and Plum in the early 1960s [2] were widely embraced as the cause of stupor and coma in patients with brain lesions. It was assumed that herniations compressed the reticular activating system in the upper brainstem, causing a depressed level of consciousness. Many post-mortem pathological examples showing a portion of the medial temporal lobe impacted between the tentorium and midbrain seemed to support uncal herniation as a mechanism of clinical deterioration, and this teaching repeatedly surfaced in textbooks [2, 10, 17, 35]. Thus, the principle that brain herniations were the cause of decreased level of consciousness in these patients was almost undisputed at the time of publication of this landmark paper [18].

Methods

Allan Ropper, a pioneering neurointensivist, personally examined patients admitted to a neurological/neurosurgical ICU with an acute supratentorial mass. He correlated clinical findings with results of CT scans performed within four hours of the neurological examination. Patients were only included if they had been examined within three days of the appearance of the mass, so that slowly enlarging masses were excluded. Patients with hydrocephalus, haemorrhage extension into the thalamus or midbrain, bilateral lesions, large or deep pre-existing lesions, or substantial intraventricular haemorrhage (IVH) were excluded. The patients' level of consciousness was classified as awake, drowsy, stuporous, or comatose. Twenty-four consecutive patients were included, of whom three deteriorated and had serial examinations and CT scans.

Results

The degree of horizontal displacement of the measured brain structures (pineal body, aqueduct, and septum pellucidum) increased as the level of alertness decreased. In other words, awake patients had the least degree of horizontal displacement while comatose patients had the greatest amount. Horizontal displacement of the pineal body was the earliest and most consistent finding associated with a depressed level of consciousness. Among eight drowsy patients, one had radiological evidence of uncal herniation. Among six stuporous patients, uncal herniations were present in two and uncertain in one. Three had distortion of the midbrain at the level of the ambient cisterns. Radiological uncal herniation was not invariably associated with a fixed dilated pupil. There were four comatose patients, two of whom had uncal herniation. Midbrain cisterns ipsilateral to the mass were widened in many patients, resulting from more rostral horizontal displacement and torquing of the mesencephalon. Central herniation (indicated by downward displacement of the pineal body) did not occur in any of the patients.

Conclusions and critique

The earliest and most consistent finding associated with a depressed level of consciousness was horizontal displacement of the pineal body. The findings of a torqued mesencephalon with ipsilateral ambient cistern widening in several patients led to the suggestion that uncal herniation may be a passive and late occurrence, and not the direct cause of impaired consciousness in all patients with acute supratentorial masses.

Ropper's findings challenged the dogma of herniation and led to reconsideration of a paradigm. It had been assumed that herniation was an active phenomenon, with the mesial temporal lobe compressing the reticular activating system in the upper brainstem to cause stupor or coma. His observation that uncal herniation may be a passive process deemphasized herniation as a clinical phenomenon and led to a re-evaluation of the mechanisms underlying acute neurological deterioration. Moreover, the close correlation of the patient's level of consciousness with the degree of lateral displacement of brain tissue, found on CT scans, had immediate and important practical implications, because it led to the understanding that a comatose patient without lateral shift may not benefit from an emergent neurosurgical procedure.

The study was followed by an MRI study that delineated the vectors of shift in a supratentorial lesion in more detail. Apart from several detailed case reports, it has been understandably difficult to amass a large series of rapidly deteriorating patients with 'enough time' to perform an MRI. Nonetheless, better understanding of deteriorating patients could come from serial MRIs before and after an intervention.

2.5 **Clarifying controversies of brain death**

Main study: Pallis C. ABC of brain stem death. From brain death to brain stem death. *BMJ* 1982; 285:1487–90.

Background

Until the twentieth century, severe brain injury led to respiratory arrest, and in a cyanotic, apneic patient, cardiac arrhythmias and circulatory arrest would quickly follow [36]. Following the introduction of endotracheal intubation and mechanical ventilation, a comatose patient's pulmonary function could be overtaken by a machine, and a patient with massive brain injury could be supported. From these circumstances, a new neurological condition characterized by irreversible coma, absent brainstem reflexes, apnea, and loss of vascular tone emerged. This condition came to be known as brain death, and clinical criteria were developed in the United States (US) [37] and, subsequently, in the United Kingdom (UK) [38]. Despite clear and comprehensive guidelines published in the UK, the British Broadcasting Corporation (BBC) aired a television programme entitled 'Transplants—are the donors really dead?' which questioned the reliability of the brainstem death criteria [39]. After the BBC refused to apologize for the alleged inaccuracies in the television show, the editor of the *British Medical Journal* commissioned neurologist Christopher Pallis to write a series of articles about brainstem death.

Methods

This article was one of a series of nine articles of the classic work *ABC of Brain Stem Death*, which were later compiled into a book. In this article, Pallis reviewed the history of the development of criteria for brain death, the implications that the criteria carried, and the mechanisms of brainstem death.

Results

Pallis briefly reviewed the historical background, beginning with a paper by the French neurologists Mollaret and Goulon that was fundamental to the development of brain death criteria [40]. In this paper, they reported 23 patients and described what are now recognized as the classic clinical features of brain death. Pallis also reviewed the report of the Ad Hoc Committee of the Harvard Medical School in 1968 [37] and the Minneapolis criteria which defined the period of apnea needed to determine brain death, emphasized the irrelevance of the electroencephalograph (EEG) in the diagnosis, and introduced the concept that irreversible damage of the brainstem was the critical component of brain death [41]. Pallis emphasized that the point that 'permanent functional death of the brainstem constitutes brain death' is highlighted in the UK guidelines and that the loss of brainstem function can be assessed clinically at the bedside. He articulated his conception of human death as: 'a state in which there is irreversible loss of the capacity for consciousness combined with irreversible loss of the capacity to breathe (and hence to maintain a heart beat)', both of which are brainstem functions. He also clarified the position that death is a process, rather than a distinct event, and used examples of the growth of hair and nails beyond the point when the heart stops, and the feasibility of using bone, arterial, or skin grafts that were collected 24–48 hours after death.

Conclusions and critique

The death of the brainstem is the necessary and sufficient component of brain death and this can be assessed and diagnosed clinically at the bedside. Death is almost always a process, rather than a single event.

The series of articles brought clarity to a topic that—thanks in part to the television programme aired by the BBC in 1980—was under considerable scrutiny and was permeated with controversy. In the US, many experts felt that the demonstration of death of the entire brain was necessary to determine brain death, while the UK criteria stated that the absence of brainstem function (including apnea testing) would suffice. Within these articles, Pallis clarified the UK position and emphasized that irreversible loss of brainstem function was the key component of brain death, and that this was almost always an infratentorial consequence of a supratentorial catastrophe. Since the publication of practice parameters by the American Academy of Neurology, there has been general understanding within the medical community that both positions are mostly similar, though there has been no unifying consensus for criteria for brain death, or brainstem death, throughout the world [39, 42–44].

Pallis' contribution to the brain death literature has been under-recognized. Pallis (and neurosurgeon Bryan Jennett) showed practicing doctors to look at the brainstem (below the tentorium rather than above the tentorium). He emphasized the importance of excluding confounders before even examining the patient and to trivialize confirmatory tests. Pallis argued that patients who are clinically dead do not need confirmation.

2.6 Definition of the persistent vegetative state

Main paper: Jennett B, Plum F. Persistent vegetative state after brain damage. A syndrome in search of a name. *Lancet* 1972; 1(7753):734–37.

Background

With the advent of ICUs and mechanical ventilation in the mid-twentieth century, an increasing number of patients were able to survive devastating brain injuries that might have earlier been fatal. Over several weeks to months after sustaining an acute brain injury, a proportion of these patients made transitions from coma to a state of occasional wakefulness but without awareness of their surroundings. As this subset of patients came to be appreciated, there grew a need to better define this clinical state to facilitate diagnosis and communication and to allow classification for research studies.

Methods

With extensive personal experience in taking care of patients with traumatic brain injury (TBI), Jennett approached Plum to write this paper together [45]. Rather than a traditional clinical study, this was an influential communication in which they explained the necessity of defining the clinical syndrome and coined the now entrenched term 'persistent vegetative state' (PVS) (Fig. 2.3).

Results

The authors described the syndrome and reviewed the previous terms used for related disorders of consciousness. The focus of the paper was to emphasize a group of patients with certain clinical characteristics. These patients showed no evidence of a 'functioning mind' which either receives or projects information. After a period of coma, survivors of severe head injury begin to open their eyes—first to noxious stimulation and, later, with longer periods of spontaneous eye opening. They do not attend to and do not appear aware of their environment. There is no consistent visual fixation or tracking, but eyes may rove. Extensor motor responses transition to slow, abnormal flexor withdrawal movements and some primitive reflexes, such as the grasp reflex, may be present. While the objective of the paper was to describe this certain clinical state, the authors did acknowledge that transitional clinical states could exist.

The authors explained why a new term was necessary by reviewing the existing names for related states of abnormal consciousness. It was felt that these terms—'coma vigil', 'akinetic mutism', and 'apallic syndrome'—did not fully capture the essence of the syndrome and sometimes erroneously implied a specific anatomical or pathological abnormality in a syndrome that, in reality, often had widely variably causative lesions. After sufficient explanations of why none of the existing terms were quite appropriate, Jennett and Plum

Points of View

PERSISTENT VEGETATIVE STATE AFTER BRAIN DAMAGE

A Syndrome in Search of a Name

BRYAN JENNETT

Institute of Neurological Sciences, Glasgow GS1 4TF

FRED PLUM

New York Hospital—Cornell Medical Center, New York City, N.Y., U.S.A.

Summary Patients with severe brain damage due to trauma or ischæmia may now survive indefinitely. Some never regain recognisable mental function, but recover from sleep-like coma in that they have periods of wakefulness when their eyes are open and move; their responsiveness is limited to primitive postural and reflex movements of the limbs, and they never speak. Such patients are best described as in a persistent vegetative state, which should be clearly distinguished from other conditions associated with prolonged unresponsiveness. What is common to these patients is the absence of function in the cerebral cortex as judged behaviourally; the lesion may be in the cortex itself, in subcortical structures of the hemisphere, or in the brain-stem, or in all of these sites. But the exact site and nature of the lesion is unknown to the bedside clinician, and the name for the syndrome should not imply more than is known.

Fig. 2.3 The term "persistent vegetative state" was suggested by Jennett and Plum in this manuscript.

Reproduced from Wijdicks Eelco, The Comatose Patient, Second edition, Copyright (2014), with permission from Oxford University Press USA

explained why the term 'persistent vegetative state' should be used instead. They preferred the word 'vegetative' because it was descriptive:

> The word vegetative itself is not obscure: vegetate is defined in the Oxford English Dictionary as 'to live a merely physical life, devoid of intellectual activity or social intercourse' and vegetative is used to describe 'an organic body capable of growth and development but devoid of sensation and thought' [45].

Furthermore, they appreciated that the term does not depend on results of ancillary tests (e.g. EEG) and that it does not imply a specific anatomical or pathological lesion. Although Jennett and Plum felt that hope for substantial clinical recovery in these patients was unrealistic, they recognized the need for more clinical studies to increase confidence in diagnosis and prognosis of this subset of patients. They also questioned how long PVS should persist before it could be declared permanent and noted that prospective studies would be needed.

Conclusion and critique

Jennett and Plum introduced the descriptive and lasting term 'persistent vegetative state' to separately classify patients with severe brain injury who are permanently unconscious. Jennett and Plum had meritable insight to separate these patients who were in such a devastating medical condition. The term 'persistent vegetative state' has become entrenched in the medical community and also is well understood by family members. The avoidance of uncommon or 'unnecessarily arcane jargon that often makes neurology needlessly difficult for others to understand' highlights the simplicity and pragmatism of the authors' word choice [45]. Still, some find that the term has a 'negative connotation' and a 'pejorative undertone' which led a European task force to recently suggest renaming the condition 'unresponsive wakefulness syndrome' [46]. The working group also felt that signs of recovery of consciousness might be missed when the term 'persistent vegetative state' is used. However, it seems unlikely that changing the term to 'unresponsive wakefulness syndrome' will prevent that from happening, and this new subjective term may lead to further confusion among medical and lay communities [47].

A widespread impression of PVS—based on the clinical description—was that it was produced by a loss of cortical function and preservation of brainstem function. A detailed neuropathological study of 49 patients later shed some light as to the locations of structural abnormalities leading to a vegetative state [48]. It was found that the structural abnormalities—regardless of the cause of injury—fundamentally consisted of extensive damage to the subcortical structures including the white matter of the cerebral hemispheres and/or the thalamus. The brainstem was damaged in only a minority of clinically vegetative patients. These pathological findings provided great insights into the pathophysiology underlying abnormal consciousness in patients with acute brain injury because it clarified the essential roles that the thalami and subcortical structures played in the maintenance of consciousness [48].

While the clinical diagnosis of PVS is straightforward for most expert neurologists, it is a rarely encountered state. Misdiagnosis is not infrequent, particularly when in the hands of non-experts [49, 50]. Since this landmark publication by Jennett and Plum, another new state of prolonged disorder of consciousness—minimally conscious state (MCS)—has been described, and some of the patients classified over the years in PVS were undoubtedly in MCS. In current practice, the assessment of PVS (or any prolonged disorder of consciousness) remains purely a clinical judgement. However, the field is evolving, and researchers are discovering new information based on modern brain imaging (e.g. functional MRI (fMRI)). Functional brain imaging cannot confirm a diagnosis of PVS, but some researchers foresee that it could potentially be used to rule out a diagnosis of PVS and possibly assist in prognosis [51]. It is possible that with the advent of these new techniques, paradigms might shift.

2.7 **The minimally conscious state defined**

Main paper: Giacino JI, Ashwal S, Childs N, et al. The minimally conscious state: definition and diagnostic criteria. *Neurology* 2002; 58:349–53.

Background

Even after considerable acute brain injury, most comatose patients who survive eventually awaken. For over thirty years, devastating neurological injury was often dichotomized into two groups: severe disability or PVS. However, in the 1990s, it had become recognized that patients in a presumed PVS sometimes showed inconsistent responsiveness, suggesting they were subtly more aware of their environment than patients in a truly vegetative state. The Aspen Consensus Conference Work Group classified these patients according to a distinct condition, the minimally conscious state (MCS), and proposed new diagnostic criteria [52].

Methods

A working group consisting of people from the fields of neurology, neuropsychology, neurosurgery, physical medicine and rehabilitation, nursing, bioethics, and allied health met nine times between the years 1995 and 2000. They initially tried to establish evidence-based guidelines for diagnosis, prognosis, and management of MCS through a literature search. Members of the group searched MEDLINE for the terms 'coma', 'vegetative state', 'minimally responsive state', 'stupor', 'slow to recover', 'severe disability', and 'Glasgow Coma Scale'. They cross-indexed these with the terms 'brain injury', 'diagnosis', and 'outcome' to find articles that included patients who did not meet criteria for a vegetative state but also were not fully conscious. However, of the 260 abstracts screened, they found only five that differentiated such patients, and the working group concluded that the data was insufficient to establish evidence-based guidelines. Consequently, consensus-based recommendations were developed for defining MCS.

Results

The working group defined MCS as 'a condition of severely altered consciousness in which minimal but definite behavioural evidence of self or environmental awareness is demonstrated' [49]. The distinguishing feature of MCS from PVS was the presence of conscious awareness. The working group listed specific behaviours—of which one or more should be seen reproducibly or on a sustained basis—to diagnose MCS. These behaviours include following simple commands, responding with verbal or gestural yes/no answers, understandable verbalization, and purposeful behaviour.

In addition to diagnostic criteria, the working group proposed criteria for emergence from the MCS to 'higher' states of consciousness, which they acknowledged is an arbitrary boundary imposed on a continuum. According to the authors, a patient is no longer considered to be minimally conscious when they reliably demonstrate functional interactive communication and/or they can functionally use two different objects. The authors pointed out the importance of excluding other neurological impairments such as aphasia, agnosia, apraxia, abulia, or sensorimotor abnormalities, as the reason for the patient's unresponsiveness. They also suggested future areas of research including the validation and interrater reliability of the diagnostic criteria for MCS and the study of the incidence, prevalence, natural history, treatment efficacy, and outcomes of MCS.

Conclusions and critique

New consensus-based diagnostic criteria were proposed to describe the 'minimally conscious state'—a subset of severely disabled patients with neurological injury who demonstrate partial awareness of the environment. Additional research is needed to validate these criteria and further define its epidemiology, pathology, natural history, and management.

Unfortunately, neither the definition of MCS nor the boundaries of this disabled state was based on prospective data in this paper. The working group emphasized that partial awareness is the feature distinguishing MCS from PVS, but aside from medicolegal implications, there was not much explanation about the consequences of this distinction between two devastating and prolonged disorders of consciousness. To some neurologists, it was not evident that a different therapeutic approach or different outcome could be expected by making this distinction. Still, the American Academy of Neurology endorsed the document and the term 'minimally conscious state' became accepted by the medical community [53].

Results of some studies have suggested that fMRI scans may be better than neurological examination to identify patients in a MCS who were previously thought to be in a PVS [54]. One study, using EEG, showed that 19% of vegetative patients were capable of following commands, despite being unable to do so by clinical behaviour [55]. In addition, a study using fMRI found preservation of large-scale cerebral networks in patients in a MCS, which has been interpreted by some to indicate that there might be residual functional capacity in some patients in a MCS [56]. There are reports of patients in a PVS 'progressing' to a MCS, and patients in a MCS further improving, even after several years [57]. Unfortunately, there have not yet been any large-scale epidemiological studies on prognosis in patients in a MCS but, most likely, there is wide heterogeneity in the type and degree of brain injury and, thus, heterogeneity in the degree of recovery.

2.8 **Detecting consciousness with magnetic resonance imaging?**

Main paper: Owen AM, Coleman MR, Boly M, et al. Detecting awareness in the vegetative state. *Science* 2006; 313:1402.

Background

After 1972, when Jennett and Plum described and separated patients in a vegetative state, the diagnosis of patients with long-term disorders of consciousness was based on clinical judgement alone [45]. Categorization of these patients was difficult at times and often required serial and careful neurological examinations. Advances in neuroimaging during the late twentieth century led to the development of functional brain imaging studies, which seemed to enticingly offer more information about patients who were not responding to their environment in a manner detectable by clinical examination [58]. In 2002, a study using structural MRI, positron emission tomography (PET), and magnetoencephalography (MEG) unexpectedly found wide variations of resting cerebral metabolism in five clinically vegetative patients, giving rise to the idea that perhaps 'islands' of preserved brain function may exist in some of these patients [56].

Methods

This influential paper was a case report of a patient who had suffered severe TBI and had been in a PVS for five months [59]. Sequences from a brain fMRI were obtained as sentences were spoken to her. The results were compared to those obtained from 34 healthy volunteers. Declarative sentences (e.g. 'There was milk and sugar in his coffee', 'The creak came from a beam in the ceiling') were spoken to the patient, delivered by an auditory stimulus delivery system with insert earplugs. The patient was then instructed to perform mental imagery tests (e.g. 'Imagine playing tennis', 'Imagine visiting the rooms in your home') which were repeated 10 times.

Results

The patient was a 23-year-old woman who had been in a traffic accident and initially had a GCS sum score of 4. During the hospitalization, she had undergone a bifrontal decompressive craniectomy and, in one month, a ventriculoperitoneal shunt was inserted. Over the next several months, a multidisciplinary team performed clinical assessments. Five months after the injury, when in a clinically vegetative state, the fMRI study was performed. In response to the declarative sentences, there was activity observed bilaterally in the middle and superior temporal gyri, the same as that observed in healthy volunteers who listened to the same sentences. When a sentence contained what the investigators thought were ambiguous words, there was additional activity seen in a left inferior frontal region that also corresponded to activity observed in normal volunteers. After being given an instruction to imagine playing tennis, fMRI activity was seen in the supplementary motor area, whereas when the instruction was to imagine walking through the patient's home, activity was seen in the parahippocampal gyrus, the posterior parietal cortex, and the lateral premotor cortex. Activity in these brain areas was the same as that seen in the healthy volunteers who were given the same instructions.

Conclusions and critique

The authors concluded that the regional activations seen on fMRI indicated that this patient, clinically vegetative five months after head injury, could understand and respond to the spoken commands.

This provocative study addressed an important question, but it probably raised more questions than it answered. The authors' interpretation of MRI activity created unease for physicians and the public alike. For the first time, it was implied that new technologies such as fMRI may be able to 'read minds' and, thus, perhaps allow communication with these patients who appear unconscious by clinical examination. This precipitated interest and further studies using fMRI and EEG to assess the brain activity of patients with clinical disorders of consciousness. Criticisms soon surfaced, however, mostly aimed at the rather dramatic interpretation of the results. The authors concluded that the patient was modulating her thoughts and made a 'decision to cooperate', but whether the activity on fMRI truly indicated actual conscious decisions was quickly questioned [60, 61], in part because brain activations can be induced in unconscious persons. In a published correspondence in response to the paper, Nachev and colleagues [61] pointed out that 'the presence of brain activation is not sufficient evidence for the associated behavior—here, supposedly consciously mediated behavior—unless one has also shown that the same activation cannot occur without it'.

It is interesting that the authors chose to perform the study 5 months after injury, since international guidelines recommended that in TBI cases, a diagnosis of permanent vegetative state should not be made until 12 months after the injury. At 6 months from the time of the injury, the chances of a patient like this one recovering consciousness was estimated to be nearly 20%. When this patient was re-examined 11.5 months after the injury, she visually fixated for more than 5 seconds and turned her eyes slowly to the right (but not to the left) when a mirror was held in front of her and moved to either side. Nevertheless, the results of this single case report sparked many researchers to attempt to detect consciousness in clinically unconscious patients, with the goal of offering objective diagnostic and prognostic tools as adjuncts to a bedside behavioural assessment.

Perhaps fMRI could be used to predict recovery, to confirm or rule out the diagnosis, or, in the future, become an instrument of communication. Communication with the patient might provide insight into their wishes, being now in this severely dependent state. Is there a 'man in the box'? What would the patient think and say? Would the patient be happy or sad? [62]

2.9 **Prognostication in comatose survivors of cardiopulmonary resuscitation**

Main paper: Levy DE, Caronna JJ, Lapinski RH, Frydman H, Plum F. Predicting outcome from hypoxic-ischemic coma. *JAMA* 1985; 253:1420–26.

Background

In the 1960s, the number of ICUs in hospitals throughout the world was increasing. The approach to the long-term care of persistently comatose patients became an important issue, and there was a need for prospective data to guide neurologists in estimating prognosis of comatose patients. Most previous studies focused on patients comatose from TBI, but there had been small studies about prognosis in comatose patients following cardiopulmonary resuscitation (CPR). Persistent coma and abnormal pupil reflexes seemed to be associated with poor outcome, but there were no large studies and no guidelines [63]. In 1981, a larger collaboration between the US and UK, studying patients in non-traumatic coma, was published [64]. From the total of 500 patients initially reported, data from the subset of 210 patients in hypoxic-ischaemic coma was analysed and presented in the current paper [65].

Methods

The study included patients over 12 years old from New York Hospital Cornell Medical Center, the Royal Victoria Infirmary in Newcastle-upon-Tyne, and San Francisco General Hospital who were comatose for at least 6 hours. The authors identified patients by attending daily neurological census rounds and visiting ICUs and emergency departments. The patients were examined at the initial evaluation and 0–1, 2–3, 4–7, and 8–14 days after coma onset. The Glasgow Outcome Scale was used to measure clinical outcome and the best functional state within the first year was used for most analyses.

Results

Of the sample of 210 patients, the cause of hypoxia-ischaemia was considered to be a primary cardiac arrest in 71%, primary respiratory failure in 11%, and something further in 18%. Most of the patients suffered the hypoxic-ischaemic event while in a hospital, while 34% were out of the hospital. An initial examination within 6 hours was obtained in 55% of patients and within 12 hours in 86% of patients. By 3 days, 25 patients had regained consciousness, which only increased to 28 after 2 weeks. Among 33 patients who were vegetative at 1 week, only three regained independence. The number of patients still comatose dropped rapidly within the first several days. After 1 day, 51% of patients remained comatose, compared to 27% at 3 days and 8% at 1 week. Of 17 patients still comatose after 1 week, only one ever regained consciousness. The overall death rate after hypoxic-ischaemic coma was high; at 1 year after the onset, only 19 patients (9%) were alive.

When analysing outcomes to the best functional neurological state attained within the first year, 78.1% were dead or vegetative, 9.5% were severely disabled and dependent on others, and 12.4% achieved independent function. None of the 52 patients with no pupillary response to light at the initial examination achieved independence, and only three of those regained consciousness. Four per cent of patients who had no corneal reflexes at the initial examination became independent within 1 year, but none who lacked corneal reflexes after the first day regained consciousness. No patients with motor posturing or lacking a motor response after 3 days of coma regained independence. While no single clinical sign could be relied on in isolation, the variable that best predicted outcome was the pupillary light reflex, followed by the motor response. The results were summarized in complex algorithms (Fig. 2.4).

Conclusions and critique

Most patients who awakened from coma due to hypoxic-ischaemic brain injury did so within the first few days. If coma persisted for 7 days, the likelihood of regaining consciousness was very poor. Absent pupil reflexes at the initial examination and a motor response worse than withdrawal on day 3 were the most reliable findings to predict a poor prognosis in these patients.

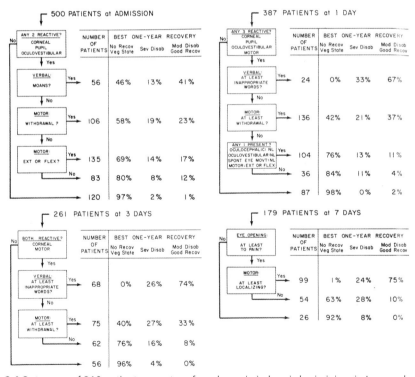

Fig. 2.4 Outcomes of 210 patients comatose from hypoxic-ischemic brain injury in Levy and colleagues' classic study.

Reproduced from Wijdicks Eelco, The Comatose Patient, Second edition, Copyright (2014), with permission from Oxford University Press USA

This study, using complex statistics, formed the basis of a more systematic approach to predicting outcome in comatose survivors of hypoxic-ischaemic brain injury. For the first time, it was shown that the clinical assessment of brainstem injury—by the testing of pupil, corneal, and oculocephalic reflexes—was crucial in estimating a prognosis in these patients. The algorithms in the paper became well accepted by neurologists over the years and several of the basic principles of prognostication in comatose patients after CPR are still used today. These include the exclusion of confounders such as prior administration of sedatives or neuromuscular blocking agents and the identification of key poor prognostic signs, including loss of brainstem reflexes and absent/extensor motor response at day 3 after cardiac arrest. These fundamentals stood the test of time and were reflected in the evidence-based review and guidelines on prognostication in comatose survivors of cardiac arrest published over 20 years later [62]. This was a notable accomplishment, considering this initial paper lacked details on level of care and information from head CT or EEG, and was largely a retrospective identification of outcome predictors.

In today's practice, induced moderate hypothermia has become standard treatment for a subset of comatose patients after CPR, and several of the clinical predictors are now more difficult to assess because of sedative and analgesic agents that are used concomitantly with induced hypothermia [67]. Specifically, the reliability of the motor response has been questioned in several recent studies, and the substantial variation in doses of sedatives and analgesics might make comparisons difficult [68, 69]. Thus, the predictors of outcome for patients with hypoxic-ischaemic brain injury are being re-evaluated in today's practice and newer predictors such as MRI—which can demonstrate evidence of diffuse laminar cortical necrosis—show promise as adjuncts to the clinical examination findings that were recognized as predictors by Levy and associates.

2.10 **Prognostication models for traumatic brain injury**

Main paper: Medical Research Council CRASH Trial Collaborators. Predicting outcome after traumatic brain injury: practical prognostic models based on large cohort of international patients. *BMJ* 2008; 336:425–29.

Background

Accurately estimating the prognosis of a patient with TBI in the acute setting has always been a tremendous challenge for clinicians. In one survey, only 37% of physicians felt their prognosis in patients with TBI was accurate, admission of a considerable amount of uncertainty despite the previous publication of several prognostic models [70]. Some potential reasons for this uneasiness were the small size and weak methodology of most of the published studies. In addition, most of the prognostic models at the time were not externally validated and were not clinically practical [71]. The Medical Research Council CRASH (Corticosteroid Randomization After Significant Head injury) trial included over 10,000 patients with TBI and was, thus, the largest clinical trial ever conducted in such patients [72, 73]. The investigators of the CRASH trial used this large population to develop and validate much needed newer prognostic models for patients with TBI [74].

Methods

The CRASH trial was a prospective, placebo-controlled randomized trial that included patients aged 16 years or older with TBI and some impairment of consciousness (GCS ≤14) within 8 hours of injury. Patients were randomized to treatment with intravenous methylprednisolone for 48 hours or placebo. Clinical outcome was assessed with the Glasgow Outcome Scale and was dichotomized into favourable (moderate disability or good recovery) and unfavourable (dead, vegetative state, or severe disability). A prognostic model was created using variables of age, sex, cause of injury, CT results, extracranial injury, and level of income in country. Analyses were adjusted for the corticosteroid treatment within the trial. The model was assessed for internal validity with the bootstrap resampling technique and was also externally validated against an external cohort of over 8500 patients with moderate and severe TBI (the IMPACT database) [75].

Results

Of the 10,008 patients, 81% were men and 75% were from low- to middle-income countries. Nearly 20% died within the first 2 weeks, 24% died within 6 months, and 37% were dead or severely disabled at 6 months. There was no association between age and the odds of death within the first 2 weeks until the age of 40, after which the relationship linearly increased. The association between GCS and mortality within 2 weeks was linear. GCS was the strongest predictor of outcome in low- to middle-income countries; age was the strongest predictor in high-income countries; and pupil non-reactivity was the third strongest predictor in both regions.

The investigators created eight prognostic models: a basic model of clinical features and a model incorporating CT results for predicting two outcomes in two settings (low- to middle-income countries and high-income countries). Four predictors were included in the basic model: age, GCS score, pupil reactivity, and the presence of major extracranial injury. Radiological characteristics on CT that were also strongly associated with outcome included the presence of petechial haemorrhages, obliteration of the basal cisterns or third ventricle, subarachnoid haemorrhage, midline shift, and haematoma. All models showed excellent discrimination with C statistics over 0.8. Models to predict 6-month outcome in patients in high-income countries were validated with the IMPACT dataset. The models were validated without the variables of extracranial injury and petechial haemorrhages because these were not available in the validation sample. Discrimination was good for the basic and CT models (C statistics 0.77 for both). The authors published a web-based calculator that allows users to enter information about individual patients with TBI to get the odds of death at 14 days and poor outcome at 6 months based on their models.

Conclusions and critique

Older age (>40 years), low GCS score, non-reactive pupils, and the presence of major extracranial injury were useful clinical variables that predicted poor prognosis in patients with TBI. CT findings that predict poor prognosis are obliteration of the third ventricle or basal cisterns and traumatic subarachnoid haemorrhage. These variables can be entered into web-based prognostic models to obtain the probability of death at 2 weeks and unfavourable outcome at 6 months.

These models, which used data from the largest clinical trial of TBI patients, are among the best available for predicting outcome early after traumatic head injury. As the authors acknowledged, the external validity of the models may be limited to some degree because the patients came from a large clinical trial rather than from the general population, but this also allowed prospective and standardized collection of data for over 10,000 patients, which increased the internal validity of the study. One of the major limitations of the study was that the investigators in the initial CRASH trial did not ask clinicians caring for the patients to report the circumstances of death. Thus, there was no information about cause of death for any of the patients. Approximately 20% of the patients in the trial died within the first 2 weeks. Whether the limitation of aggressive medical or surgical care—or withdrawal of life-sustaining treatments—was associated with the presence of the prognostic variables later studied (older age, lower GCS score, non-reactive pupils, major extracranial injury, etc.) is not known. In addition, it can be difficult to apply a general probability to an individual patient in clinical practice, but this same problem is encountered with the use of any prognostic model.

A degree of uncertainty in prognostication very early after head injury is unavoidable, but the results of this study have greatly assisted clinicians in making therapeutic decisions and counselling patients and their relatives. Furthermore, TBI is a leading cause of death and disability worldwide and prognostic models such as these can be valuable in regard to healthcare spending and allocation of resources, which are under ever-increasing scrutiny.

Key unanswered questions

1 What specific mechanisms produce a fixed unilateral pupil in patients with acute neurological deterioration?

2 How do hyperosmolar therapy and hyperventilation work to acutely lower intracranial hypertension?

3 Can we reach a global unifying consensus for the criteria for brain death?

4 Do areas of brain activation on fMRI indicate true consciousness?

5 Does early prognostication in clinical practice impact on outcome?

References

1 **Fisher CM.** The neurological examination of the comatose patient. *Acta Neurologica Scandinavica* 1969; **45**(Suppl 36):31–56.

2 **McNealy DE, Plum F.** Brainstem dysfunction with supratentorial mass lesions. *Arch Neurol* 1962; **7**:10–32.

3 **Eckenhoff JE.** The care of the unconscious patient. *JAMA* 1963; **186**:541–3.

4 **Fisher CM.** *Memoirs of a Neurologist.* Rutland, VT: Academy Books; 1992.

5 **Posner JB, Saper CB, Schiff ND,** *Plum and Posner's Diagnosis of Stupor and Coma,* **4**th **ed.** New York: Oxford University Press; 2007.

6 **Wijdicks EFM.** *Famous First Papers for the Neurointensivist.* New York: Springer; 2013.

7 **Jefferson G.** The tentorial pressure cone. *Arch Neurol Psychiat* 1938; **40**:857–76.

8 **Reid WL, Cone WV.** The mechanism of fixed dilatation of the pupil resulting from ipsilateral cerebral compression. *JAMA* 1939; **112**:2030–4.

9 **Sunderland S, Bradley KC.** Disturbances of oculomotor function accompanying extradural haemorrhage. *J Neurol Neurosurg Psychiat* 1953; **16**:35–46.

10 **Schwarz GA, Rosner AA.** Displacement and herniation of hippocampal gyrus through the incisura tentorii: a clinicopathologic study. *Arch Neurol Psychiat* 1941; **46**:297–321.

11 **Jaeckle KA, Digre KB, Jones CR, Bailey PL, McMahill PC.** Central neurogenic hyperventilation: pharmacologic intervention with morphine sulfate and correlative analysis of respiratory, sleep, and ocular motor dysfunction. *Neurology* 1990; **40**:1715–20.

12 **Howell DA.** Upper brain-stem compression and foraminal impaction with intracranial space-occupying lesions and brain swelling. *Brain* 1959; **82**:525–50.

13 **Johnson RT, Yates PO.** Clinicopathological aspects of pressure changes at the tentorium. *Acta Radiologica* 1956; **46**:242–9.

14 **Fisher-Brugge E.** Das 'Klivuskanten syndrom' Zugleich ein beitrag uber du entstehung der gleichseitigen pupillen erweitering und starre. *Acta Neurochirurg* 1951; **2**:36–8.

15 **Ropper AH, Cole D, Louis DN.** Clinicopathologic correlation in a case of pupillary dilation from cerebral hemorrhage. *Arch Neurol* 1991; **48**:1166–9.

16 **Koehler PJ, Wijdicks EF.** Fixed and dilated: the history of a classic pupil abnormality. *J Neurosurg* 2015; **122**:453–463.

17 **Munro D, Sisson WR.** Hernia through the incisura of the tentorium cerebelli in connection with craniocerebral trauma. *N Engl J Med* 1952; **247**:699–708.

18 **Ropper AH.** Lateral displacement of the brain and level of consciousness in patients with an acute hemispheral mass. *N Engl J Med* 1986; **314**:953–8.

19 **Koehler PJ, Wijdicks EF.** Historical study of coma: looking back through medical and neurological texts. *Brain* 2008; **131**:877–89.

20 **Jennett B.** The history of the Glasgow Coma Scale: an interview with professor Bryan Jennett. Interview by Carole Rush. Int J Trauma Nurs 1997; **3**:114–8.

21 **Teasdale G, Jennett B.** Assessment of coma and impaired consciousness. A practical scale. *Lancet* 1974; **2**:81–4.

22 **Teasdale G, Jennett B, Murray L, Murray G.** Glasgow Coma Scale: to sum or not to sum. *Lancet* 1983; **2**:678.

23 **Rowley G, Fielding K.** Reliability and accuracy of the Glasgow Coma Scale with experienced and inexperienced users. *Lancet* 1991; **337**:535–8.

24 **Riechers II RG, Ramage A, Brown W, et al.** Physician knowledge of the Glasgow Coma Scale. *J Neurotrauma* 2005; **22**:1327–34.

25 Wijdicks EF, Bamlet WR, Maramattom BV, Manno EM, McClelland RL. Validation of a new coma scale: the FOUR score. *Ann Neurol* 2005; **58**:585–93.

26 Benzer A, Mitterschiffthaler G, Marosi M, et al. Prediction of non-survival after trauma: Innsbruck Coma Scale. *Lancet* 1991; **338**:977–8.

27 Stanczak DE, White III JG, Gouview WD, et al. Assessment of level of consciousness following severe neurological insult. A comparison of the psychometric qualities of the Glasgow Coma Scale and the Comprehensive Level of Consciousness Scale. *J Neurosurg* 1984; **60**:955–60.

28 Sugiura K, Muraoka K, Chishiki T, Baba M. The Edinburgh-2 Coma Scale: a new scale for assessing impaired consciousness. *Neurosurgery* 1983; **12**:411–5.

29 Kramer AA, Wijdicks EF, Snavely VL, et al. A multicenter prospective study of interobserver agreement using the Full Outline of Unresponsiveness score coma scale in the intensive care unit. *Crit Care Med* 2012; **40**:2671–6.

30 Marcati E, Ricci S, Casalena A, Toni D, Carolei A, Sacco S. Validation of the Italian version of a new coma scale: the FOUR score. *Intern Emerg Med* 2012; 7:145–52.

31 Wolf CA, Wijdicks EF, Bamlet WR, McClelland RL. Further validation of the FOUR Score Coma Scale by intensive care nurses. *Pro Mayo Clinic* 2007; **82**:435–8.

32 Iyer VN, Mandrekar JN, Danielson RD, Zubkov AY, Elmer JL, Wijdicks EF. Validity of the FOUR Score Coma Scale in the medical intensive care unit. *Pro Mayo Clinic* 2009; **84**:694–701.

33 Idrovo L, Fuentes B, Medina J, et al. Validation of the FOUR Score (Spanish version) in acute stroke: an interobserver variability study. *Eur Neurol* 2010; **63**:364–9.

34 Wijdicks EF, Kramer AA, Rohs T Jr, et al. Comparison of the Full Outline of UnResponsiveness score and the Glasgow Coma Scale in predicting mortality in critically ill patients. *Crit Care Med* 2015; **43**: 439–444.

35 Myer A. Herniation of the brain. *Arch Neurol Psychiatry* 1920; **4**:387–400.

36 Wijdicks EF. *Brain Death*, 2nd ed. New York: Oxford University Press; 2011.

37 A definition of irreversible coma. Report of the Ad Hoc Committee of the Harvard Medical School to Examine the Definition of Brain Death. *JAMA* 1968; **205**:337–40.

38 Criteria for the diagnosis of brain stem death. Review by a working group convened by the Royal College of Physicians and endorsed by the Conference of Medical Royal Colleges and their Faculties in the United Kingdom. *J Royal Coll Physicians Lond* 1995; **29**:381–2.

39 Wijdicks EF. The transatlantic divide over brain death determination and the debate. *Brain* 2012; **135**:1321–31.

40 Mollaret P, Goulon M. The depassed coma (preliminary memoir). *Revue Neurologique* 1959; **101**:3–15.

41 Mohandas A, Chou SN. Brain death. A clinical and pathological study. *J Neurosurg* 1971; **35**:211–8.

42 Wijdicks EF. Practice parameters for determining brain death in adults (summary statement). The Quality Standards Subcommittee of the American Academy of Neurology. *Neurology* 1995; **45**:1012–4.

43 Wijdicks EF, Varelas PN, Gronseth GS, Greer DM. Evidence-based guideline update: determining brain death in adults: report of the Quality Standards Subcommittee of the American Academy of Neurology. *Neurology* 2010; **74**:1911–8.

44 Wijdicks EF. Brain death worldwide: accepted fact but no global consensus in diagnostic criteria. *Neurology* 2002; **58**:20–5.

45 Jennett B, Plum F. Persistent vegetative state after brain damage. A syndrome in search of a name. *Lancet* 1972; **1**:734–7.

46 Laureys S, Celesia GG, Cohadon F, et al. Unresponsive wakefulness syndrome: a new name for the vegetative state or apallic syndrome. *BMC Medicine* 2010; **8**:68.

47 Wijdicks E. Being comatose: why definition matters. *Lancet Neurol* 2012; **11**:657–8.

48 **Adams JH, Graham DI, Jennett B.** The neuropathology of the vegetative state after an acute brain insult. *Brain* 2000; **123**(Pt 7):1327–38.

49 **Childs NL, Mercer WN, Childs HW.** Accuracy of diagnosis of persistent vegetative state. *Neurology* 1993; **43**:1465–7.

50 **Schnakers C, Vanhaudenhuyse A, Giacino J, et al.** Diagnostic accuracy of the vegetative and minimally conscious state: clinical consensus versus standardized neurobehavioral assessment. *BMC Neurology* 2009; **9**:35.

51 **Monti MM, Laureys S, Owen AM.** The vegetative state. *BMJ* 2010; **341**:c3765.

52 **Giacino JT, Ashwal S, Childs N, et al.** The minimally conscious state: definition and diagnostic criteria. *Neurology* 2002; **58**:349–53.

53 **Wijdicks EF.** Minimally conscious state vs. persistent vegetative state: the case of Terry (Wallis) vs. the case of Terri (Schiavo). *Pro Mayo Clinic* 2006; **81**:1155–8.

54 **Monti MM, Vanhaudenhuyse A, Coleman MR, et al.** Willful modulation of brain activity in disorders of consciousness. *N Engl J Med* 2010; **362**:579–89.

55 **Cruse D, Chennu S, Chatelle C, et al.** Bedside detection of awareness in the vegetative state: a cohort study. *Lancet* 2011; **378**:2088–94.

56 **Schiff ND, Ribary U, Moreno DR, et al.** Residual cerebral activity and behavioural fragments can remain in the persistently vegetative brain. *Brain* 2002; **125**:1210–34.

57 **Schiff ND, Giacino JT, Kalmar K, et al.** Behavioural improvements with thalamic stimulation after severe traumatic brain injury. *Nature* 2007; **448**:600–3.

58 **Hannawi Y, Lindquist MA, Caffo BS, Sair HI, Stevens RD.** Resting brain activity in disorders of consciousness: A systematic review and meta-analysis. *Neurology* 2015; **84**:1272–1280.

59 **Owen AM, Coleman MR, Boly M, Davis MH, Laureys S, Pickard JD.** Detecting awareness in the vegetative state. *Science* 2006; **313**:1402.

60 **Greenberg DL.** Comment on 'Detecting awareness in the vegetative state'. *Science* 2007; **315**:1221; author reply 1221.

61 **Nachev P, Husain M.** Comment on 'Detecting awareness in the vegetative state'. *Science* 2007; **315**:1221; author reply 1221.

62 **Wijdicks EFM.** Being comatose: why definition matters. *Lancet Neurol* 2012; **11**:657–8.

63 **Willoughby JO, Leach BG.** Relation of neurological findings after cardiac arrest to outcome. *BMJ* 1974; **3**:437–9.

64 **Levy DE, Bates D, Caronna JJ, et al.** Prognosis in nontraumatic coma. *Ann Intern Med* 1981; **94**:293–301.

65 **Levy DE, Caronna JJ, Singer BH, Lapinski RH, Frydman H, Plum F.** Predicting outcome from hypoxic-ischemic coma. *JAMA* 1985; **253**:1420–6.

66 **Wijdicks EF, Hijdra A, Young GB, Bassetti CL, Wiebe S.** Practice parameter: prediction of outcome in comatose survivors after cardiopulmonary resuscitation (an evidence-based review): report of the Quality Standards Subcommittee of the American Academy of Neurology. *Neurology* 2006; **67**:203–10.

67 **Fugate JE, Wijdicks EF, White RD, Rabinstein AA.** Does therapeutic hypothermia affect time to awakening in cardiac arrest survivors? *Neurology* 2011; **77**:1346–50.

68 **Rossetti AO, Oddo M, Logroscino G, Kaplan PW.** Prognostication after cardiac arrest and hypothermia: a prospective study. *Ann Neurol* 2010; **67**:301–7.

69 **Al Thenayan E, Savard M, Sharpe M, Norton L, Young B.** Predictors of poor neurologic outcome after induced mild hypothermia following cardiac arrest. *Neurology* 2008; **71**:1535–7.

70 **Perel P, Wasserberg J, Ravi RR, Shakur H, Edwards P, Roberts I.** Prognosis following head injury: a survey of doctors from developing and developed countries. *J Eval Clin Pract* 2007; **13**:464–5.

71 **Perel P, Edwards P, Wentz R, Roberts I.** Systematic review of prognostic models in traumatic brain injury. *BMC Med Inform Decis Mak* 2006; **6**:38.

72 **Roberts I, Yates D, Sandercock P, et al.** Effect of intravenous corticosteroids on death within 14 days in 10008 adults with clinically significant head injury (MRC CRASH trial): randomised placebo-controlled trial. *Lancet* 2004; **364**:1321–8.

73 **Edwards P, Arango M, Balica L, et al.** Final results of MRC CRASH, a randomised placebo-controlled trial of intravenous corticosteroid in adults with head injury—outcomes at 6 months. *Lancet* 2005; **365**:1957–9.

74 **Perel P, Arango M, Clayton T, et al.** Predicting outcome after traumatic brain injury: practical prognostic models based on large cohort of international patients. *BMJ* 2008; **336**:425–9.

75 **Maas AI, Marmarou A, Murray GD, Teasdale SG, Steyerberg EW.** Prognosis and clinical trial design in traumatic brain injury: the IMPACT study. *J Neurotrauma* 2007; **24**:232–8.

Chapter 3

Headache

Peter J. Goadsby

3.0 **Introduction**

At first blush, selecting the top 10 papers on headache in the last 150 years, and writing about them, seemed perhaps a simple matter. However, the task quickly turned Herculean as one understands how much has been written and how many truly excellent papers will not be mentioned. Since the authors have been tasked to discuss influence and single out specific papers, what follows is certainly personal, thus slanted to the mechanisms rather than, for example, the substantial and important contributions to epidemiology and disability of headache [1, 2]. Coverage is restricted to primary headaches, and that is in many ways to make the task manageable. One hopes the perspective is thought provoking and, to maintain interest, is written to be just a *little* controversial.

The considerations are divided into those affecting migraine and then those affecting other headache disorders. Specific people are mentioned because history is very much more colourful for the characters it throws into the fray; and all comments are to be taken in their historical context. About 150 years ago, Gowers (1845–1915; Fig. 3.1) had written on migraine: the clinical description, laterality, sensitivity to stimuli, allodynia, cranial autonomic and premonitory symptoms are all there [3]. Indeed, migraine is presented as a brain disorder, so the many re-descriptions of what the nineteenth-century neurologists knew do not seem to represent progress to this writer. The reappearance, for example, of chronic or frequent migraine [4] would be an excellent example of reinventing the wheel. What follows, from a mainly mechanistic perspective, is the important story of how we lost the way but, most recently, found it again. It is the unfolding story of how to develop therapies, and the need to know the target organ.

Migraine is probably the main disorder referred to neurologists and, therefore, must be included here. After migraine, the trigeminal autonomic cephalalgias (TACs) are the next most troublesome disorder that one sees in referral practice. Some might argue that tension-type headache (TTH) should be covered first. Suffice to say, however, that according to the second edition of the *International Classification of Headache Disorders* (ICHD-II) [5], TTH is a rare problem in referral practice, at least in Australia, the United Kingdom, or the United States.

We would probably all agree that important steps have been taken with regard to TACs in the last 150 years, and that describing them is a worthy thing. The term TAC was developed as a way of placing emphasis on a crucial aspect of the phenotype of cluster headache, paroxysmal hemicrania, short-lasting unilateral neuralgiform headache attacks with conjunctival injection and tearing/cranial autonomic features (SUNCT/SUNA), and hemicrania continua [6]. The concept emphasizes the group and has two broad bases. First, the clinical picture shares much in the phenotype—particularly laterality of symptoms, be they cranial autonomic symptoms when compared to migraine [7], even at any age [8], or migrainous-type symptoms, such as photophobia [9]. Secondly, functional imaging outcomes suggest some part of the dicenphalon in the posterior region of the hypothalamus

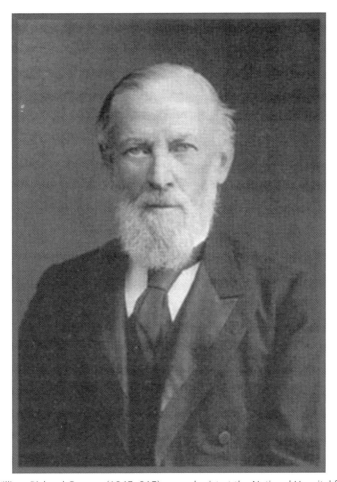

Fig. 3.1 Sir William Richard Gowers (1845–915), neurologist at the National Hospital for the Paralysed and Epileptics, Queen Square.

or adjacent brain is involved in the syndromes [10]. Perhaps even more than migraine, these headache types have yielded to greater understanding in the last century and a half. The oldest described syndrome is probably cluster headache [11], and it is certainly the most common of these disorders.

3.1 **The vascular theory**

Main paper: Graham JR, Wolff HG. Mechanism of migraine headache and action of ergotamine tartrate. *Archives of Neurology and Psychiatry* 1938; 39:737–63.

Background

While it was clear to Gowers, and indeed others such as Lieving [12] and Critchley (personal communication), that migraine was primarily a brain disorder, the introduction into therapeutic use of ergot derivatives [13] and their well-known vascular effects triggered a series of studies and concepts that dominated migrainology from the 1930s until perhaps the end of the twentieth century [14]. The logic of Graham and Wolff was clear and plainly stated, 'because ergotamine tartrate predominantly affects smooth muscle, inquiry concerning . . . migraine headache . . . centered on the cranial blood vessels' [15].

Methods

The study was of 32 attacks of migraine in 16 subjects. Migraine was defined as unilateral, often preceded by visual disturbance and accompanied by nausea. For controls, 46 subjects contributed 50 observations. Pulsations of the temporal and occipital branches of the external carotid were recorded by a reflectance system using tambours placed over the vessels. Blood pressure was recorded, as was skin temperature; the latter in 10 experiments. Headache was recorded by patients on a '1–10+ ' score with 10+ being severe headache. Three baseline measurements were taken before treatment. It is not clear from the methods how the reflectance data were measured. Ergotamine was administered intravenously in doses from 0.37 to 0.5 mg.

Results

In 20 experiments, there was an average decrease in vessel diameter of 50%, range 18–84%, with 16 of these experiments having a close relationship between headache resolution and tambour signal change. The reductions were usually immediate, although in an unspecified number it was 10–15 minutes after administration, while the maximum drop occurred 30–40 minutes later. Controls were also reported to have an average 50% reduction in vessel signal. No signal change was seen in three patients whose retinas were observed, although in one there was venous change. The authors also reported on manual compression of the common carotid artery in 24 migraine attacks in 10 patients, claiming all had some degree of improvement.

Conclusions and critique

It is hard to overstate the influence of this work or emphasize the limits of the presentation. The patient group is unclear, there is no mention of blinding, no mention of either an inactive placebo or active non-vascular treatment, nor any statistical assessment. It is hard to imagine the overall design being published in the modern era, which is not to detract from the technologically clever way of asking the questions. The authors set out with a view and 'proved' it. It was nearly 50 years before the field began to question the vascular dogma. It became widely accepted that migraine aura was a vasoconstrictor phenomenon and migraine pain, a vasodilator phenomenon. The work placed migraine in the periphery, the cranial vessels, and, thus, directed experimentation to such mechanisms. The explanation had the virtue of simplicity and, consequently, arrested thinking for half a century. To paraphrase Glaxo's Pat Humphrey: 'if the real complexity of serotonin receptors, and I suspect migraine, had been know, Pharma interest may never have developed toward the triptans.'

3.2 **Migraine aura and the cortical spreading depression of Leão**

Main paper: Leão AAP. Spreading depression of activity in cerebral cortex. *Journal of Neurophysiology* 1944; 7:359–90.

Background

The visual disturbance of migraine aura is so typical of the syndrome that when the slow march of symptoms is elicited [5], the clinician is usually on familiar territory. While Graham and Wolff [15] were careful to note their studies had 'no bearing on preheadache phenomenon', it was not long before the logic of vasodilation and pain had been extended to the concept that migraine aura was due to vasoconstriction [16]. However, even as speculation of a vasospastic nature to migraine to explain the aura was rife, a very careful Brazilian neurophysiologist, Aristides de Azevedo Pacheco Leão (1914–1993), was at work and evolving a much better explanation. Attempting to study epilepsy, he happened on what he called 'an interesting response' in rabbit cortex with stimulation [17]. Even as the reader considers this, someone, somewhere in the world, is likely to be linking migraine aura with this response; it could be widely agreed it was at least *interesting*.

Methods

Rabbits were anaesthetized, laid prone, and their cortices exposed. The cortex was stimulated electrically and changes recorded with pial placement of fine chlorided silver wires. Tracings were made on a six-channel Grass ink recorder (which the writer reminisces were still in use 40 years later when they began laboratory work).

Results

The very first result in the paper is an 'enduring depression' of spontaneous cortical activity that progressed over about 90 seconds under the recording electrodes and lasted up to 10 minutes in some regions. Interestingly, it spread in all directions. Leão reported that mechanical stimulation could have the same effect. Remarkably, the effect was most consistent in the frontal pole and not so consistent in the occipital pole. He confirmed it was not anaesthetic dependent (using chloralose) and not species specific (using pigeons and cats). The latter had had brainstem transection, confirming the effect did not necessarily involve bulbar structures.

Conclusions and critique

Other papers on the subject soon followed. Shortly after, Leão [18] published that the wave of depression of electrical activity was accompanied by pial vessel dilation of between 50% and 100% and probably secondary to activity in 'nervous elements'. By the next paper, he had deduced the essential relationship: 'the slow march of scotomata . . . is suggestively similar to the experimental phenomenon of cortical spreading depression' [19]. It was a little over 10 years later until others had begun to share Leão's speculation [20]. It took many years for the evidence to accumulate: for example, Olesen and colleagues' early blood flow studies in migraine aura [21], Cutrer and colleagues' perfusion-weighted blood flow work [22], and the elegant functional magnetic resonance imaging (fMRI)/blood oxygenation level-dependent (BOLD) work of Hadjikani and colleagues [23]. Although much is understood, even more nuances are being identified [24, 25], and the basic observation is still playing a validating role in studying other advances, such as the effects of the familial hemiplegic mutation in the CACNA1A gene (see section 3.8 and [26]) whose knock-in animal model has altered cortical spreading depression (CSD) properties [27], perhaps as Leão might have predicted.

3.3 **Classification**

Main paper: Headache Classification Committee of The International Headache Society. Classification and diagnostic criteria for headache disorders, cranial neuralgias and facial pain. *Cephalalgia* 1988; 8:1–96.

Background

Prior to 1988, headache classification was not terribly well organized, with the diagnosis largely dependent on the most senior person offering a view. Graham and Wolff [15] (described in section 3.1) is an excellent example—the clinical description is simply impossible to replicate. An ad hoc classification developed under the auspices of the American National Institutes of Health (NIH) [28] but was imprecise and unsuitable for any scientific endeavour, mirroring well the National Institute of Neurological Disorders and Stroke's (NINDS's) modern-day efforts in the field. Two things were happening in the mid-1980s to conspire in favour of a better system. First, The International Headache Society had been formed and was starting to think about the science of headache and how that might be approached. Secondly, Glaxo's Pat Humphrey (to be discussed in section 3.4)was hot on the trail of a new therapy for acute migraine [29].

Methods

The International Headache Society formed a classification committee, chaired by Jes Olesen, and charged them to develop a system for classifying headache. Olesen assembled the team: André Bes (France), Robert Kunkel (USA), James W. Lance (Australia), Guiseppe Nappi (Italy), Volker Pfaffenrath (Germany), Frank Clifford Rose (UK), Bruce S. Schoenberg (USA), Diether Soyka (Germany), Peer Tfelt-Hansen (Denmark), K. Micheal A. Welch (USA), and Marica Wilkinson (UK). The members met on several occasions, formed sub-committees for the various sections, and drafted a document. An important underlying philosophy was to have operational criteria, rather like the *Diagnostic and Statistical Manual of Psychiatric Disorders*. The authors wanted the patients so classified to be comparable wherever they were seen. This would standardize diagnosis and, thus, facilitate both clinical translational and clinical trial research.

Results

The outcome was the first edition of the *International Classification of Headache Disorders* (ICHD-I) [30] and its subsequent iterations, ICHD-II [5] and ICHD-III [31].

Conclusions and critique

This publication simply revolutionized every aspect of headache. The ICHD has been used to teach, to treat, to understand, and to develop new therapies in many areas, with migraine especially benefiting by its development. Much of what follows in this chapter relies on studies that use ICHD as a basis for patient definition. It is frightening to consider what would have happened had the ad hoc criteria been used and a great mercy that it was abandoned completely for the ICHD.

3.4 **Triptans: serotonin 5-HT$_{1B/1D}$ receptor agonists**

Main paper: Humphrey PPA, Feniuk W, Marriott AS, Tanner RJN, Jackson MR, Tucker ML. Preclinical studies on the anti-migraine drug, sumatriptan. *European Neurology* 1991; 31:282–90.

Background

The mid-1980s saw one of the two great therapeutic advances in headache of the last 150 years. Arguably, the development and introduction into clinical use, with the attendant pharmacological purity, of triptans [32] brought the promise and then the reality of science to migraine therapeutics [33]. While the 1991 paper of Humphrey and colleagues [34] is cited here as the main work, one could argue that the earlier pharmacology paper of Feniuk and colleagues [35] is an equally valid contender. Indeed, Humphrey, with the great modesty that excellence often brings, always credited the team [29], and particularly Wasyl Feniuk. It is notable that the first reference in the 1991 paper [34] is to Graham and Wolff [15], which shows something of the lineage of these things. An earlier molecule is noted here for completeness [36] but was not pursued.

Methods

The 1991 paper is a review of the preclinical studies that underpinned the development and clinical trial programme for sumatriptan. The preclinical programme was based around the notion of constricting a dilated vessel, although by the time of its writing, the concept of neurogenic inflammation in the dura mater was beginning to gain ground [37] (see section 3.5). The pursuit of the 5-HT$_1$-like receptor is outlined.

Results

Binding studies *in vitro* very clearly showed how much more specific sumatriptan (GR43175) was than dihydroergotamine. Studies at the 5-HT$_2$ receptor, using greyhound and pig coronary vessels, and at the 5-HT$_3$ receptor, using an assay involving the vagus nerve, were clearly unreactive. Beagle dogs were used to characterize the carotid effects of sumatriptan with 50% of maximum vasoconstriction with 39 mcg/kg intravenously—an effect attenuated by methiothepin, a 5-HT$_1$-like receptor antagonist. There was an important effect on arterio-venous shunts, building on the very careful pharmacological studies of Saxena and colleagues [38]. The pharmacokinetics, absorption, excretion, and metabolism of sumatriptan are discussed, which, knowingly or unknowingly, set the parameters for all that was to come in the development of the newer triptans. One very telling section is that on the haemodynamic effects of sumatriptan, where the choice of greyhound coronaries perhaps left a degree of concern unexplored that has turned out to be the Achilles' heel of the class [39]. No important toxicology was observed, and this statement remains true 20 years later.

Conclusions and critique

It is hard to overstate how useful triptans have been to patients. I have vivid memories and many lovely letters from patients whose lives were transformed beyond their imagination when they began to use these medicines. It is hard to now recall a time when we questioned if we needed more treatments [40, 41]. Another important aspect of the development of sumatriptan was the clinical trial programme. The sumatriptan development programme, pursued with scientific discipline by Pilgrim and colleagues [42], gave great impetus to the development of broader guidelines [43] and was, in many ways, as important, as its consequences have influenced acute medicine development in the field, well beyond the triptans. The authors summarize work showing how sumatriptan could attenuate dural plasma protein extravasation (PPE) in rats [44], and this provides a bridge from Graham and Wolff, through the discovery of sumatriptan, to the PPE story that shall be tackled in section 3.5. I am sure any author would have selected a paper involving sumatriptan for inclusion in this book.

3.5 **Neurogenic inflammation in migraine**

Main paper: Markowitz S, Saito K, Moskowitz MA. Neurogenically mediated leakage of plasma proteins occurs from blood vessels in dura mater but not brain. *Journal of Neuroscience* 1987; 7:4129–36.

Background

With the development of the triptans and a relatively specific acute migraine treatment, the opportunity to employ their very discrete pharmacology to study the biology of migraine was on offer. Presented as selective cranial vasoconstrictors, this explanation seemed unlikely to many. Even as industry, perhaps for convenience, pushed on with the mechanism view, competing views were being debated [45]. Two alternate views emerged, both with profound implications for understanding the disorder—one, a neurogenic dural inflammatory hypothesis involving plasma protein extravasation (PPE) (discussed here), and the second, a neural theory (discussed in section 3.6). Was migraine pain due to a sterile inflammatory change in the dura mater, and did triptans work to reverse this? The demonstration that trigeminal ganglion stimulation resulted in a leakage of plasma proteins into the dura mater initiated a concept that still remains, to some, an option to explain migraine [37], and sumatriptan worked in that model [44].

Methods

Anaesthetized rats were studied to determine leakage of plasma proteins after chemical, electrical, or immunological stimulation, as measured by extravasation of Evans blue or ^{125}I-bovine serum albumin (BSA). The basis for the concept was that peripheral nerve stimulation could produce an inflammatory response altered by capsaicin [46].

Results

Intravenous capsaicin produced extravasation in the dura mater and conjunctiva, but not in the temporalis muscle. Electrical stimulation of the trigeminal ganglion produced extravasation in the ipsilateral dura mater, eyelids, lips, and gingival mucosa. Substance P and neurokinin A, when administered intravenously, caused dural extravasation, whereas calcitonin gene-related peptide (CGRP) did not. C fibres were considered the likely basis for the responses to capsaicin, and extravasation was not seen in the brain.

Conclusions and critique

The effect of the paper was profound. The Harvard Group that had described the neurogenic dural PPE quickly determined that sumatriptan blocked the effect [44], as did other drugs used in migraine, such as dihydroergotamine [47]. The effect was dramatic and PPE became a standard model with which to check new approaches.

The study clearly predicted that other anti-PPE compounds would work in migraine, such as substance P-neurokinin 1 receptors and that CGRP receptors were not. Herein was the cul-de-sac reached by those in the field. PPE was blocked by newly described substance P-neurokinin 1 receptor antagonists. However, four acute attack studies [48–51] and one preventive study [52] all failed. Not to be hampered by the data, an endothelin antagonist, effective in blocking PPE [53], was studied and again shown to be ineffective in acute migraine [54]. A neurosteroid, ganaxolone, was again studied in migraine and failed [55]. To round off the published failures, it was speculated that inhibition of inducible nitric oxide synthase (iNOS)—a form of nitric oxide synthase activated in dura mater with inflammation [56]—would be effective in migraine. So, a potent iNOS inhibitor [57] was again tested in the acute [58] and preventive [59] management of migraine: both studies failed. The prominence of capsaicin mechanisms and, thus, the TRPV-1 receptor [60], led to a study of that target [61] now reported as negative [61a]; model systems other than PPE predicted this would have failed [62].

Given there is no evidence for dural inflammation in migraine and with the failure of ten studies reported, the cul-de-sac of neurogenic inflammation in migraine is a landmark in misdirection and part of the rich tapestry of the development of the field. The CGRP story in section 3.6 illustrates how, by simply giving greatest emphasis to human data in migraine [63], this could have been avoided, reinforcing the importance of translational research to therapeutical development.

3.6 **Neural approaches to migraine: calcitonin gene-related peptide based mechanisms**

Main paper: Goadsby PJ, Edvinsson L, Ekman R. Vasoactive peptide release in the extra-cerebral circulation of humans during migraine headache. *Annals of Neurology* 1990; 28: 183–7.

Background

As the 1980s began, the vascular theory had dominated migraine for nearly half a century, and it seemed the mechanisms could all be traced to blood vessel changes. An advantage to distance is that one can allow non-mainstream ideas to develop without censorship. So, Lance had started to think about migraine in the context of neural mechanisms. Trained as a classical neurologist in the Sherringtonian tradition [64], his laboratory began to explore how the central nervous system may be responsible for important parts of migraine. Brainstem structures seemed obvious from a clinical perspective [65] and, with the publication of an alternate way to consider aura [21], a central nervous system concept began to emerge [66].

There is a recurrent issue in each of the cases in this chapter which have a translational aspect—how does one link 'bench' and 'bedside'? Lambert and colleagues had commenced exploring the trigeminovascular system [67], and the beginnings of the study of the cranial autonomic pathway were also at the 'bench' [68, 69]. Yet was this all relevant in humans? At that point, this author attended a Neural Control of the Cerebral Circulation Meeting in Sweden, in the mid-summer of 1985, and heard Edvinsson and colleagues [70] describe a protective function for the trigeminovascular system that seemed largely dependent on CGRP (Fig. 3.2). We talked and evolved a series of experiments to explore if these trigemi-novascular mechanisms were relevant in humans. Initially, we studied if substance P and CGRP could be measured in cats and humans, with trigeminal stimulation, and found that the cat data predicted the outcome in humans; both were raised during stimulation [71]. However, was this important in migraine?

Methods

Measurements were made on venous blood samples from the cubital fossa and external jugular vein of 22 patients with severe acute migraine, with and without aura [63].

Results

Increases in CGRP were observed (about double the level of the cubital fossa or of the controls during migraine), with no change in substance P or neuropeptide Y. The negative results served as a control for the sampling, lest the change was a volume of collection effect. In the cat, CGRP, but not substance P, was elevated when the superior sagittal sinus was stimulated [72].

Conclusions and critique

The initial result of the publication was to evoke angst, since it suggested substance P had no role—a fact borne out by the many subsequent failed studies of neurokin-1 receptor

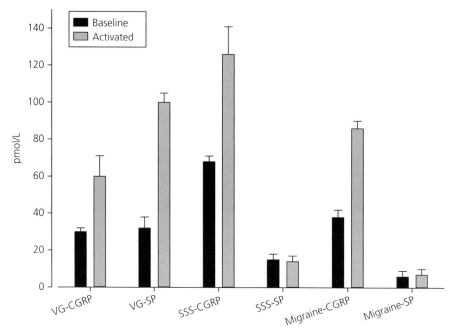

Fig. 3.2 Calcitonin gene-related peptide (CGRP) and substance P (SP) levels (pmol/L) were elevated in the cranial circulation in humans after trigeminal ganglion (VG) stimulation (VG-CGRP/VG-SP; [71]). In cats, superior sagittal sinus (SSS) stimulation elevated CGRP but not SP levels in the cranial circulation (SSS-CGRP/SSS-SP; [72]), an effect mirrored in migraine, where CGRP and not SP levels were elevated (Migraine-CGRP/Migraine-SP; [63]), thus predicting a role for CGRP in migraine.

antagonists [73]. The subsequent work in showing that sumatriptan and dihydroergotamine could block CGRP release in cats and that sumatriptan attenuated CGRP levels in humans as it controlled migraine [74], presented a fundamental challenge to received wisdom and direction for therapy. First, if CGRP was important and substance P not, then not only would neurokinin-1 receptor antagonists fail, and they did [73], but also dural neurogenic inflammatory mechanisms would not be important and their blockade would not be useful, and it was not [75]. Secondly, the work predicted that CGRP receptor antagonists would be useful in migraine, and they were [76]. Lastly, and most fundamentally, since CGRP receptor antagonists would not have vasoconstrictor effects, and they do not [77], the Graham-Wolff diversion of the vascular theory was, in essence, wrong. Non-vascular drugs would work, and they do (e.g. the CGRP receptor antagonists [78a], monoclonal antibodies [78b,c] or 5-HT$_{1F}$ receptor agonists [79]), and vasodilation is indeed not important as a generator of migraine pain. Vasodilation is neither necessary [80], sufficient [81], nor predictive [82] of migraine. The brain, and neural mechanisms, are regained [83] as the organ of the disorder and, thus, direction of translational medicine became clearer.

3.7 **Brain imaging**

Main paper: Weiller C, May A, Limmroth V, et al. Brain stem activation in spontaneous human migraine attacks. *Nature Medicine* 1995; 1:658–60.

Background

The most fundamental key to rationale medicine development, indeed understanding a disorder, is to be sure what organ is the target of the problem. It can be argued that from a macro- and integrated physiological perspective, brain imaging has done more than other human studies to elucidate fundamental aspects [10]. Here, two groups of observations vie for mention. The beginning of the end for the Wolffian [16] concept of migraine aura as a vasoconstrictor phenomenon was the imaging work of Olesen and colleagues [21] showing a progressive, slowly propagating wave of reduced brain blood flow traversing the cerebral cortex. The change was reminiscent of the cortical spreading depression of Leão [17] described in section 3.2, the link to which others had already speculated upon [20]. Given aura in that form only affects one-quarter of migraineurs and is neither necessary nor essential for migraine [84], one can argue that it is functional imaging of migraine itself that has really made the crucial contribution, and if that is accepted, then Weiller and colleagues [85] would be considered to have made the great leap.

Methods

Nine patients with migraine without aura [30] were studied during spontaneous right-sided attacks. Patients were studied within 6 hours of onset, with ^{15}C-O_2 inhalational positron emission tomography (PET), in three states: in pain during the attack; after relief from sumatriptan 6 mg; and in a headache-free interval some 3 days to 4 months later. The analysis was done with statistical parametric mapping (SPM) [86] which, parenthetically, would be in anyone's list of methodological top 10 neuroscience contributions.

Results

The authors reported activations in the cingulate cortex (pain and attention) and auditory and parieto-occipital cortices (phonophobia and photophobia). These results were not surprising. What was extraordinary was the appearance of activations in the brainstem in the dorsal midbrain and dorsolateral pons (Fig. 3.3). The cortical activations were not present after successful treatment with sumatriptan, while the brainstem activation persisted.

Conclusions and critique

Again, it is hard to overstate how revolutionary this paper was at the time. While electrophysiological evidence on brain involvement had been accumulating over some period [87, 88], and should have been afforded more attention, imaging seemed somehow more concrete. The new findings were consistent with dicencephalic and brainstem involvement as a unifying concept for the variety of symptoms in migraine [89]; hitherto, only bench

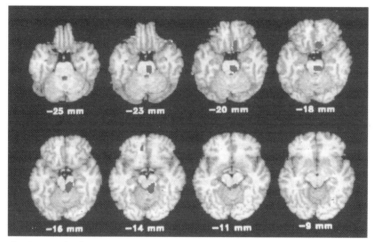

Fig. 3.3 Activations in the brain comparing interval and acute migraine attacks in nine patients showing brainstem changes that did not abate when the attack was controlled with sumatriptan. Reproduced from *Nature Medicine*, 1, Weiller C, May A, Limmroth V, Jüptner M, Kaube H, et al. Brain stem activation in spontaneous human migraine attacks, p. 658–660, Copyright (1995), with permission from Macmillan.

data existed from experimental animals [65, 90]. Subsequent studies have largely reproduced the initial finding of brainstem activation in migraine [91, 92] and reinforced that the changes are associated with lateralization of symptoms [93]. The findings are consistent with observations of brain perturbation [94, 95] and with the results from the more recently developed connectivity methods [96]. Moreover, the long-standing question of whether the brainstem changes are due to pain or are part of the underlying disorder has now been settled by the observation of their presence in the premonitory phase before pain is present [97].

Migraine is fundamentally a brain disorder, so functional brain imaging results must stand as among the crucial findings during the last 150 years. How these changes relate to each other and whether ligand imaging methods can address the next great question—the site of action of medicines—will no doubt form crucial papers in the coming years.

3.8 Familial hemiplegic migraine: a biologically defined disorder

Main paper: Ophoff RA, Terwindt GM, Vergouwe MN, et al. Familial hemiplegic migraine and episodic ataxia type-2 are caused by mutations in the Ca^{2+} channel gene CACNL1A4. *Cell* 1996; 87:543–52.

Background

There seems little doubt, from clinical practice [98] or from an epidemiological perspective [99], that genetic influences play a role in migraine. The molecular age offered the tools to begin to take this clinical observation and explore the biological bounty. Lieving [12] described cases of hemiplegic migraine, and Clarke [100], the first family. A rather prescient comment was that of Whitty [101], in the syndrome-defining paper for familial hemiplegic migraine (FHM), remarking on Symonds' [102] case in which the first cerebral angiography was done in hemiplegic migraine and seen to be normal: 'it is difficult to envisage a primary arterial spasm sufficient to cause an ischaemia which results in motor and sensory loss which may persist for days and yet recover completely.' Clarke [100] had originally suggested that the group be treated specially, and it was not until the end of the twentieth century that chromosome 19 was identified to carry the gene [103] and the very special nature of the syndrome was revealed by the Leiden Group, led by Frants and Ferrari [26].

Methods

Sixteen patients from six families with FHM, including six patients with sporadic hemiplegic migraine, were studied [26]. In addition, four subjects from four unrelated families with episodic ataxia type-2 (EA-2) were also studied.

Results

The subjects with FHM had been mapped to chromosome 19p13 and the authors characterized the gene for the alpha-1 subunit of the P/Q-type Ca^{2+} CACNL1A4. Four different missense mutations were found in FHM of which one mutation was seen in two different unrelated cases. The authors demonstrated that EA-2 is an allelic disorder to what is now called FHM-I.

Conclusions and critique

The paper was, again, truly a landmark in migraine research. As with any ground-breaking work, it has spurred much discussion and many other studies. Certainly, the paper marked the encroachment of the molecular age into the migraine arena. Important other clinical–molecular data have followed, with other mutations involving the ATP1A2 gene, FHM-II [104], and the SCN1A gene, FHM-III [105]. The unifying theme has been effects on channels. In turn, bench research has benefited with the FHM-I knock mouse whose phenotype includes increased susceptibility to cortical spreading depression [27]. Importantly, the FHM-II mouse also has that susceptibility [106], so that the importance of this line of enquiry is certain. It is disappointing that the mutations in FHM do not map easily to a clinical phenotype in detail [107], although the S218L mutation [108] did solve the puzzle of migraine coma [109]. Much has been validated; for example, it is clear that glutamatergic mechanisms are at play in cortical spreading depression [110], just as they are at play in migraine aura [111]. Whatever happens in migraine genetics, the identification of the FHM-I gene will certainly stand the test of time.

3.9 **Cluster headache—brain or not?**

Main paper:May A, Bahra A, Buchel C, Frackowiak RS, Goadsby PJ. Hypothalamic activation in cluster headache attacks. *Lancet* 1998; 352:275–8.

Background

As one approached the mid-twentieth century, most authors considered cluster headache to be due to local dilation of branches of the external carotid [112]. Even astute observers had considered it basically a type of migraine [113, 114]. Horton and colleagues [115] described most of the salient features, while the term 'cluster' was introduced by Kunkle and colleagues [116], although again, the latter did not insist on differentiation from migraine. Ekbom [117] set out the differences nicely, as did Lance and Anthony [118], both concluding cluster headache was a different syndrome from migraine. In the late 1980s, the pericarotid plexus was implicated [119], while, as inflammatory mechanisms became the flavour *du jour* of the early 1990s, cluster headache became implicated in such mechanisms [120]. From a clinical perspective, this seemed very unlikely to this author, and so, when the chance to study the brain in cluster headache arose, it was grasped.

Methods

Nine males with chronic cluster headache were studied during a nitroglycerin (NTG)-induced attack [121]. NTG triggering had been observed to activate cluster headache many years earlier [122] and this seemed, and continues to seem, a useful approach. The triggered attacks were phenotypically identical in terms of lateralization and cranial autonomic features. The control group was eight patients with episodic cluster headache who were out of their bout. PET using $H_2^{15}O$ was utilized, having tried, without success, to capture attacks in MRI in the preceding months.

Results

When the baseline headache-free versus NTG-induced headache period was compared, activations were found in the region of the ipsilateral posterior hypothalamus (Fig. 3.4), the anterior cingulate cortex bilaterally, the contralateral posterior thalamus, ipsilateral basal ganglia, and bilateral insulae.

Conclusions and critique

From the authors' point of view, it seemed very reasonable to find activations in the cingulate cortex, insulae, and contralateral thalamus as part of the expression of the pain. Possibly basal ganglia activation had some part to play in the restlessness that is so characteristic of the phenotype. The hypothalamic region held much possibility in terms of the endocrine disturbances in the syndrome [123] and the circadian aspects. Perhaps the most remarkable aspect of the outcome was the successful use of the posterior hypothalamic region as a target for deep brain stimulation (DBS) in medically refractory cluster headache, as reported by Leone and colleagues [124]. Large series have followed [125] and have

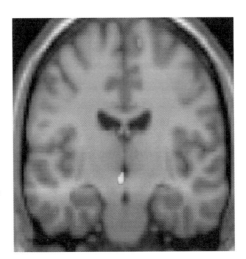

Fig. 3.4 Activations in the brain in a region adjacent to the third ventricle and behind the region of the posterior hypothalamus marked cluster headache as a disorder of the brain.

Reproduced from *The Lancet*, 352(9124), May A, Bahra A, Buchel C, Frackowiak RS, Goadsby PJ. Hypothalamic activation in cluster headache attacks, p. 275–8, Copyright (1998), with permission from Elsevier.

confirmed a more than chance effect, although a recent clinical trial with a short observation period was negative. The technique has been used for other trigeminal autonomic cephalalgias (TACS), such as SUNCT [126], since their functional imaging also involves the same part of the brain [127]. Were it not for the obvious morbidity issues [128], there would probably be more studies done. Certainly, further studies with PET activations [129, 130] and fluoro-deoxyglucose [131] have confirmed the initial finding.

It is remarkable that the same region has been known to neurosurgeons to produce restlessness and agitation when stimulated in other settings [132] and, thus, may even provide insights into a notable part of the cluster headache phenotype. More broadly, DBS work initiated thinking about neuromodulation in cluster headache as a plausible option, and drove initial studies of occipital nerve stimulation [133–135] as a means to avoid the potential morbidity of DBS.

3.10 **Indomethacin-sensitive headaches**

Main paper: Sjaastad O, Dale I. Evidence for a new (?) treatable headacheentity. *Headache* 1974; 14:105–8.

Background

Although not common, indomethacin-sensitive headaches, such as paroxysmal hemicrania (PH) and hemicrania continua (HC), are the stuff of clinical legend. They are defined clearly in ICHD-II [5], and there are reasonable large case series of each [136, 137]. Any headache medicine trainee is soon taught about them and waits almost breathless for the first patient. The initial response is as magical as it was when first described, indeed defining both syndromes and providing both a treatment and an invitation to understand its mechanism to make the long term outcomes better.

Methods and results

The authors reported two cases: one they had observed for 12 years and the other, for 5 years. Both patients were female and had had the problem for 20 years. One patient initially had clustering, and both had suffered with more or less daily pain for over a decade. The attacks were lateralized, frequent, six to eighteen a day, without a circadian pattern, and short compared to more usual cluster headaches (at 15–45 minutes). There was some inter-paroxysmal discomfort. Cranial autonomic symptoms were homolateral to the pain. Ergotamine, chlorpromazine, beta-blockers, antidepressants, and carbamazepine were not useful, yet salicylates were somewhat helpful. Indomethacin was not helpful to 10 patients with cluster headache, yet made the new headache 'fade away' within 24 hours of 50–75 mg per day and stay away at 5 and 7 months' follow-up.

Conclusions and critique

The authors had indeed identified a 'new treatable headache entity' which they subsequently named 'chronic paroxysmal hemicrania' [138]. Sometime later, Kudrow and colleagues [139] reported the episodic version—episodic paroxysmal hemicrania—and large series are now available [137]. Sjaastad recognized the other major indomethacin-sensitive TAC some years later, as hemicrania continua [140]; Medina and Diamond [141] having tripped over it a few years earlier and not realizing that it was more than cluster headache [136]. It is hard to overstate how important the first observation was. Not a teaching course goes by without the attendees being advised to seek indomethacin-sensitive headaches.

Sadly, in the nearly 40 years since its description, the unique mechanism of action of indomethacin is yet to be resolved. Functional brain imaging has reinforced that the syndromes of paroxysmal hemicrania [142] and hemicrania continua [143] are unique from cluster headache [121], and, indeed, Sjaastad's comment that indomethacin is not helpful for cluster headache rings true over time. Some recent data suggest a role for nitrergic mechanisms in the effect of indomethacin [144, 145], and this may provide a clue going forward. Neuromodulation has proved useful in hemicrania continua [134], since when indomethacin is not tolerated, the way forward is seldom easy.

Remarkably, the entire indomethacin-sensitive headache story arises from two patients, and could be described as a case report, standing a very good chance of rejection were it submitted today to any major neurological journal. This is not because it was not interesting or impactful, but because case reports have become so little valued. This particular story encapsulates the meta-message from the 10 papers in this chapter: when confronted with clinical observations that seem compelling and laboratory science that contradicts and seems persuasive, choose the clinic—it is our best laboratory for translational medicine.

Key unanswered questions

1 When will we identify the first gene(s) for migraine without aura?
   In terms of pathogenesis, this is the most pressing unanswered question. Such information will transform, beyond recognition, our understanding of the molecular pathogenesis and how to approach the development of new preventives.

2 Is the blood–brain barrier altered in migraine?
   From a therapeutic viewpoint, this now well-rehearsed question is important since, if the brain is the target organ, the integrity of the blood–brain barrier will inform how to develop new therapeutics.

3 What is the nature of the noxious stimulus in migraine?
   This remains a very great intellectual problem. Is there a noxious event that is key to the pathophysiology or is the nociceptive aspect of migraine simply an extension of the other sensory modality dysfunctions (i.e. as light, sound, and smells, perceived to be unpleasant and whose input is normally ignored for optimal function, now synchronized by a dysfunction in habituation mechanisms)?

4 What is the precise region that is dysfunctional in cluster headache and how does its change in behaviour drive the attacks?
   Understanding the brain regions involved in cluster headache will no doubt facilitate management of the problem.

5 What is the mechanism of indomethacin?
   As indicated in section 3.10, a crucial question to help the move forward with new therapeutics in the area of indomethacin-sensitive headaches is what is the special, differentiating effect of indomethacin that makes it so effective in the patients who respond so clearly?

References

1 Lipton RB, Stewart WF, Diamond S, Diamond ML, Reed M. Prevalence and burden of migraine in the United States: data from the American Migraine Study II. *Headache* 2001; **41**:646–57.

2 Lipton RB, Stewart WF, Sawyer J, Edmeads JG. Clinical utility of an instrument assessing migraine disability: the migraine disability assessment (MIDAS) questionnaire. *Headache* 2001; **41**:854–61.

3 Gowers WR. *A Manual of Diseases of the Nervous System*. Philadelphia: P. Blakiston, Son & Co; 1899.

4 Olesen J, Bousser MG, Diener HC, et al. New appendix criteria open for a broader concept of chronic migraine. *Cephalalgia* 2006; **26**:742–6.

5 Headache Classification Committee of the International Headache Society. The International Classification of Headache Disorders, 2nd ed. *Cephalalgia* 2004; **24**:1–160.

6 Goadsby PJ, Lipton RB. A review of paroxysmal hemicranias, SUNCT syndrome and other short-lasting headaches with autonomic features, including new cases. *Brain* 1997; **120**:193–209.

7 Lai T-H, Fuh J-L, Wang S-J. Cranial autonomic symptoms in migraine: characteristics and comparison with cluster headache. *Journal of Neurology, Neurosurgery and Psychiatry* 2009; **80**:1116–9.

8 Gelfand AA, Reider AC, Goadsby PJ. Cranial autonomic symptoms in pediatric migraine are the rule, not the exception. *Neurology* 2013; **81**:431–6.

9 Irimia P, Cittadini E, Paemeleire K, Cohen AS, Goadsby PJ. Unilateral photophobia or phonophobia in migraine compared with trigeminal autonomic cephalalgias. *Cephalalgia* 2008; **28**:626–30.

10 Sprenger T, Goadsby PJ. What has functional neuroimaging done for primary headache . . . and for the clinical neurologist? *Journal of Clinical Neuroscience* 2010; **17**:547–53.

11 Isler H. Episodic cluster headache from a textbook of 1745: Van Swieten's classic description. *Cephalalgia* 1993; **13**:172–4.

12 Lieving E. *On Megrim, Sick-Headache, and Some Allied Disorders. A Contribution to the Pathology of Nerve-storms*. London: Arts & Boeve Nijmegen; 1873.

13 Maier HW. L'ergotamine inhibiteur du sympathique etudie en clinque, comme moyen d'exploration et comme agent therapeutique. *Revue Neurologie* 1926; **33**:1104–8.

14 Tfelt-Hansen P, Saxena PR, Dahlof C, et al. Ergotamine in the acute treatment of migraine—a review and European consensus. *Brain* 2000; **123**:9–18.

15 Graham JR, Wolff HG. Mechanism of migraine headache and action of ergotamine tartrate. *Archives of Neurology and Psychiatry* 1938; **39**:737–63.

16 Wolff HG. *Headache and Other Head Pain*. New York: Oxford University Press; 1948.

17 Leão AAP. Spreading depression of activity in cerebral cortex. *Journal of Neurophysiology* 1944; **7**:359–90.

18 Leão AAP. Pial circulation and spreading activity in the cerebral cortex. *Journal of Neurophysiology* 1944; **7**:391–6.

19 Leão AP, Morison RS. Propagation of spreading cortical depression. *Journal of Neurophysiology* 1945; **8**:33–45.

20 Marshall WH. Spreading cortical depression of Leão. *Physiological Reviews* 1959; **39**:239–88.

21 Olesen J, Larsen B, Lauritzen M. Focal hyperemia followed by spreading oligemia and impaired activation of rCBF in classic migraine. *Annals of Neurology* 1981; **9**:344–52.

22 Cutrer FM, Sorensen AG, Weisskoff RM, et al. Perfusion-weighted imaging defects during spontaneous migrainous aura. *Annals of Neurology* 1998; **43**:25–31.

23 Hadjikhani N, Sanchez del Rio M, Wu O, et al. Mechanisms of migraine aura revealed by functional MRI in human visual cortex. *Proceedings of the National Academy of Sciences (USA)* 2001; **98**:4687–92.

24 Brennan KC, Beltran-Parrazal L, Lopez Valdes HE, Theriot J, Toga A, Charles AC. Distinct vascular conduction with cortical spreading depression. *Journal of Neurophysiology* 2007; **97**:4143–51.

25 Hansen JM, Baca SM, VanValkenburgh P, Charles A. Distinctive anatomical and physiological features of migraine aura revealed by 18 years of recording. *Brain* 2013; **136**:3589–95.

26 Ophoff RA, Terwindt GM, Vergouwe MN, et al. Familial hemiplegic migraine and episodic ataxia type-2 are caused by mutations in the Ca^{2+} channel gene CACNL1A4. *Cell* 1996; **87**:543–52.

27 van den Maagdenberg AMJM, Pietrobon D, Pizzorusso T, et al. A Cacna1a knock-in migraine mouse model with increased susceptibility to cortical spreading depression. *Neuron* 2004; **41**:701–10.

28 Ad Hoc Committee on Classification of Headache of the NIH. Classification of headache. *Journal of the American Medical Association* 1962; **179**:717–8.

29 Humphrey PPA, Feniuk W, Perren MJ, Beresford IJM, Skingle M, Whalley ET. Serotonin and migraine. *Annals of the New York Academy of Sciences* 1990; **600**:587–98.

30 Headache Classification Committee of the International Headache Society. Classification and diagnostic criteria for headache disorders, cranial neuralgias and facial pain. *Cephalalgia* 1988; **8**:1–96.

31 Headache Classification Committee of the International Headache Society. The International Classification of Headache Disorders, 3rd ed. (beta version). *Cephalalgia* 2013; **33**:629–808.

32 Goadsby PJ. The pharmacology of headache. *Progress in Neurobiology* 2000; **62**:509–25.

33 Goadsby PJ, Lipton RB, Ferrari MD. Migraine—current understanding and treatment. *New England Journal of Medicine* 2002; **346**:257–70.

34 Humphrey PPA, Feniuk W, Marriott AS, Tanner RJN, Jackson MR, Tucker ML. Preclinical studies on the anti-migraine drug, sumatriptan. *European Neurology* 1991; **31**:282–90.

35 Feniuk W, Humphrey PPA, Perren MJ. The selective carotid arterial vasoconstrictor action of GR43175 in anaesthetised dogs. *British Journal of Pharmacology* 1989; **96**:83–90.

36 Doenicke A, Siegel E, Hadoke M, Perrin VL. Initial clinical study of AH25086B (5-HT$_1$-like agonist) in the acute treatment of migraine. *Cephalalgia* 1987; **7**:437–8.

37 Markowitz S, Saito K, Moskowitz MA. Neurogenically mediated leakage of plasma proteins occurs from blood vessels in dura mater but not brain. *Journal of Neuroscience* 1987; **7**:4129–36.

38 Johnston BM, Saxena PR. The effect of ergotamine on tissue blood flow and the arteriovenous shunting of radioactive microspheres in the head. *British Journal of Pharmacology* 1978; **63**:541–9.

39 Dodick D, Lipton RB, Martin V, et al. Consensus statement: cardiovascular safety profile of triptans (5-HT$_{1B/1D}$ agonists) in the acute treatment of migraine. *Headache* 2004; **44**:414–25.

40 Ferrari MD, Roon KI, Lipton RB, Goadsby PJ. Oral triptans (serotonin, 5-HT$_{1B/1D}$ agonists) in acute migraine treatment: a meta-analysis of 53 trials. *The Lancet* 2001; **358**:1668–75.

41 Goadsby PJ. A triptan too far. *Journal of Neurology, Neurosurgery and Psychiatry* 1998; **64**:143–7.

42 Pilgrim AJ. Methodology of clinical trials of sumatriptan in migraine and cluster headache. *European Neurology* 1991; **31**:295–9.

43 International Headache Society Committee on Clinical Trials in Migraine. Guidelines for controlled trials of drugs in migraine. *Cephalalgia* 1991; **11**:1–12.

44 Buzzi MG, Moskowitz MA. The antimigraine drug, sumatriptan (GR43175), selectively blocks neurogenic plasma extravasation from blood vessels in dura mater. *British Journal of Pharmacology* 1990; **99**:202–6.

45 **Humphrey PPA, Goadsby PJ.** Controversies in headache. The mode of action of sumatriptan is vascular? A debate. *Cephalalgia* 1994; **14**:401–10.

46 **Jancso N, Jancso-Gabor A, Szolcsanyi J.** Direct evidence for neurogenic inflammation and its prevention by denervation and by pretreatment with capsaicin. *British Journal of Pharmacology* 1967; **31**:138–51.

47 **Buzzi MG, Moskowitz MA.** Evidence for 5-HT$_{1B/1D}$ receptors mediating the antimigraine effect of sumatriptan and dihydroergotamine. *Cephalalgia* 1991; **11**:165–8.

48 **Connor HE, Bertin L, Gillies S, Beattie DT, Ward P, the GR205171 Clinical Study Group.** Clinical evaluation of a novel, potent, CNS penetrating NK$_1$ receptor antagonist in the acute treatment of migraine. *Cephalalgia* 1998; **18**:392.

49 **Diener H-C, the RPR100893 Study Group.** RPR100893, a substance-P antagonist, is not effective in the treatment of migraine attacks. *Cephalalgia* 2003; **23**:183–5.

50 **Goldstein DJ, Wang O, Saper JR, Stoltz R, Silberstein SD, Mathew NT.** Ineffectiveness of neurokinin-1 antagonist in acute migraine: a crossover study. *Cephalalgia* 1997; **17**:785–90.

51 **Norman B, Panebianco D, Block GA.** A placebo-controlled, in-clinic study to explore the preliminary safety and efficacy of intravenous L-758,298 (a prodrug of the NK1 receptor antagonist L-754,030) in the acute treatment of migraine. *Cephalalgia* 1998; **18**:407.

52 **Goldstein DJ, Offen WW, Klein EG, et al.** Lanepitant, an NK-1 antagonist, in migraine prevention. *Cephalalgia* 2001; **21**:102–6.

53 **Clozel M, Breu V, Gray AG, et al.** Pharmacological characterisation of bosentan, a new potent orally active nonpeptide endothelin receptor antagonist. *Journal of Pharmacology and Experimental Therapeutics* 1994; **270**:228–35.

54 **May A, Gijsman HJ, Wallnoefer A, Jones R, Diener HC, Ferrari MD.** Endothelin antagonist bosentan blocks neurogenic inflammation, but is not effective in aborting migraine attacks. *Pain* 1996; **67**:375–8.

55 **Data J, Britch K, Westergaard N, et al.** A double-blind study of ganaxolone in the acute treatment of migraine headaches with or without an aura in premenopausal females. *Headache* 1998; **38**:380.

56 **Reuter U, Bolay H, Jansen-Olesen I, et al.** Delayed inflammation in rat meninges: implications for migraine pathophysiology. *Brain* 2001; **124**:2490–502.

57 **Alderton WK, Angell AD, Craig C, et al.** GW274150 and GW273629 are potent and highly selective inhibitors of inducible nitric oxide synthase in vitro and in vivo. *British Journal of Pharmacology* 2005; **145**:301–12.

58 **Palmer JE, Guillard FL, Laurijssens BE, Wentz AL, Dixon RM, Williams PM.** A randomised, single-blind, placebo-controlled, adaptive clinical trial of GW274150, a selective iNOS inhibitor, in the treatment of acute migraine. *Cephalalgia* 2009; **29**:124.

59 **Hoye K, Laurijssens BE, Harnisch LO, et al.** Efficacy and tolerability of the iNOS inhibitor GW274150 administered up to 120 mg daily for 12 weeks in the prophylactic treatment of migraine. *Cephalalgia* 2009; **29**:132.

60 **Caterina MJ, Schumacher MA, Tominaga M, Rosen TA, Levine JD, Julius D.** The capsaicin receptor: a heat-activated ion channel in the pain pathway. *Nature* 1997; **389**:816–24.

61 **Rami HK, Thompson M, Stemp G, et al.** Discovery of SB-705498: a potent, selective and orally bioavailable TRPV1 antagonist suitable for clinical development. *Bioorganic & Medicinal Chemistry Letters* 2006; **16**:3287–91.

61a **Chizh B, Palmer AJ, Lai RY, Guillard F, Bullman J, Baines A, et al.** A randomised, two-period cross-over study to investigate the efficacy of the TRPV1 antagonist SB-705498 in acute migraine. http://www.efic-congress.org/showabstract.php?abstract=702: EFIC Pain in Europe VI; 2009.

62 **Summ O, Akerman S, Holland PR, Goadsby PJ.** TRPV1 receptor blockade is ineffective in different in vivo models of migraine. *Cephalalgia* 2011; **31**:172–80.

63 **Goadsby PJ, Edvinsson L, Ekman R.** Vasoactive peptide release in the extracerebral circulation of humans during migraine headache. *Annals of Neurology* 1990; **28**:183–7.

64 **Lance JW.** The control of muscle tone, reflexes, and movement: Robert Wartenberg Lecture. *Neurology* 1980; **30**:1303–13.

65 **Goadsby PJ, Lambert GA, Lance JW.** Differential effects on the internal and external carotid circulation of the monkey evoked by locus coeruleus stimulation. *Brain Research* 1982; **249**:247–54.

66 **Lance JW, Lambert GA, Goadsby PJ, Duckworth JW.** Brainstem influences on cephalic circulation: experimental data from cat and monkey of relevance to the mechanism of migraine. *Headache* 1983; **23**:258–65.

67 **Lambert GA, Bogduk N, Goadsby PJ, Duckworth JW, Lance JW.** Decreased carotid arterial resistance in cats in response to trigeminal stimulation. *Journal of Neurosurgery* 1984; **61**:307–15.

68 **Goadsby PJ, Lambert GA, Lance JW.** Effects of locus coeruleus stimulation on carotid vascular resistance in the cat. *Brain Research* 1983; **278**:175–83.

69 **Goadsby PJ, Lambert GA, Lance JW.** The peripheral pathway for extracranial vasodilatation in the cat. *Journal of the Autonomic Nervous System* 1984; **10**:145–55.

70 **McCulloch J, Uddman R, Kingman TA, Edvinsson L.** Calcitonin gene-related peptide: functional role in cerebrovascular regulation. *Proceedings of the National Academy of Sciences (USA)* 1986; **83**:1–5.

71 **Goadsby PJ, Edvinsson L, Ekman R.** Release of vasoactive peptides in the extracerebral circulation of man and the cat during activation of the trigeminovascular system. *Annals of Neurology* 1988; **23**:193–6.

72 **Zagami AS, Goadsby PJ, Edvinsson L.** Stimulation of the superior sagittal sinus in the cat causes release of vasoactive peptides. *Neuropeptides* 1990; **16**:69–75.

73 **May A, Goadsby PJ.** Substance P receptor antagonists in the therapy of migraine. *Expert Opinion in Investigational Drugs* 2001; **10**:1–6.

74 **Goadsby PJ, Edvinsson L.** The trigeminovascular system and migraine: studies characterizing cerebrovascular and neuropeptide changes seen in humans and cats. *Annals of Neurology* 1993; **33**:48–56.

75 **Peroutka SJ.** Neurogenic inflammation and migraine: implications for therapeutics. *Molecular Interventions* 2005; **5**:306–13.

76 **Olesen J, Diener HC, Husstedt IW, et al.** Calcitonin gene-related peptide receptor antagonist BIBN 4096 BS for the acute treatment of migraine. *New England Journal of Medicine* 2004; **350**:1104–10.

77 **Petersen KA, Birk S, Lassen LH, et al.** The CGRP-antagonist, BIBN4096BS does not affect cerebral or systemic haemodynamics in healthy volunteers. *Cephalalgia* 2005; **25**:139–47.

78a **Ho TW, Edvinsson L, Goadsby PJ.** CGRP and its receptors provide new insights into migraine pathophysiology. *Nature Reviews Neurology* 2010; **6**:761–6.

78b **Dodick DW, Goadsby PJ, Spierings ELH, Scherer JC, Sweeney SP, Grayzel DS.** CGRP Monoclonal Antibody LY2951742 for the Prevention of Migraine: A Phase 2, Randomized, Double-Blind, Placebo-Controlled Study. Lancet Neurology. 2014; **13**:885–92.

78c **Dodick DW, Goadsby PJ, Silberstein SD, Lipton RB, Olesen J, Ashina M, et al.** Randomized, Double-blind, Placebo-controlled, Phase II Trial of ALD403, an anti-CGRP peptide antibody in the prevention of frequent episodic migraine. Lancet Neurology. 2014; **13**:1100–7.

79 **Farkkila M, Diener HC, Geraud G, et al.** Efficacy and tolerability of lasmiditan, an oral 5-HT(1F) receptor agonist, for the acute treatment of migraine: a phase 2 randomised, placebo-controlled, parallel-group, dose-ranging study. *Lancet Neurology* 2012; **11**:405–13.

80 **Schoonman GG, van der Grond J, Kortmann C, van der Geest RJ, Terwindt GM, Ferrari MD.** Migraine headache is not associated with cerebral or meningeal vasodilatation—a 3T magnetic resonance angiography study. *Brain* 2008; **131**:2192–200.

81 **Amin FM, Asghar MS, Hougaard A, et al.** Magnetic resonance angiography of intracranial and extracranial arteries in patients with spontaneous migraine without aura: a cross-sectional study. *Lancet Neurology* 2013; **12**:454–61.

82 **Rahmann A, Wienecke T, Hansen JM, Fahrenkrug J, Olesen J, Ashina M.** Vasoactive intestinal peptide causes marked cephalic vasodilatation but does not induce migraine. *Cephalalgia* 2008; **28**:226–36.

83 **Akerman S, Holland P, Goadsby PJ.** Diencephalic and brainstem mechanisms in migraine. *Nature Reviews Neuroscience* 2011; **12**:570–84.

84 **Goadsby PJ.** Parallel concept of migraine pathogenesis. *Annals of Neurology* 2002; **51**:140.

85 **Weiller C, May A, Limmroth V, et al.** Brain stem activation in spontaneous human migraine attacks. *Nature Medicine* 1995; **1**:658–60.

86 **Friston KJ, Holmes AP, Worsley KP, Proline JB, Frith CD, Frackowiak RSJ.** Statistical parametric maps in functional imaging: a general linear approach. *Human Brain Mapping* 1995; **2**:189–210.

87 **Bocker KB, Timsit-Berthier M, Schoenen J, Brunia CH.** Contingent negative variation in migraine. *Headache* 1990; **30**:604–9.

88 **Maertens de Noordhout A, Timsit-Berthier M, Schoenen J.** Contingent negative variation (CNV) in migraineurs before and during prophylactic treatment with beta-blockers. *Cephalalgia* 1985; **5**:34–5.

89 **Lance JW, Lambert GA, Goadsby PJ.** A unifying hypothesis for migraine. *Annals of Neurology* 1982; **12**:83.

90 **Goadsby PJ, Lance JW.** Brainstem effects on intra- and extracerebral circulations. Relation to migraine and cluster headache. In: Olesen J, Edvinsson L, eds. *Basic Mechanisms of Headache.* Amsterdam: Elsevier Science Publishers; 1988: 413–27.

91 **Afridi S, Giffin NJ, Kaube H, et al.** A PET study in spontaneous migraine. *Archives of Neurology* 2005; **62**:1270–5.

92 **Denuelle M, Fabre N, Payoux P, Chollet F, Geraud G.** Brainstem and hypothalamic activation in spontaneous migraine attacks. *Cephalalgia* 2004; **24**:775–814.

93 **Afridi S, Matharu MS, Lee L, et al.** A PET study exploring the laterality of brainstem activation in migraine using glyceryl trinitrate. *Brain* 2005; **128**:932–9.

94 **Raskin NH, Hosobuchi Y, Lamb S.** Headache may arise from perturbation of brain. *Headache* 1987; **27**:416–20.

95 **Veloso F, Kumar K, Toth C.** Headache secondary to deep brain implantation. *Headache* 1998; **38**:507–15.

96 **Mainero C, Boshyan J, Hadjikhani N.** Altered functional magnetic resonance imaging resting-state connectivity in periaqueductal gray networks in migraine. *Annals of Neurology* 2011; **70**:838–45.

97 **Maniyar FH, Sprenger T, Monteith T, Schankin C, Goadsby PJ.** Brain activations in the premonitory phase of nitroglycerin triggered migraine attacks. Brain. 2014; **137**:232–42.

98 **Lance JW, Goadsby PJ.** *Mechanism and Management of Headache.* New York: Elsevier; 2005.

99 **Russell MB, Iselius L, Olesen J.** Investigation of the inheritance of migraine by complex segregation analysis. *Human Genetics* 1995; **96**:726–30.

100 **Clarke JM.** On recurrent motor paralysis in migraine. *British Medical Journal* 1910; **1**:1534–8.

101 **Whitty CW.** Familial hemiplegic migraine. *Journal of Neurology, Neurosurgery & Psychiatry* 1953; **16**:172–7.

102 **Symonds C.** Migrainous variants. *Transactions of the Medical Society of London* 1952; **67**:237–50.

103 **Joutel A, Bousser MG, Biousse V, et al.** A gene for familial hemiplegic migraine maps to chromosome 19. *Nature Genetics* 1993; **5**:40–5.

104 De Fusco M, Marconi R, Silvestri L, et al. Haploinsufficiency of ATP1A2 encoding the Na^{+}/K^{+} pump a2 subunit associated with familial hemiplegic migraine type 2. *Nature Genetics* 2003; **33**:192–6.

105 Dichgans M, Freilinger T, Eckstein G, et al. Mutation in the neuronal voltage-gated sodium channel *SCN1A* causes familial hemiplegic migraine. *The Lancet* 2005; **366**:371–7.

106 Leo L, Gherardini L, Barone V, et al. Increased susceptibility to cortical spreading depression in the mouse model of familial hemiplegic migraine type 2. *PLoS Genetics* 2011; **7**:e1002129.

107 Ducros A, Denier C, Joutel A, et al. The clinical spectrum of familial hemiplegic migraine associated with mutations in a neuronal calcium channel. *New England Journal of Medicine* 2001; **345**:17–24.

108 Kors EE, Terwindt GM, Vermeulen FLMG, et al. Delayed cerebral edema and fatal coma after minor head trauma: role of CACNA1A calcium channel subunit gene and relationship with familial hemiplegic migraine. *Annals of Neurology* 2001; **49**:753–60.

109 Fitzsimons RB, Wolfenden WH. Migraine coma—meningitic migraine with cerebral edema associated with a new form of autosomal dominant cerebellar-ataxia. *Brain* 1985; **108**:555–7.

110 Lauritzen M, Hansen AJ. The effect of glutamate receptor blockade on anoxic depolarization and cortical spreading depression. *Journal of Cerebral Blood Flow and Metabolism* 1992; **12**:223–9.

111 Afridi S, Giffin NJ, Kaube H, Goadsby PJ. A randomized controlled trial of intranasal ketamine in migraine with prolonged aura. *Neurology* 2013; **80**:642–7.

112 Friedman AP, Mikropoulos HE. Cluster headache. *Neurology (Minneapolis)* 1958; **8**:653–63.

113 Harris W. Ciliary (migrainous) neuralgia and its treatment. *British Medical Journal* 1936; **1**:457–60.

114 Symonds CP. A particular variety of headache. *Brain* 1956; **79**:217–32.

115 Horton BT, MacLean AR, Craig WM. A new syndrome of vascular headache; results of treatment with histamine; a preliminary report. *Proceedings of the Mayo Clinic* 1939; **14**:250–7.

116 Kunkle EC, Pfieffer JB, Wilhoit WM, Hamrick LW. Recurrent brief headache in cluster pattern. *Transactions of the American Neurological Association* 1952; **27**:240–3.

117 Ekbom K. A clinical comparison of cluster headache and migraine. *Acta Neurologica Scandinavica* 1970; **46**:1–48.

118 Lance JW, Anthony M. Migrainous neuralgia or cluster headache? *Journal of the Neurological Sciences* 1971; **13**:401–14.

119 Moskowitz MA. Cluster headache—evidence for a pathophysiologic focus in the superior pericarotid cavernous sinus plexus. *Headache* 1988; **28**:584–6.

120 Hardebo JE. How cluster headache is explained as an intracavernous inflammatory process lesioning sympathetic fibres. *Headache* 1994; **34**:125–31.

121 May A, Bahra A, Buchel C, Frackowiak RS, Goadsby PJ. Hypothalamic activation in cluster headache attacks. *The Lancet* 1998; **352**:275–8.

122 Ekbom K. Nitroglycerin as a provocative agent in cluster headache. *Archives of Neurology* 1968; **19**:487–93.

123 Leone M, Partuno G, Vescovi A, Bussone G. Neuroendocrine dysfunction in cluster headache. *Cephalalgia* 1990; **10**:235–9.

124 Leone M, Franzini A, Bussone G. Stereotatic stimulation of the posterior hypothalamic gray matter in a patient with intractable cluster headache. *New England Journal of Medicine* 2001; **345**:1428–9.

125 Leone M, Franzini A, Broggi G, Bussone G. Hypothalamic stimulation for intractable cluster headache: long-term experience. *Neurology* 2006; **67**:150–2.

126 Leone M, Franzini A, D'Andrea G, Broggi G, Casucci G, Bussone G. Deep brain stimulation to relieve drug-resistant SUNCT. *Annals of Neurology* 2005; **57**:924–7.

127 **May A, Bahra A, Buchel C, Turner R, Goadsby PJ.** Functional MRI in spontaneous attacks of SUNCT: short-lasting neuralgiform headache with conjunctival injection and tearing. *Annals of Neurology* 1999; **46**:791–3.

128 **Schoenen J, Di Clemente L, Vandenheede M, et al.** Hypothalamic stimulation in chronic cluster headache: a pilot study of efficacy and mode of action. *Brain* 2005; **128**:940–7.

129 **May A, Bahra A, Buchel C, Frackowiak RSJ, Goadsby PJ.** PET and MRA findings in cluster headache and MRA in experimental pain. *Neurology* 2000; **55**:1328–35.

130 **Sprenger T, Boecker H, Tolle TR, Bussone G, May A, Leone M.** Specific hypothalamic activation during a spontaneous cluster headache attack. *Neurology* 2004; **62**:516–7.

131 **Magis D, Bruno MA, Fumal A, et al.** Central modulation in cluster headache patients treated with occipital nerve stimulation: an FDG-PET study. *British Medical Council Neurology* 2011; **11**:25.

132 **Bejjani BP, Houeto JL, Hariz M, et al.** Aggressive behavior induced by intraoperative stimulation in the triangle of Sano. *Neurology* 2002; **59**:1425–7.

133 **Burns B, Watkins L, Goadsby PJ.** Successful treatment of medically intractable cluster headache using occipital nerve stimulation (ONS). *The Lancet* 2007; **369**:1099–106.

134 **Burns B, Watkins L, Goadsby PJ.** Treatment of hemicrania continua by occipital nerve stimulation using the novel bion device: long term follow up of six patients. *The Lancet Neurology* 2008; **7**:1001–12.

135 **Magis D, Allena M, Bolla M, De Pasqua V, Remacle JM, Schoenen J.** Occipital nerve stimulation for drug-resistant chronic cluster headache: a prospective pilot study. *The Lancet Neurology* 2007; **6**:314–21.

136 **Cittadini E, Goadsby PJ.** Hemicrania continua: a clinical study of 39 patients with diagnostic implications. *Brain* 2010; **133**:1973–86.

137 **Cittadini E, Matharu MS, Goadsby PJ.** Paroxysmal hemicrania: a prospective clinical study of thirty-one cases. *Brain* 2008; **131**:1142–55.

138 **Sjaastad O, Dale I.** A new (?) clinical headache entity 'chronic paroxysmal hemicrania'. *Acta Neurologica Scandinavica* 1976; **54**:140–59.

139 **Kudrow L, Esperanca P, Vijayan N.** Episodic paroxysmal hemicrania? *Cephalalgia* 1987; **7**:197–201.

140 **Sjaastad O, Spierings EL.** Hemicrania continua: another headache absolutely responsive to indomethacin. *Cephalalgia* 1984; **4**:65–70.

141 **Medina JL, Diamond S.** Cluster headache variant: spectrum of a new headache syndrome. *Archives of Neurology* 1981; **38**:705–9.

142 **Matharu MS, Cohen AS, Frackowiak RSJ, Goadsby PJ.** Posterior hypothalamic activation in paroxysmal hemicrania. *Annals of Neurology* 2006; **59**:535–45.

143 **Matharu MS, Cohen AS, McGonigle DJ, Ward N, Frackowiak RSJ, Goadsby PJ.** Posterior hypothalamic and brainstem activation in hemicrania continua. *Headache* 2004; **44**:747–61.

144 **Akerman S, Holland PR, Summ O, Lasalandra MP, Goadsby PJ.** A translational *in vivo* model of trigeminal autonomic cephalalgias—therapeutic characterization. *Brain* 2012; **135**:3664–75.

145 **Summ O, Andreou AP, Akerman S, Goadsby PJ.** A potential nitrergic mechanism of action for indomethacin, but not of other COX inhibitors—relevance to indomethacin-sensitive headaches. *Journal of Headache and Pain* 2010; **11**:477–83.

Chapter 4

Functional neurological symptoms

Alan Carson and Jon Stone

4.0 **Introduction**

Functional neurological symptoms are common, disabling, distressing, and tend to persist. They are known by a variety of synonyms including hysteria, conversion disorder, somatoform disorders, non-organic and psychogenic symptoms. They are characterized by the complaint of physical symptoms which, on examination, display inconsistency or incongruity with recognised neurological disease.

They were among the first medical conditions ever described, dating back to Egyptian medicine. The initial belief was of an exclusively female disorder connected to some disruption of uterine function (hence 'hysterical'). This view held sway throughout Greco-Roman medicine and was endorsed with the Hippocratic School and by Galen. It was maintained through the Dark Ages but, as the Renaissance came, doubts were increasingly articulated about the theory. The pre-eminent British physician, Thomas Willis (1621–1675), wrote extensively on it, describing it as a neurological disorder caused by small cerebral explosions. But a shift in opinion followed over the course of the next century, leading to a view that was much more challenging: some form of disorder of 'psyche'. This brought its own problems. Psyche does not have a direct translation for secular societies and is as suggestive of 'soul' as it is of a 'mind'. It was to be questioned whether this was a matter for doctors at all or one for priests. Either way, it was clear that patients did not fancy the label much. The alternate label of 'malingerers', that gradually emerged in the eighteenth and nineteenth century, offered little attraction either. The tensions between the two labels continue to the current day.

In this chapter, we describe the 10 papers that we think embodied key periods in the development of scientific ideas on the topic. They are certainly not the 10 most cited, or in some cases most laudable studies, but each serves, we believe, to represent a chapter in the story. As we move to modern times, selection of topics has been harder, and many papers we would like to have included have been omitted, and to these authors we apologize. Even when we settled on a topic, the decision on which paper to use to illustrate it, particularly on the use of videotelemetry for diagnosis of non-epileptic attacks and functional imaging of motor symptoms, was difficult. However, if nothing else, we hope our choices will be a source of discussion and attract interest.

4.1 **The first case control cohort study**

Main paper: Briquet P. *Traité Clinique et Thérapeutique de l'Hysterie* (Treatise on Hysteria). Paris: J.B. Ballière; 1859.

Background, methods, and results

French physician, Paul Briquet's (1796–1881) *Treatise on Hysteria* heralded a modern era of research in the field [1]. He described a clinical and epidemiological study of 430 patients attending his unit at the Hôpital de la Charité in Paris over a 10-year period.

It was an exhaustive monograph detailing specific symptoms, tabulating features that distinguished hysterical seizures from epilepsy, describing pain as a central feature, inconsistency and fluctuation in clinical signs, and an association with emotional instability. He noted an increased rate in first-degree relatives.

A dominant view of the time was that both the psychological and physical strain of sexual continence was a causal factor in the development of hysterical symptoms—indeed, Parisian physicians frequently used digital and hydro-genital massage, and began, by the 1870s, to experiment with the vaginal vibrator, as therapeutic options. Briquet was not convinced. In his cohort, he noted that married woman were more likely to present with hysterical symptoms than unmarried (whom he, perhaps naively, assumed to be virgins). However, to his credit, he sought out three comparison cohorts—nuns, house servants, and prostitutes. He concluded that the rate of hysteria increased with increasing sexual activity. He went further though and measured other confounding factors, considering it unlikely that it was the sexual activity itself but, rather, the increased rates of distress, fears, and life difficulties that were causal.

Briquet was clear that psychogenic factors were of aetiological significance and considered that marital or family afflictions were the most common precipitating cause (25% of his series). However, he also recognized a role for panic (14%) and for physical illness (5%) as a precipitant. In contrast to a popular view of the time, he was dismissive of any role of ovarian disease as a precipitant. He opined that the course of the disease:

> . . . is under the influence of two causes, those resulting from the idiosyncrasies of the subject, the others depending on the environmental circumstances in which the hysteric is living [2].

He recognized a poor prognosis. Interestingly, he identified that recognition of the precipitant was an important predictor, with those developing the condition after a slight cause having poorer prognosis as this indicated a strong predisposition. He noted that over half affected patients failed to recover.

Conclusions and critique

But what was special about this work? It was not his theories on hysteria. Although he made some novel points, his views were unremarkable for the era:

> I consider the facts from a different perspective and for me hysteria is a neurosis of the brain, whose apparent phenomena are primarily a disruption of vital acts that serve as a manifestation of the affective sensations and passions . . . not all of them, only those which are manifested by painful

sensations, affections and sad or violent passions. Finally these events, by their frequent repetition, eventually lead to lesions, either dynamic or material, in the affected organs, which add new complications that complement the hysterical symptoms [1].

In that regard, it would be difficult to argue that he moved the field on from other notable writers such as British physician, Thomas Sydenham (1624–1689), over a century earlier.

What was unique about Briquet's treatise was that he not only described his views and thoughts but that he also attempted to objectively test them quantitatively by examining his own cohort and, crucially, by finding comparison groups in order to test specific hypotheses.

It was not the theories that were missing but the facts, it is necessary to study these last: this is what I did [1].

In a footnote to the story, Mai and Merskey, who have highlighted Briquet's work in the English language [2–4], suggest that his name was in fact 'Pierre', following identification of his grave in the Père Lachaise cemetery in Paris (Fig. 4.1) (personal communication). This is one area that the treatise cannot help us with—it was simply signed 'P. Briquet'.

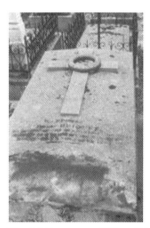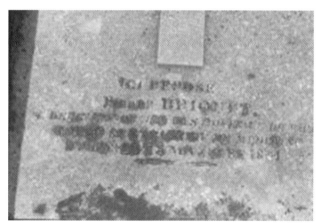

Fig. 4.1 The grave of 'Pierre' (Paul) Briquet.
Photos courtesy of Francois Mai [3].

4.2 **A 'dissociative' model of functional symptoms involving physiological and psychological factors**

Main paper: Janet P. *The Major Symptoms of Hysteria*. London: Macmillan; 1907.

Background, methods, and results

The French psychologist, Pierre Janet (1859–1947), wrote several books on hysteria including *État Mental Des Hystériques* (The Mental State of Hysterics) (1894) and *Névroses et Idées Fixes* (1898). However, *The Major Symptoms of Hysteria* [5] was a more readable summary of lectures given to Harvard University in 1906 and, as such, reached a wider audience.

Janet has been one of the lasting influences on the topic of hysteria over the twentieth century, predominantly through his ideas about dissociation and its relationship to trauma. Janet was medically trained but was one of the key early figures in the development of psychology as a discipline.

The Major Symptoms of Hysteria represented a summation of Janet's work on hysteria at that time and dealt with motor and sensory symptoms, 'attacks', speech problems, and fugue states as well as gastrointestinal symptoms, breathing, amnesia, and double personalities. As a clinical handbook, one of the authors of this chapter has come back to it more than any other text of the time (as evidenced by all the bookmarks sticking out of it).

Truly new clinical observations in hysteria are rare, since the problem has been around so long and so many people have looked carefully at it, but many have been forgotten. Janet is a good place to find them again. For example, Janet described how hysteria could affect the face [5; p.132], whereas Charcot thought it did not. If you see enough patients with functional symptoms, you do start to see patients with contraction of orbicularis and platysma causing facial asymmetry—a problem that was recognized in the past [6] and more recently [7].

Janet's many clinical observations and tips suggest that he spent a lot of time listening to and examining patients with hysteria. He counts 124 in his first book [8]. He also references others generously and avoids the pomposity that was common in that era. It was Janet, for example, who summed up the nature of localized sensory loss in hysterical anaesthesia as a consequence of:

> . . . the popular conception of the organ rather than to its anatomic conception . . . for the common people the hand terminates at the wrist. They don't care if all the principal muscles that animate the hand and forearm are lodged beyond in the forearm [5]. (see Fig. 4.2)

Another appealing aspect of Janet, for the modern reader, is his refusal to let the problem of hysteria be pigeonholed as either arising from the brain or the mind. On the subject of astasia-abasia (when the patient can move their legs on the bed but cannot walk), for example, he suggested there was a disruption in what would now be called a motor programme in the brain but which he called a 'system of images and movements'. In answering critics who suggested this sounded like a dangerously neurological interpretation, his comment was: 'I do not deny it; the fact that a system is psychological should not cause us to conclude that it is not at the same time anatomical.'

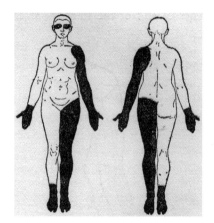

Fig. 4.2 Map of hysterical anaesthesia demonstrating sharp cut-offs at the wrist, groin, and shoulder.
Reproduced from Pierre Janet *Major Symptoms of Hysteria* (1907)

Janet also highlighted the importance of an 'accident' in triggering hysterical symptoms—so called 'traumatic neurosis'—of which there had been quite a long history before him. He elucidated it further though and brought in a psychological model to help understand such symptoms. He writes that the accident would typically be 'very slight in itself' but 'accompanied by a violent moral emotion and disturbance of the imagination'. It is worth looking at what he meant using his own examples:

- Minor injuries to the buttock or back leading to lower limb paralysis;
- Fatigue of a limb from playing a musical instrument or painting a ceiling leading gradually on to paralysis;
- An 'accident' which was not an actual accident at all but one that was imagined to have happened, for example:

  A man travelling by train had done an imprudent thing: while the train was running, he had got down on the step in order to pass from one door to the other, when he became aware that the train was about to enter a tunnel. It occurred to him that his left side, which projected, was going to be knocked slantwise and crushed against the arch of the tunnel. This thought caused him to swoon away but happily for him, he did not fall on the track, but was taken back inside the carriage, and his left side was not even grazed. In spite of this, he had a left hemiplegia [5].

- A woman who developed hand paralysis at the moment of having to play the piano in public;
- After profound sleep;
- After a 'convulsive fit';
- A nurse who thought she saw a ghost was frightened and felt her legs shake. Her legs then 'gave way' and she became paraplegic.

This mixture of physical and psychological triggers start to give a mechanism for the symptom which is truly biopsychosocial, rather than the extreme psychogenic model found in the conversion hypothesis (see section 4.3), and forms the inspiration for at least one of our studies of similar triggers in twenty-first-century patients with functional paralysis [9].

In the example of the man on the train previously mentioned, the idea of paralysis, brought on by terror of an imminent injury, has become dissociated from the patient's consciousness and is acting independently as a '*fixed idea*' (*idée fixe*). Janet was keen to point out, however, that it is not necessarily the idea itself that is the cause of the symptom, but the action of that idea on a biologically and psychologically vulnerable individual. His conception of the 'idée fixe' could also be more sophisticated than 'I am paralysed' or 'I am numb'. He thought, in many cases, that the 'idée fixe' could be something less immediately related to the symptom—for example, the fixed idea of a mother's death or the departure of a spouse.

Janet ambitiously placed his theories within general theories of consciousness. He referred to the principle process in hysteria as a 'retraction of the field of personal consciousness and a tendency to the dissociation and emancipation of the system of ideas and functions that constitute personality' [5].

Conclusions and critique

Janet's ideas were seminal to the concept of dissociation and psychological trauma but, in the field of hysteria, they were overshadowed by Freudian conversion theory. In recent years, however, there has been renewed interest in his notion that functional neurological symptoms arise as a disorder of attention [10], based on beliefs. One of the key differences in newer ideas is that the disorder is not one of decreased attention—what Janet called the absent mindedness of hysteria—but of increased attention to symptoms based on a self-fulfilling expectation that 'something is wrong' [11].

4.3 **The first description of the conversion hypothesis on aetiology and of treatment by cathartic psychotherapy**

Main paper: Breuer JE, Freud S. *Studien über Hysterie* (Studies in Hysteria). Leipzig and Vienna: Deuticke; 1895.

Background

The Austrian neurologist, Sigmund Freud's (1856–1939) first major work is probably rivalled only by Hippocrates as the most famous medical textbook of all time. It has had an impact on Western culture far beyond its scope as a medical text. *Studies in Hysteria*, written collaboratively between Freud and Josef Breuer (1842–1925), had its origins in Breuer's treatment of Anna O between 1880 and 1882 [12]. Breuer at the time was an eminent Viennese physician; Freud, by contrast, had just qualified, but the two had been friends for some time. It is a difficult manuscript to assess as Freud's views have become so entrenched in popular and academic culture that everyone has an opinion on what they believe was said. As a consequence, people tend to approach the manuscript through the optic of preconceived ideas, so much so that it is easier to consider *Studies in Hysteria* in terms of what was not said. Critically, Freud did not articulate his (ideas on) seduction theory (child sexual abuse) or his later retreat to ideas of infantile sexuality and the Oedipal complex. Nor did he articulate his structural ideas of mind based on id, ego, and superego. In fact, *Studies in Hysteria* might be considered relatively prosaic, were it not a herald for what was to come.

Methods

It contains five case histories and a number of theoretical considerations on the aetiology and treatment of hysterical states.

Results

At the time of writing, Freud had relied on the treatments of the era for hysterical symptoms; hydrotherapy, electrotherapy, massage, and the Weir Mitchell rest cure. However, Breuer's treatment of Anna O made a substantive impression on him 'from the very first' and he began to experiment with hypnosis, not in the manner of suggestion that it had been traditionally used for, but as a method of inducing light trance in which a cathartic exploration of psychic worries could be made.

It was with the fifth case in the book, Elizabeth von R (1892), that Freud felt he had conducted his 'first full length analysis of a hysteria'. Elizabeth von R was a 24-year-old woman with a two-year history of unexplained leg pains and abasia, accompanied by a cheerful air—'the belle indifference of the hysteric I could not help thinking' (a phrase he attributed to Charcot). Freud initially treated her with massage and faradization but then moved to a process of abreaction, at first under hypnosis, but later, just with his hand pressed firmly on her forehead: 'From the beginning it seemed to me probable that Fräulien Elizabeth was conscious of the basis of her illness, that what she had in her consciousness was only a secret and not a foreign body' [12]. As treatment progressed, however, he changed his opinion and concluded that Elizabeth von R had indeed a guilty secret—she had fallen in love with her brother-in-law and felt so ashamed of this that she had unconsciously repressed all such notions.

> The recovery of this repressed idea had a shattering effect on the poor girl. She cried aloud when I put the situation drily before her with the words: 'so for a long time you had been in love with your brother-in-law'. She complained at this moment of the most frightful pains, and made one last desperate effort to reject the explanation: it was not true . . . she was incapable of such wickedness [12].

The authors opined:

> But the causal relationship between the determining psychical trauma and the hysterical phenomena is not of a kind implying that the trauma merely acts like an agent provocateur in releasing the symptom, which thereafter leads an independent existence. We must presume rather that the psychical trauma—or more precisely the memory of the trauma—acts like a foreign body which long after its entry must continue to be regarded as an agent that is still at work . . . we found that each individual hysterical symptom immediately and permanently disappeared when we succeeded in bringing clearly to light the memory of the event by which it was provoked and in arousing its accompanying affect [12].

Freud acknowledged that, at this stage, 'I cannot, I must confess, give any hint of how a conversion of this kind is brought about', although in the preface to the second edition, 10 years later, he commented that the:

> attentive reader will be able to detect in the present book the germs of all that has since been added to the theory of catharsis: for instance, the part played by psychosexual factors and infantilism, the importance of dreams and of unconscious symbolism [12].

Conclusions and critique

Limitations aside, the conversion hypothesis was born. Treatment was to be by a talking cure involving catharsis. It took the Western world by storm. It is fair to say that not all in the neurological world were impressed or convinced by Freud's ideas, but there is little to suggest they offered alternate competing theories. Rather, it seems that they withdrew from treating such patients and viewed the problem with increasing distaste. (Although, it might be reasonable to assume that it was not a popular condition to treat even before that.)

The influence of Freud's ideas hold in popular culture to the current day. As for their influence on functional symptoms, while the majority, certainly within the medical world, but also including many practitioners of psychodynamic psychotherapy, have rejected the additional ideas of infantile sexuality, dreams, and symbolism, many still hold that this initial description of cathartic articulation of distressing thoughts and desires remains the mode of treatment for functional symptoms.

4.4 **Extreme physical treatment for hysteria, with relevance for today**

Main paper: Adrian E, Yealland L. The treatment of some common war neuroses. *Lancet* 1917; 189:867–72.

Background

Hysteria, with its origins in the uterus, was a woman's disease. Although clinicians since Willis and Sydenham, in the 1680s, had noted that men sometimes developed hysterical symptoms, they were generally said to have hypochondria (and later, neurasthenia), even if the symptoms were often similar to those of hysteria [13]. Charcot notably observed, in the 1880s, that men did not have to be effeminate or aristocratic to develop hysterical symptoms but, even at that time, this was a controversial view [14]. But to those that doubted that hysteria was a condition that could also affect men, the First World War provided overwhelming evidence to the contrary. Large numbers of men with dramatic paralyses, mutism, and movement disorders, mixed with physical injury and psychological trauma, provided a lot of material for the neurologists and psychiatrists of the day.

There are many names attached to the study of shell shock or war neurosis. These include those studying pathology in patients who died near exploding shells, such as British neuropathologist, Frederick Mott (1853–1926), and those providing treatment for men whose symptoms began even before the shell exploded, such as Tom Pear and G. Elliott Smith [15]. Treatments ranged from physical treatments such as rest, massage, and balneotherapy, to psychological treatments. Physicians such as Mott, practicing at the Institute of Psychiatry in London [16], and Major Arthur Hurst [17], recorded their experience of treating war neurosis using a mixture of persuasion, suggestion, and, sometimes, electricity (faradization).

We have chosen this paper by Adrian and Yealland [18] partly because it has gained a certain notoriety over time and partly because, in its failure to inspire others despite apparent success, it symbolizes a last 'hurrah' for the medical model of treating hysteria at that time. Similar treatments must have continued but Yealland's methods in particular, often using electricity, came to be regarded as brutal and inhumane, standing in stark dramatic contrast to the lengthy empathetic approach of psychoanalysis. It is this dramatic contrast that has been so appealing to historians and novelists of the First World War such as Pat Barker. In the first book of her *Regeneration* trilogy [19], there is a re-enactment of a session of faradization for mutism in an apparently terrified soldier which models very closely that described by Yealland.

Methods

Lewis Yealland (1884–1954) was resident medical officer at Queen Square during most of the First World War. He developed a particular interest in treatment of the more 'neurological' war neuroses and this paper describes his experience of 250 of them, with symptoms such as paralysis (n = 99), mutism (n = 82), gait disturbance (n = 18), and deafness (n = 34), who were sent to him by others practicing at the hospital and further afield. He expanded further on his ideas in his book, *Hysterical Disorders of Warfare* [20]. The book recounts, almost like a screenplay, the conversations that he had with his patients, which is perhaps why it is such good material for historians and dramatists. Edgar Douglas Adrian (1889–1977, and joint winner of the Nobel Prize for Physiology with Sir Charles Sherrington) was his boss and, because of the similarities of this paper to the book, we assume that most of the writing of the *Lancet* paper [18] was Yealland's.

Yealland's method was recommended only for patients with obvious motor or sensory symptoms. It was based on the idea that the patient with hysteria had a 'weak will and intellect' and had a 'fixed idea' about the nature of their symptom. They did not attempt to treat the vulnerability which they regarded as permanent, but simply remove the symptom which they regarded as the main cause of distress and disability.

The first principle of treatment was suggestion, stating to the patient that they have a routine problem for which the treatment is quick and effective. Yealland was keen to advise that the patient should *not* be encouraged to speak during this process: 'The barest statement should suffice and the patient should be silenced at once if he attempts to air his own views on the subject.' The second principle of 're-education' described restoring function until the 'bad habit is lost'. This was achieved by demonstrating to the patient that their symptom was reversible by, for example, tickling the back of the throat in mutism or using a strong electrical stimulus to make a paralysed limb move (Fig. 4.3). Yealland was aware that most of the effect of this may reside in the confidence and personality of the operator rather than the electricity itself, but he had no hesitation in using 'extremely painful' currents which appear to have been the main physical treatment to remove symptoms:

> The current can be made extremely painful if it is necessary to supply the disciplinary element which must be invoked if the patient is one of those who prefer not to recover [18].

The third principle was of discipline—breaking down the 'unconscious resistance of the patient to the idea of recovery' and, in a military setting, 'commanding' the patient to get better.

Results

In terms of immediate response to treatment, his methods appeared startlingly effective although, like many papers of the era, numerical data are hard to assess. Yealland would spend several hours, if necessary, treating an individual until he produced a breakthrough in symptoms. While the process certainly appears brutal and must have been traumatic for many, what also comes across is an intense desire to improve these men's symptoms. In some cases, he documents that the recovered men became emotional and profoundly grateful, but Yealland cautioned against any emotional response in the doctor.

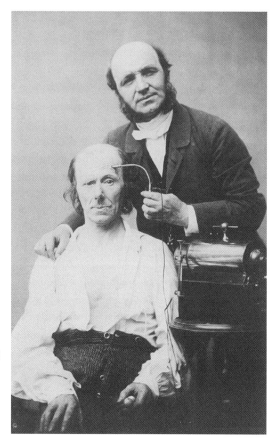

Fig. 4.3 Faradism was a commonly used treatment and investigation for many types of neurological disorders in the nineteenth and early twentieth century. This famous photograph shows Duchenne de Boulogne (1806–1875) stimulating frontalis.
Reproduced from George Eastman House, New York (1862).

Yealland's *Lancet* paper [18] and his book only report outcome at discharge. He does not specifically suggest that men are sent back to the front—most seem to end up in jobs at home, such as in a munitions factory. One reason why he did not see them again may have been what he told them would happen if they relapsed:

> If the patient's manner suggests that he is likely to relapse as soon as he leaves the hospital, he is told that this is very unlikely, but that if it should occur he should report sick at once and come back for treatment with a current far stronger than that already used [18].

He reported failure with four or five cases that would now be regarded as fixed dystonia and also mentioned suggestion under anaesthetic as an alternative.

Conclusions and critique

Such vigorous and punitive treatments appear to have fallen by the wayside after the First World War, in favour of longer and more sympathetic psychological treatments. While no one today could condone many aspects of the treatment, there is, however, much of interest in Yealland's approach. In particular, his focus on physical treatments to remove the symptom (as the main cause of psychological distress), the explicit use of diagnostic confidence, demonstration of reversibility, and producing an atmosphere of recovery has more relevance now than at any time since the First World War. Recent preliminary studies of physiotherapy [21] and transcranial magnetic stimulation [22] for functional motor symptoms suggest they may be at least as good, if not better than, psychotherapeutic approaches.

4.5 **A new data-based system of classification in psychiatry**

Main paper: Guze SB. The diagnosis of hysteria: what are we trying to do? *American Journal of Psychiatry* 1967; 124:491–8.

Background

The psychodynamic school of thinking held influence over psychiatry through the first half of the twentieth century. The idea of diagnoses drifted, judgements were made about patients on the basis of an individual analysis of the psychological processes, which effectively allowed clinicians to describe someone having a disease if they thought the person showed evidence of such thought processes. This mode of assessment became so extreme, at one stage, that one could have functional symptoms without actually having any physical complaints but just by thinking in the manner of someone who might.

Samuel Guze (1923–2000), however, was a man ahead of his time. He practiced psychiatry from the perspective of his background; his medical training looking for features of commonality between individual clinical presentations. In this seminal paper for psychiatry in general, he outlined his view that psychiatric diagnosis could be described by operationalized criteria according to the following underlying principles. He thought that a reliable and valid classification was the essential foundation for communication, teaching, comparison, and evaluation. He set out to describe this approach using hysteria as a model [23].

> The diagnosis of a functional psychiatric illness may be considered if the patients do not develop features of a different illness, if they have a similar course, and if an increased prevalence of the same disorder is encountered among their relatives [20].

This seemingly obvious approach was considered heretical when the dominant view of psychiatric disorder was of a highly idiosyncratic reaction to the particular circumstances of an individual's life.

Methods

In this paper, Guze summarizes his group's work and proposes a novel classificatory system. They started with a 6–8-year follow-up study based on a retrospective case series of attendees at psychiatric clinics over an 18-month period. They conducted detailed structured interviews seeking symptoms that appeared to discriminate patients with a diagnosis of hysteria. They then tested the reliability and validity of these criteria on a separate cohort of patients attending neurology clinics over a 7-year period. Finally, they conducted family studies on these two cohorts.

Results

They proposed a definition based solely on clinical features of multiple unexplained symptomatology: a minimum of 25 symptoms distributed across a range of body systems with onset before age 35. They demonstrated that such diagnoses could be made accurately between clinicians and were stable over time. They found a familial aggregation and noted an association with antisocial personality disorder in familial clusters. They paid homage to Briquet's influential work and named the disorder after him, although Briquet himself never distinguished between mono- and poly-symptomatic presentations of hysteria.

Conclusions and critique

The classification proposed by Guze has remained reliable but it is now recognized that 'Briquet's syndrome' is a relatively rare and severe form of presentation of somatoform symptoms occurring in only 0.1–0.2% of the population, compared to a general population prevalence of somatoform symptoms of between 5–15%, depending on what definition is used.

The problem for epidemiologists with Guze's approach is where cut-offs should be set. At the milder end of the spectrum, functional symptoms start to merge with normal function—we have all stood outside an exam hall with our stomach tied in knots (highly unpleasant), but few of us would think of this as a clinical disorder. What about a newly qualified doctor, anxious at their new responsibilities, who has diarrhoea for 3 months and has some investigations? Should that be considered a disorder? Or do we wait for the most extreme case of a patient who has 15 episodes of diarrhoea a day and cannot leave the house without planning a route around public toilets? Does it matter which bodily system the symptom occurs in? Can functional paralysis ever be considered normal? In its pure form, probably not, but what about mild collapsing weakness and a voluntary protective flexed posture secondary to an injury in an arm? It may be functional but do we really class it as morbidity? This remains unresolved and attempts have been made to solve it by counting the number of different symptoms suffered or by looking at the disability associated with an individual symptom or by combinations of the two—with no universally accepted solution emerging [24, 25].

The importance of Guze's contribution to the field was not, however, his actual definition of Briquet's syndrome but the underlying principle of his approach that patients could be objectively measured in terms of the presenting symptoms and clustered into groups in a meaningful way to allow quantitative measurement—a head-on collision with the psychodynamic zeitgeist of the era.

The influence of Guze's work extended far beyond functional symptoms and has come to dominate psychiatric practice. The methods he laid out for an operationalized approach to psychiatric diagnosis changed the landscape and, along with similar work he subsequently conducted on schizophrenia [26] and the UK–US diagnostic study on schizophrenia [27] based on the same methods, led directly to the *Diagnostic and Statistical Manual of Mental Disorders*, third edition (DSM-III) and a whole new and, in our opinion, improved era of psychiatric diagnosis.

Guze's influence on operationalized diagnosis for functional symptoms remains into the current revisions for DSM-V, but unfortunately, it did not significantly affect the medical approach to the condition over the second part of the twentieth century. Shortly after Guze's work on reliability of diagnosis of Briquet's syndrome, the whole field of hysteria, including Guze's work, came under attack in a now infamous study and lecture given by Eliot Slater [28].

4.6 **A highly influential but critical cohort study that held back progress for half a century**

Main paper: Slater ET. Diagnosis of 'hysteria'. *British Medical Journal* 1965; i:1395–9.

Background

> The malady of the wandering womb began as a myth, and a myth it yet survives. But, like all unwarranted beliefs which still attract credence, it is dangerous. The diagnosis of "hysteria" is a disguise for ignorance and a fertile source of clinical error. It is in fact not only a delusion but also a snare [28].

British psychiatrist, Eliot Trevor Oakeshott Slater's (1904–1983) scathing attack, in 1965, on the concept of hysteria, held a dominant sway over the views of the condition held by psychiatrists (at least in the UK) throughout the remainder of the twentieth century [28, 29]. At the time, the article drew a stinging rebuke from Sir Francis Walshe, neurologist [30]. It continues to provoke strong feeling to this day. Slater had resigned from the National Hospital at Queen Square the year before, when his neurology colleagues had failed to support a benefaction from the Mental Health Research Fund to set up a Chair in Psychiatry [31]. Responding to the lack of support with a high-profile lecture in which he accused his neurological colleagues of ignorance and incompetence did little to improve relations.

Methods

But what did the paper actually show? This is a surprisingly difficult puzzle to decipher. As an exercise in scientific epidemiology, it was poor for such a well-known study—so much so that almost every reader reaches a different conclusion on the actual numbers. The study was based on in-patients with a diagnosis of hysteria at the National Hospital for Nervous Diseases in 1951, 1953, and 1955. A total of 112 patients were identified, and they attempted to contact 99 of them.

Results

Some assessment was possible on 85 patients, comprising in-patients (n = 5), out-patients (n = 35), home visits (n = 30), and GP information (n = 15); 12 patients had died. Of these 85, it is reported that there were very high rates of misdiagnosis, but here the description breaks down. What is actually being counted as a misdiagnosis is far from clear in some circumstances.

Slater described comorbidity of hysteria with disease at the time of diagnosis where 'in the long run the course of the illness was that of the basic disease process'; for example, 'The glioma was recognized at the time of the diagnosis, which was in fact that of "left temporal lobe glioma plus hysteria"'. His discussion mixes this type of diagnostic change with other more obvious errors. In some cases, one simply cannot know from the information presented if misdiagnosis occurred; for example, 'a woman with atypical migrainous headaches, later rediagnosed as a basilar vessel migraine'. In other cases, there is no evidence at all of misdiagnosis; for example, 'a girl of 23 has subsequently developed the radiological picture of cortical atrophy' [28].

Conclusions and critique

The paper came at the end of an era when British psychiatry was dominated by big personalities espousing strongly held views largely based on strength of their own conviction. Sadly, Slater's polemic lasted and influenced a generation of clinicians: an apparent moratorium on making a diagnosis of a functional disorder became part of standard medical teaching for several decades. It probably also contributed to a sense of separation between neurology and psychiatry that is only now starting to be reversed.

Slater's claims have not stood the test of time. An attempted replication of the study conducted by Crimlisk et al in 1998, but using superior epidemiological techniques of a clearly defined consecutive series and defined outcome, identified 73 patients with motor conversion disorder admitted to the National Hospital at Queen Square over a 2-year period [32]. Six-year follow-up data, including face-to-face neurological reassessment, was obtained on 66 subjects and only three diagnostic revisions were noted. In two of these, significant communication problems may have hindered the initial assessment, and in the third case, a diagnosis of paroxysmal hemidystonia was made to explain the gait disturbance of a 68-year-old man which, as an accompanying editorial by O'Brien [33] states, is 'always a difficult diagnosis and a condition not fully characterized at the time of the original presentation'. In a systematic review of the literature reported in 2005, we found 27

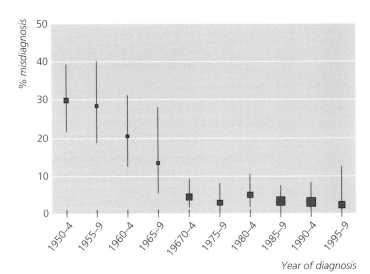

Fig. 4.4 Systematic review of the misdiagnosis of hysteria and conversion symptoms showing a rate of around 4% since 1970 (27 studies, n = 1466, mean duration follow up 5 years) [34].

Reproduced from the *BMJ*, 331, Stone J, Smyth R, Carson A, et al, Systematic review of misdiagnosis of conversion symptoms and 'hysteria', p. 989, Copyright (2005), with permission from BMJ Publishing Group Ltd.

Table 4.1 Diagnostic change does not have to mean diagnostic error. A list of reasons why diagnoses can change in patients with functional symptoms [35].

Type of diagnostic revision		Example	Degree of clinician error
1	Diagnostic error	Patient presented with symptoms that were plausibly due to multiple sclerosis. The diagnosis of multiple sclerosis had not been considered and was unexpected at follow-up.	Major
2	Differential diagnostic change	Patient presented with symptoms that were plausibly related to a number of conditions. Doctor suggested chronic fatigue syndrome as most likely but considered multiple sclerosis as a possible diagnosis. Appropriate investigations and follow-up confirmed multiple sclerosis.	None to minor
3	Diagnostic refinement	Doctor diagnosed epilepsy but at follow-up the diagnosis is refined to juvenile myoclonic epilepsy.	Minor
4	Comorbid diagnostic change	Doctor correctly identified the presence of both epilepsy and non-epileptic seizures in the same patient. At follow-up, one of the disorders has remitted.	None
5	Prodromal diagnostic change	Patient presented with an anxiety state. At follow-up the patient has developed a dementia. With hindsight, anxiety was a prodromal symptom of dementia but the diagnosis could not have been made at the initial consultation as the dementia symptoms (or findings on examination or investigation) had not developed.	None
6	De *novo* development of organic disease	Patient is correctly diagnosed with chronic fatigue syndrome. During the period of follow-up, the patient develops subarachnoid haemorrhage as a completely new condition.	None
7	Disagreement between doctors – without new information at follow-up	Patient is diagnosed at baseline with chronic fatigue syndrome and at follow-up with chronic Lyme disease by a different doctor even though there is no new information. However, if the two doctors had both met the patient at follow-up, they could still arrived at the same diagnoses. This would be reflected in similar divided opinion among their peers.	None
8	Disagreement between doctors – with new information at follow-up	Patient is diagnosed at baseline with chronic fatigue syndrome and at follow-up with fatigue due to a Chiari malformation by a different doctor because of new information at follow-up, (in this case an MRI scan ordered at the time of the first appointment). However, the first doctor seeing the patient again at follow-up continues to diagnose chronic fatigue syndrome believing the Chiari malformation to be an incidental finding. This would be reflected in divided opinion among their peers.	None

eligible studies including a total of 1466 patients with a median duration of follow-up of 5 years. Since 1970, the mean misdiagnosis rate has been 4%. This rate was not influenced by the introduction of new imaging techniques and is similar to misdiagnosis rates in other neurological and psychiatric disorders [34] (see Fig. 4.4).

We went on to conduct a large prospective cohort study, the Scottish Neurological Symptoms Study. Of 3781 new neurology out-patients, we identified 1144 with symptoms poorly explained by organic disease [35]. We were able to follow up 1030 for a period of 18 months. In 111 cases, we felt there was a possible better explanation for the original presenting symptoms. However, in only four of these cases did any misdiagnosis seem likely and much more common was differential diagnosis change, diagnostic refinement, and the development of new incidental pathology. We also noted that there were many reasons for diagnostic revision which did not imply clinical error (Table 4.1).

The conclusions are clear: the diagnosis of a functional neurological disorder can be made with sufficient reliability to be clinically useful but, as in all branches of medicine, some errors will occur, and clinicians should be mindful of this.

4.7 **One of the best early clinical case series of non-epileptic attacks, heralding a new scientific approach**

Main paper: Meierkord H, Will B, Fish D, Shorvon S. The clinical features and prognosis of pseudoseizures diagnosed using video-EEG telemetry. *Neurology* 1991; 41:1643–6.

Background

By the 1970s and 1980s, functional neurological symptoms had hit serious doldrums. Although neurologists continued to recognize the problem, little was published on it. Weighed down by the twin opposing concerns of misdiagnosis, so forcefully voiced by Eliot Slater in 1965, and malingering, which remains a concern for many neurologists today [36], it seems that this was not an area for the young neurologist to develop an interest in.

We chose this paper by neurologists at Queen Square in London (Hartmut Meierkord, Bob Will, David Fish, and Simon Shorvon) [37] as the best and largest of the early published case series of 'pseudoseizures' which heralded proper recognition of this subtype of functional neurological symptom. There had been other case series with 30 or fewer patients [38–45], including one by Gates [46], who subsequently went on to edit a book about non-epileptic attacks [47]. Many of these early series were published to highlight simply that the problem existed and that video electroencephalography (EEG) could help identify it. Studies by Lempert et al. [48] (n = 50) and Krumholz et al. [49] (n = 41) had more patients and clinical and prognostic data, and vied for this slot as a landmark paper. The particular series we have chosen had the distinction of being the largest at the time and also of defining all cases using new 'video cable telemetry' for more reliable diagnosis.

As the authors commented on in their introduction, the state of the literature 20 years ago was considerably different to now:

> In spite of the common occurrence, disabling nature and management difficulties of pseudoseizures, there are little reported data on their clinical presentation, long-term outcome, or associated prognostic factors [37].

Methods

This was a retrospective follow-up study with clinical description of 110 patients with a diagnosis of pseudoseizures who had come through video EEG and data on follow up.

Results

The majority (78%) of the patients were female, with a median age of onset of 25 years. The age range was large though, with patients as young as 7 years and as old as 71 years, anticipating later studies highlighting a subset of patients who develop non-epileptic attacks later in life, often in response to comorbid health anxiety [50]. A small group (14%) also had epilepsy, 33% had motionless unresponsive episodes, and the rest had 'thrashing'. Although attempts have subsequently been made to divide non-epileptic attacks in a more fine-grained way [51], in practice these remain the two main types. The presence of stereotyped attacks (n = 82), physical injury (n = 19), and incontinence (n = 7), and the lack of additional psychopathology in the majority of patients (n = 58), provided myth-busting data that may still be a surprise to many.

A total of 70 patients were followed up 'for 12 months or more', and 42 of them were still having attacks. None of them had an alternative diagnosis, in contrast to Slater's study in the same hospital 25 years earlier [29]. Being male, not having received psychological treatment, and having coexistent epilepsy all conferred worse prognosis. The authors advocated patient and humane explanation, and suggested psychological treatment was worthwhile, making their comments on diagnosis via psychological assessment particularly interesting: 'We did not find the presence or absence of abnormal personality traits helpful in making a distinction between epilepsy and pseudoepilepsy.'

Twenty-two years later, many groups, especially US-based, are still trying to prove this wrong using tools such as Minnesota Multiphasic Personality Inventory (MMPI) or other scales [52], but none, in our opinion, have been successful in substituting for diagnosis based on the nature of the attack. Attempts to use conversation analysis have been more successful at distinguishing groups and warrant further study in normal clinical settings [53].

Conclusions and critique

These early studies of non-epileptic attacks, of which this is one of the best examples, were vital in delineating the third most common cause of blackouts in the general population in the era of video EEG. The problem needed delineating again, not because it had ever gone away, but because neurological interest in it had declined so dramatically over the course of the twentieth century [54]. These early studies, led almost exclusively by epileptologists, paved the way for subsequent more careful definition of other functional symptoms in neurology and an increased interest, generally, in the topic.

4.8 **One of the best early clinical case series of psychogenic movement disorder**

Main paper: Koller W, Lang A, Vetere-Overfield B, et al. Psychogenic tremors. *Neurology* 1989; 39:1094–9.

Background

Publications about psychogenic (functional) movement disorders lagged behind those on non-epileptic attacks, which had been gathering in pace since the early 1980s.

It was not until American neurologist, Stanley Fahn, described five cases in abstract form in 1983 [55] and then 21 cases of psychogenic dystonia in 1988 [56], that a trickle of papers started to appear from the movement disorders community describing, in case series format, other types of psychogenic movement disorder. Fahn, himself, has described how reluctantly neurologists made the diagnosis of psychogenic movement disorder at that time [57], and especially David Marsden (1938–1998), working at the Institute of Neurology, who had done so much to change psychological views on task-specific dystonia. Marsden did, nonetheless, write an insightful paper on hysteria in 1985 [58] and, in 1998, was an author on the key study of misdiagnosis [32] which included many patients who did have psychogenic movement disorder at follow up, suggesting his opinion had changed over time.

It is hard to single out one study at this time, but we have chosen the 1989 description of psychogenic tremor by Koller et al [59]. in *Neurology* partly because it was the first delineation of this most common type of functional movement disorder, and also because the authors included Tony Lang and Stewart Factor, who authored several other important papers at that time describing psychogenic dystonia, psychogenic parkinsonism, and co-morbidity of psychogenic with 'organic' movement disorders [60–63]. Other notable early papers on psychogenic movement disorders include descriptions of psychogenic myoclonus [64] and hemifacial symptoms [65] by Joe Jankovic and colleagues, as well as a paper by Günther Deuschl's group demonstrating that tremor in reflex sympathetic dystrophy has psychogenic features [66].

Methods

This study by Koller et al. [59] defined key characteristics of psychogenic (functional) tremor. The paper itself is simply a case series describing 25 patients (9 men) with a diagnosis of psychogenic tremor.

Results

The authors described abrupt onset, distractibility, inconsistency, atypical tremorgraphic features, unusual handwriting, association with other 'somatizations', and recovery with psychotherapy as some of the clinical features. They made the particularly useful observation that tremor frequency variability is more important than amplitude variability (Fig. 4.5).

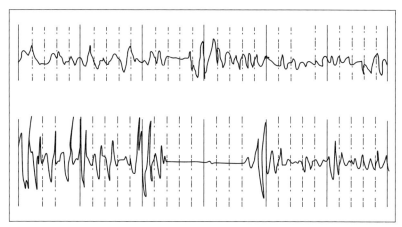

Fig. 4.5 Tremorgrams showing changing amplitude and frequency (top) and transient disappearance of tremor during distraction (bottom).
Reproduced from *Neurology*, 39, Koller W, Lang A, Vetere-Overfield B, Findley L, Cleeves L, Factor S, Singer C, Weiner W, Psychogenic tremors, p. 1094–9, Copyright (1989), with permission from Wolters Kluwer.

Conclusions and critique

As with the early 'pseudoseizure' studies, many of these features identified in this study had individually been observed in the past, but this particular case series, and those like it at the time, were crucial in defining psychogenic movement disorders clinically, as an entity which could be diagnosed positively, and also as a legitimate area of neurological research. Without any positive criteria for diagnosis, the whole field was likely to have continued to languish in a 'no mans land' between neurology and psychiatry, that seemed to have been the case for decades.

From the last decade, Anette Schrag's 2004 paper on 103 patients with fixed/psychogenic dystonia (with colleagues Michael Trimble in neuropsychiatry and Niall Quinn and Kailash Bhatia from movement disorders neurology) [67] was also a close runner-up for us as a landmark paper in this book. Its balanced exploration of the overlap between fixed dystonia and complex regional pain syndrome is in contrast to some of the more polarized debates on this topic that continue to wear on. The whole debate about whether complex regional pain syndrome (CRPS) is a psychogenic disorder would benefit from more respect and understanding of functional symptoms as a legitimate problem on the one hand, but also more appreciation, from those that see it as purely 'psychogenic', that there are biological dimensions to functional symptoms too.

The whole field of psychogenic movement disorders took an important step forward with a meeting in 2003 in Atlanta, and subsequent book [68], organized by the Movement Disorders Society. A second conference in 2009, and book [69], has kept momentum going and the number of publications, as well as co-operation between neurologists and psychiatrists, is slowly growing.

4.9 An early high-quality functional imaging study exploring possible neural mechanisms underpinning functional symptom production

Main paper: Vuilleumier P, Chicherio C, Assal F, Schwartz S, Slosman D, Landis T. Functional neuroanatomical correlates of hysterical sensorimotor loss. *Brain* 2001; 124:1077–90.

Background

The gradual evolution in the consideration of hysterical symptoms that occurred during the Renaissance, from disorders of the uterus to disorders of the mind, created a substantive explanatory problem in terms of the actual mechanism of symptom production. For all its faults, the uterine model at least 'explained' how the symptoms came to be, whether by direct pressure or release of noxious gas within the body cavity. Intermediary theories, such as Willis's description of micro 'explosions' in the cerebral cortex, at least offered some continuation of this, and Charcot's suggestion of functional or dynamic lesion continued this tradition. But the shift to psychodynamic theories, although offering a passing nod with the description of conversion disorder, never really grappled with what the mechanics would actually be. Moves in the second half of the twentieth century to a more atheoretical but, nonetheless, explicitly psychogenic understanding, continued this tradition. The 'elephant in the room' was the notable lack of any plausible explanation of why distress caused paralysis of an upper limb in one person and a psychogenic seizure in another, and how these symptoms actually came to pass.

The development of functional imaging studies offered the potential to directly examine functional brain correlates of conversion disorders. Early case studies [70, 71] suggested the failure of motor activity was associated with increased activation in prefrontal regions, implying excessive inhibition of sensorimotor action.

Methods

However, it was a study by Vuilleumier and colleagues [72] of seven patients with unilateral hysterical hemisensorimotor loss that really opened up the possibilities of the technique, with two novel aspects to the design. First, cerebral activity was measured via single photon emission computed tomograpy (SPECT), using ^{99m}-Tc-ECD, both at rest and during active sensory stimulation. Second, subjects were imaged while unwell and following recovery.

Results

Fascinatingly, the authors found a consistent decrease of regional cerebral blood flow in the thalamus and basal ganglia contralateral to the deficit (Fig. 4.6). The hypoactivation resolved on recovery, although the interpretation must be treated cautiously as only four of the seven actually recovered. However, the degree of deactivation in the caudate was predictive of the extent of recovery. They were intrigued to note that the same subcortical premotor circuits are also involved in unilateral motor neglect.

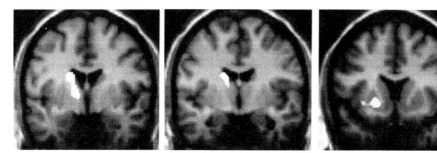

Fig. 4.6 SPECT of four patients with unilateral functional motor and sensory symptoms, comparing the symptomatic state to the recovered state. The figures show hypoactivity in thalamus, caudate, and putamen [72].

Reproduced from *Brain*, 124, Vuilleumier P, Chicherio C, Assal F, et al, Functional neuroanatomical correlates of hysterical sensorimotor loss, p. 1077–90, Copyright (2001), with permission from Oxford University Press.

Conclusions and critique

The authors accepted that this study was essentially a mechanistic study of 'how' symptoms came to be and did not necessarily enlighten us as to 'why' they happened in the first place. The patients in the study were a group who had suffered a number of psychologically traumatic life events including sexual assault and death of a child. The authors hypothesized a potential link between emotional and situational cues from the limbic system being processed in the basal ganglia, in particular the caudate, and modulating motor processes. They close by commenting that newer techniques, in particular functional connectivity analysis, may be of interest in pursuing this relationship.

Voon et al. picked up this challenge in a magnetic resonance imaging (MRI) functional connectivity study comparing 16 patients with a mixture of conversion disorders to healthy control subjects [73]. They used an emotional Stroop task involving fearful, neutral, and happy faces. As one would predict, the healthy controls showed greater right amygdala activity for the fearful faces, decreasing through the neutral and happy ones. The patients with conversion disorder, by contrast, failed to have any valence differences between the images (i.e. they showed a fearful response to happy faces). In functional connectivity analyses, the patients with conversion disorder showed greater functional connectivity between the right amygdale and right supplementary motor cortex in response to both the fearful and the happy images, compared to controls, and the response was less likely to habituate. In normal function, the amygdala plays a critical role in evaluating the initial relevance of sensory stimuli and rapidly habituates with repeated presentations, thus allowing for a shift of attentional resources to more salient stimuli. This failure in conversion disorder offers the potential to explain why psychological or physiological stressors can trigger or exacerbate the condition.

However, there is a long way to go. Functional imaging investigations in the field are in their infancy. The studies are small and often mutually contradictory. It is too early to claim that a comprehensive theory is emerging but one possibility is that there are overly sensitive amygdala fear responses (i.e. abnormal responses to stimuli, even objectively neutral stimuli), possibly conditioned by previous learning experiences, that drive changes in networks mediating perceptual experiences and/or movement plans. These changes, in the presence of abnormal self-directed attention [11] (cf. prefrontal activations in functional imaging studies), are capable of producing movements or perceptual experiences which are not associated with a normal sense of self-agency [74] and are, therefore, interpreted by patients as involuntary symptoms of an underlying disease [24].

4.10 **A landmark randomized controlled trial of treatment for non-epileptic attacks**

Main paper: Goldstein LH, Chalder T, Chigwedere C, et al. Cognitive-behavioral therapy for psychogenic nonepileptic seizures: a pilot RCT. *Neurology* 2010; 74:1986–94.

Background

The treatment of hysteria is a topic that features in the very first medical document, the Kahun papyrus from around 1800BC. That particular document suggested that aching eyes, lack of vision, and neck pains could be treated with the liver of an ass and fumigation of the vulva with incense (to bring back the wandering womb).

It took a long time from the Kahun papyrus (Fig. 4.7), and indeed the first randomized controlled trial (RCT) in medicine (1948 trial of streptomycin for tuberculosis [75]), to see RCTs for functional neurological symptoms. Franny Moene and colleagues in the Netherlands reported two well-designed RCTs to evaluate the additional effect of hypnosis on rehabilitation in in-patients (n = 44) [76] and on out-patients versus waiting list controls (n = 45) [77] with functional motor symptoms. The in-patient trial showed no additive effect of hypnosis, probably because both arms of the trial did well with multidisciplinary rehabilitation. Despite a mean duration of 4 years, 84% of patients were better at 6-month follow up. Hypnosis did confer an advantage for out-patients, compared to waiting list controls. Since then, there have been scattered other trials for functional neurological symptoms, including our own of guided self-help [78, 79].

We have chosen for our final landmark paper though, a trial of cognitive behavioural therapy (CBT) for psychogenic or dissociative non-epileptic attacks by Laura Goldstein and colleagues at the Institute of Psychiatry in London [80]. Although relatively modest

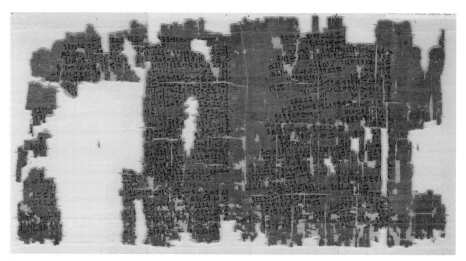

Fig. 4.7 The Kahun papyrus, the first medical document (c.1800BC), contained treatment advice for functional neurological symptoms.

in size (33 participants in each arm), the trial still represents a milestone in the history of scientific endeavour in 'hysteria' and clearly shows that high-quality trials can be done in this area.

The basis of psychotherapy for functional neurological symptoms goes back not only to Freud and Breuer's psychoanalysis but also to Paul Dubois, whose talking treatment for nervous disorders like neurasthenia involved 'rational persuasion', a forerunner to CBT [81]. However, during the twentieth century, if a patient found their way to a psychiatrist (and it seems likely that many did not [54]), psychodynamic therapy fitted best with the prevailing hypothesis about the cause of the symptoms.

Increasing evidence for CBT for physical symptoms like chronic fatigue syndrome and irritable bowel syndrome, along with the attraction of a therapy that could be manualized more easily than psychodynamic therapy, has led to successful RCTs in those conditions [82]. In an earlier study, Goldstein and colleagues showed that panic symptoms were common prior to non-epileptic attacks in many patients [83], a conclusion that naturally led to a cognitive behavioural treatment similar to that used for panic disorder. They described the treatment in a promising pilot series [84], placing heavy emphasis on engaging the patient, repeatedly emphasizing the genuine nature of the condition, and describing the attack as their brain or mind 'switching off'. Treatment then moved to simple distraction techniques to try to gain some control and graded exposure to avoided situations or activities. Later on, only once these basics had been established, did they suggest more typical psychotherapeutic activities such as looking at self-esteem, life difficulties, and relationships with others.

Methods

The trial randomized 33 patients to 12 one-hour cognitive behavioural treatments using these principles. The 33 controls received 'standard medical care' consisting of meetings with a neuropsychiatrist in which further discussion of the diagnosis took place and anticonvulsant medication was reduced but no CBT elements were given.

Results

The result was a clear difference in median seizure frequency at the end of treatment with CBT (12 to 1.5 per month) compared to standard care (8 to 5). The number of treatments required for seizure freedom was five. At 3-month follow up, the effect was attenuating, but scrutiny of the data suggests that the small size of the trial was partly to blame.

Conclusions and critique

Given the small size of the trial and unusually long mean duration of the seizures in the trial entrants (4 years), this study gave significant optimism that a larger trial could show conclusively that therapy for non-epileptic attacks can be devised, taught, and delivered in a cost-effective way.

Among neurologists, attitudes to treatment of patients with functional neurological symptoms are not always helpful. With respect to treatment, there is sometimes a tendency among neurologists either to believe that the problem is basically untreatable and to give up or, conversely, to consider that it is best to leave the patient alone and not make the problem worse by providing medical 'attention'. Evidence like that of the Goldstein trial, and others [85], shows that treatment does work, and that some treatments are better than others. This places an evidence-based responsibility on clinicians to work with those providing treatment to do things better.

Key unanswered questions

We think the future looks bright for functional disorders; there is a renewed sense of interest in the scientific and clinical community. The very inclusion, in a textbook of landmark papers in neurology, of this chapter, unthinkable 30 years ago, illustrates this. We now know that functional symptoms exist, that we diagnose them accurately, that they cause substantive disability and distress, and that they tend to persist. This makes them a topic ripe for clinical research to understand the mechanisms underpinning these disorders and to trial of better treatments to help the patients who suffer from them. We need more integration from across the spread of neurosciences, collaboration between different disciplines, and the application of new techniques and ideas from outside the traditional paradigms. We hope that if there is a request for a second or third edition of this book, that our choice of landmark papers will be different and will include at least one definitive treatment trial. Do we have any ideas for what may be a landmark paper of the future? One bet might be a 2012 publication by Edwards et al. entitled 'A Bayesian account of hysteria' [11]. This paper offers an integrative hypothesis explaining the neurophysiological mechanisms, based on strategies to minimize prediction error in the context of strong but incorrect illness beliefs that might underpin functional neurological symptoms. It is too early to say if it will stand the test of time and become a landmark paper, but undoubtedly it is one to read and consider.

References

1 **Briquet P.** *Traité Clinique et Thérapeutique de l'Hysterie.* Paris: J.B. Ballière; 1859.

2 **Mai FM.** Pierre Briquet: 19th century savant with 20th century ideas. *Can J Psychiatry* 1983; **28**:418–21.

3 **Mai FM, Merskey H.** Briquet's treatise on hysteria. A synopsis and commentary. *Arch Gen Psychiatry* 1980; **37**:1401–5.

4 **Mai F, Merskey H.** Pierre Briquet. *Arch Gen Psychiatry* 1983; **40**:223.

5 **Janet P.** *The Major Symptoms of Hysteria.* London: Macmillan; 1907.

6 **Purves-Stewart J, Worster-Drought C.** The psychoneuroses and psychoses. In: *Diagnosis of Nervous Diseases.* Baltimore: The Williams and Wilkins Company 1952; 661–758.

7 **Fasano A, Valadas A, Bhatia KP, et al.** Psychogenic facial movement disorders: clinical features and associated conditions. *Mov Disord* 2012; **27**:1544–51.

8 **Janet P.** *The Mental State of Hystericals.* New York: Putnams; 1901.

9 **Stone J, Warlow C, Sharpe M.** Functional weakness: clues to mechanism from the nature of onset. *J Neurol Neurosurg Psychiatry* 2012; **83**:67–9.

10 **Roelofs K, Van Galen GP, Eling P, Keijsers GP, Hoogduin CA.** Endogenous and exogenous attention in patients with conversion disorders. *Cog Neuropsych* 2003; **20**:733–45.

11 **Edwards MJ, Adams RA, Brown H, Parees I, Friston KJ.** A Bayesian account of 'hysteria'. *Brain* 2012; **135**:3495–512.

12 **Breuer JE, Freud S.** *Studien über Hysterie.* Leipzig and Vienna: Deuticke; 1895.

13 **Micale M.**S. *Hysterical Men: The Hidden History of Male Nervous Illness.* Cambridge, Massachusetts: Harvard University Press; 2008.

14 **Charcot JM.** A propos de six cas d'hysterie chez l'homme. In: *Clinical Lectures on Diseases of the Nervous System (Volume 3).* London: New Sydenham Society; 1889.

15 **Pear T, Smith E.** *Shell Shock and its Lessons.* Manchester: University of Manchester; 1917.

16 **Mott FW.** *War Neuroses and Shell Shock.* London: Henry Frowde, Hodder & Stoughton, Oxford University Press; 1919.

17 **Hurst A.** *The Psychology of the Special Senses and their Functional Disorders.* London: Henry Frowde, Hodder & Stoughton, Oxford University Press; 1920.

18 **Adrian ED, Yealland LR.** The treatment of some common war neuroses. *Lancet* 1917; **189**:867–72.

19 **Barker P.** *Regeneration.* London: Viking; 1991.

20 **Yealland LR.** *Hysterical Disorders of Warfare.* London: Macmillan; 1918.

21 **Czarnecki K, Thompson JM, Seime R, Geda YE, Duffy JR, Ahlskog JE.** Functional movement disorders: successful treatment with a physical therapy rehabilitation protocol. *Parkinsonism Relat Disord* 2012; **18**:247–51.

22 **Chastan N, Parain D.** Psychogenic paralysis and recovery after motor cortex transcranial magnetic stimulation. *Mov Disord* 2010; **25**:1501–4.

23 **Guze SB.** The diagnosis of hysteria: what are we trying to do? *Am J Psychiatry* 1967; **124**:491–8.

24 **Carson AJ, Brown R, David AS, et al.** Functional (conversion) neurological symptoms: research since the millennium. *J Neurol Neurosurg Psychiatry* 2012; **83**:842–50.

25 **Lang AE.** General overview of psychogenic movement disorders: epidemiology, diagnosis and prognosis. In: Hallett M, Fahn S, Jankovic J, Lang AE, Cloninger CR, Yudofsky SC, eds. *Psychogenic Movement Disorders.* Philadelphia: Lippincott, Williams and Wilkins 2006; 35–41.

26 **Feighner JP, Robins E, Guze SB, Woodruff RA, Winokur G, Munoz R.** Diagnostic criteria for use in psychiatric research. *Arch Gen Psych* 1972; **26**:57–62.

27 **Cooper J.** The diagnosis and psychopathology of schizophrenia in New York and London. *Schizoph Bull* 1974; **1**:80–102.

28 **Slater ET.** Diagnosis of 'hysteria'. *BMJ* 1965; i:1395–9.

29 **Slater ET, Glithero E.** A follow-up of patients diagnosed as suffering from 'hysteria'. *J Psychosom Res* 1965; **9**:9–13.

30 **Walshe F.** Diagnosis of hysteria. *BMJ* 1965; **2**:1451–4.

31 **Barraclough B.** In conversation with Eliot Slater. *Psychiat Bull* 1981; **5**:178–81.

32 **Crimlisk HL, Bhatia K, Cope H, David A, Marsden CD, Ron MA.** Slater revisited: 6 year follow up study of patients with medically unexplained motor symptoms. *BMJ* 1998; **316**:582–6.

33 **O'Brien MD.** Medically unexplained neurological symptoms. *BMJ* 1998; **316**:564–5.

34 **Stone J, Smyth R, Carson A, Lewis S, Prescott R, Warlow C, Sharpe M.** Systematic review of misdiagnosis of conversion symptoms and 'hysteria'. *BMJ* 2005; **331**:989.

35 **Stone J, Carson A, Duncan R, et al.** Symptoms 'unexplained by organic disease' in 1144 new neurology out-patients: how often does the diagnosis change at follow-up? *Brain* 2009; **132**: 2878–88.

36 **Kanaan R, Armstrong D, Barnes P, Wessely S.** In the psychiatrist's chair: how neurologists understand conversion disorder. *Brain* 2009; **132**:2889–96.

37 **Meierkord H, Will B, Fish D, Shorvon S.** The clinical features and prognosis of pseudoseizures diagnosed using video-EEG telemetry. *Neurology* 1991; **41**:1643–6.

38 **Wilkus RJ, Dodrill CB, Thompson PM.** Intensive EEG monitoring and psychological studies of patients with pseudoepileptic seizures. *Epilepsia* 1984; **25**:100–7.

39 **Guberman A.** Psychogenic pseudoseizures in non-epileptic patients. *Can J Psychiatry* 1982; 27:401–4.

40 **King DW, Gallagher BB, Murvin AJ, et al.** Pseudoseizures: diagnostic evaluation. *Neurology* 1982; **32**:18–23.

41 **Gulick TA, Spinks IP, King DW.** Pseudoseizures: ictal phenomena. *Neurology* 1982; **32**:24–30.

42 **Luther JS, McNamara JO, Carwile S, Miller P, Hope V.** Pseudoepileptic seizures: methods and video analysis to aid diagnosis. *Ann Neurol* 1982; **12**:458–62.

43 **Roy A.** Hysterical fits previously diagnosed as epilepsy. *Psychol Med* 1977; **7**:271–3.

44 **Roy A.** Hysterical seizures. *Arch Neurol* 1979; **36**:447.

45 **Lesser RP, Lueders H, Dinner DS.** Evidence for epilepsy is rare in patients with psychogenic seizures. *Neurology* 1983; **33**:502–4.

46 **Gates JR, Ramani V, Whalen S, Loewenson R.** Ictal characteristics of pseudoseizures. *Arch Neurol* 1985; **42**:1183–7.

47 **Gates JR, Rowan JA.** *Non-epileptic attacks.* Boston: Butterworth-Heinemann; 1993.

48 **Lempert T, Schmidt D.** Natural history and outcome of psychogenic seizures: a clinical study in 50 patients. *J Neurol* 1990; **237**:35–8.

49 **Krumholz A, Niedermeyer E.** Psychogenic seizures: a clinical study with follow-up data. *Neurology* 1983; **33**:498–502.

50 **Duncan R, Oto M, Martin E, Pelosi A.** Late onset psychogenic nonepileptic attacks. *Neurology* 2006; **66**:1644–7.

51 **Hubsch C, Baumann C, Hingray C, et al.** Clinical classification of psychogenic non-epileptic seizures based on video-EEG analysis and automatic clustering. *J Neurol Neurosurg Psychiatry* 2011; **82**:955–60.

52 **Purdom CL, Kirlin KA, Hoerth MT, et al.** The influence of impression management scales on the Personality Assessment Inventory in the epilepsy monitoring unit. *Epilepsy Behav* 2012; **25**: 534–8.

53 **Reuber M, Monzoni C, Sharrack B, Plug L.** Using interactional and linguistic analysis to distinguish between epileptic and psychogenic nonepileptic seizures: a prospective, blinded multirater study. *Epilepsy Behav* 2009; **16**:139–44.

54 **Stone J, Hewett R, Carson A, Warlow C, Sharpe M.** The 'disappearance' of hysteria: historical mystery or illusion? *J R Soc Med* 2008; **101**:12–8.

55 **Fahn S, Williams DT, Reches A, Lesser RP, Jankovic J.** Hysterical dystonia, a rare disorder: report of five documented cases. *Neurology* 1983; **33(suppl 2)**:161.

56 **Fahn S, Williams DT.** Psychogenic dystonia. *Adv Neurol* 1988; **50**:431–55.

57 **Fahn S.** The history of psychogenic movement disorders. In: Hallett M, Lang AE, Fahn S, Cloninger CR, Jankovic J, Yudofsky SC, eds. *Psychogenic Movement Disorders*. Philadelphia: Lippincott, Williams, and Wilkins and the American Academy of Neurology; 2005:24–34.

58 **Marsden CD.** Hysteria—a neurologist's view. *Psychol Med* 1986; **16**:277–88.

59 **Koller W, Lang A, Vetere-Overfield B, et al.** Psychogenic tremors. *Neurology* 1989; **39**:1094–9.

60 **Factor SA, Podskalny GD, Molho ES.** Psychogenic movement disorders: frequency, clinical profile, and characteristics. *J Neurol Neurosurg Psychiatry* 1995; **59**:406–12.

61 **Ranawaya R, Riley D, Lang A.** Psychogenic dyskinesias in patients with organic movement disorders. *Mov Disord* 1990; **5**:127–33.

62 **Lang AE, Koller WC, Fahn S.** Psychogenic parkinsonism. *Arch Neurol* 1995; **52**:802–10.

63 **Lang AE.** Psychogenic dystonia: a review of 18 cases. *Can J Neurol Sci* 1995; **22**:136–43.

64 **Monday K, Jankovic J.** Psychogenic myoclonus. *Neurology* 1993; **43**:349–52.

65 **Tan EK, Jankovic J.** Psychogenic hemifacial spasm. *J Neuropsychiatry Clin Neurosci* 2001; **13**:380–4.

66 **Deuschl G, Blumberg H, Lucking CH.** Tremor in reflex sympathetic dystrophy. *Arch Neurol* 1991; **48**:1247–52.

67 **Schrag A, Trimble M, Quinn N, Bhatia K.** The syndrome of fixed dystonia: an evaluation of 103 patients. *Brain* 2004; **127**:2360–72.

68 **Hallett M, Fahn S, Jankovic J, Lang AE, Cloninger CR, Yudofsky S.** *Psychogenic Movement Disorders*. Philadelphia: Lippincott, Williams & Wilkins; 2006.

69 **Hallett M, Lang AE, Jankovic J, et al.** *Psychogenic Movement Disorders and Other Conversion Disorder*. Cambridge: Cambridge University Press; 2011.

70 **Tiihonen J, Kuikka J, Viinamaki H, Lehtonen J, Partanen J.** Altered cerebral blood flow during hysterical paresthesia. *Biol Psychiatry* 1995; **37**:134–5.

71 **Marshall JC, Halligan PW, Fink GR, Wade DT, Frackowiak RS.** The functional anatomy of a hysterical paralysis. *Cognition* 1997; **64**:B1–B8.

72 **Vuilleumier P, Chicherio C, Assal F, Schwartz S, Slosman D, Landis T.** Functional neuroanatomical correlates of hysterical sensorimotor loss. *Brain* 2001; **124**:1077–90.

73 **Voon V, Brezing C, Gallea C, et al.** Emotional stimuli and motor conversion disorder. *Brain* 2010; **133**:1526–36.

74 **Voon V, Gallea C, Hattori N, Bruno M, Ekanayake V, Hallett M.** The involuntary nature of conversion disorder. *Neurology* 2010; **74**:223–8.

75 **Medical Research Council— Streptomycin in Tuberculosis Trials Committee.** Streptomycin treatment of pulmonary tuberculosis. *BMJ* 1948; **ii**:769–83.

76 **Moene FC, Spinhoven P, Hoogduin KA, Van Dyck R.** A randomised controlled clinical trial on the additional effect of hypnosis in a comprehensive treatment programme for in-patients with conversion disorder of the motor type. *Psychother Psychosom* 2002; **71**:66–76.

77 **Moene FC, Spinhoven P, Hoogduin CA, Van Dyck R.** A randomized controlled clinical trial of a hypnosis-based treatment for patients with conversion disorder, motor type. *Int J Clin Exp Hypn* 2003; **51**:29–50.

78 **Sharpe M, Walker J, Williams C, et al.** Guided self-help for functional (psychogenic) symptoms: a randomized controlled efficacy trial. *Neurology* 2011; **77**:564–72.

79 **LaFrance Jr WC, Keitner GI, Papandonatos GD, et al.** Pilot pharmacologic randomized controlled trial for psychogenic nonepileptic seizures. *Neurology* 2010; **75**:1166–73.

80 **Goldstein LH, Chalder T, Chigwedere C, et al.** Cognitive-behavioral therapy for psychogenic nonepileptic seizures: a pilot RCT. *Neurology* 2010; **74**:1986–94.

81 **Dubois P.** *The Psychic Treatment of Nervous Disorders.* New York: Funk & Wagnalls; 1909.

82 **White PD, Goldsmith KA, Johnson AL, et al.** Comparison of adaptive pacing therapy, cognitive behaviour therapy, graded exercise therapy, and specialist medical care for chronic fatigue syndrome (PACE): a randomised trial. *Lancet* 2011; **377**:823–36.

83 **Goldstein LH, Mellers JD.** Ictal symptoms of anxiety, avoidance behaviour, and dissociation in patients with dissociative seizures. *J Neurol Neurosurg Psychiatry* 2006; **77**:616–21.

84 **Goldstein LH, Deale AC, Mitchell-O'Malley SJ, Toone BK, Mellers JD.** An evaluation of cognitive behavioral therapy as a treatment for dissociative seizures: a pilot study. *Cogn Behav Neurol* 2004; **17**:41–9.

85 **Sharpe M, Walker J, Williams C, et al.** Guided self-help for functional (psychogenic) symptoms: a randomized controlled efficacy trial26. *Neurology* 2011; **77**:564–72.

Chapter 5

Stroke

Charles Warlow and Jan van Gijn

5.0 **Introduction**

Looking back over the last 50 years, when we were both in the business of medicine, and then over the 50 and more years before that, it is difficult indeed to select the landmark papers that most changed medical thinking or practice, or both simultaneously. There have been very few instant 'breakthroughs'. Medical researchers have worked away patiently on problems, their thoughts and results emerging in a series of papers over many years. No single paper was necessarily the landmark, at least not at the time, although it may possibly have become so later—indeed, some of our landmark papers were rediscoveries, probably because they were published in obscure journals. Also, it is quite common for the same idea to emerge in different places at the same time, and even to be published in the same year, making any decision about which deserves landmark status even more troubling. We have chosen 10 papers that, as part of a longer story and bigger picture, can be regarded as very influential, if not *the* most influential in the development of ideas about the causes and management of stroke.

5.1 **The carotid artery**

Main paper: Chiari H. Über das Verhalten des Teilungswinkels des Carotis Communis bei der Endarteritis chronica deformans [About the role of the bifurcation of the common carotid artery in chronic atherosclerosis]. *Verh Ddtsch Path Ges* 1905; 9:326–30.

Background

In the 1820s, Léon Rostan (1790–1866) identified cerebral softening ('ramollissement') as a separate category of stroke ('apoplexy') which, until then, had been largely synonymous with cerebral haemorrhage, but its pathogenesis still escaped him [1]. Many of his contemporaries had little doubt that 'inflammation' was the cause. The first inkling of a relationship between arterial disease and brain softening had been voiced by Abercrombie [2]. He drew an analogy with gangrene, caused by 'failure of circulation', this in turn being secondary to 'ossification of arteries'. Rudolph Virchow (1821–1902) firmly established that thrombosis of arteries was caused not by inflammation but by fatty metamorphosis of the vessel wall, for which he revived the term 'arteriosclerosis'. In addition, Virchow observed thrombosis as the result of atherosclerosis and also embolism (his newly coined term) of clots from the heart in patients with gangrene of the lower limbs. He extrapolated these events to the cause of cerebral softening [3], while cerebral infarction in patients without heart disease remained more or less synonymous with 'cerebral thrombosis', that is, intracranial atherosclerosis complicated by thrombosis.

Methods and results

Hans Chiari (1851–1916) was an Austrian-born physician who was professor of pathological anatomy at the German University in Prague [4]. He contributed several observations to medicine, such as hepatic vein thrombosis, aorto-oesophageal fistula, pneumocephaly, pituitary adenomas, and malformations in the posterior fossa in which parts of the cerebellum and medulla oblongata descend into the spinal canal. About a series of postmortem observations in patients with cerebral softening he wrote:

> . . . I would like to draw attention to two special issues concerning the role of the carotid bifurcation in endarteriitis chronica deformans, which in my opinion have received too little consideration. This is on the one hand the relative frequency of *thrombosis* secondary to endarteritis chronica deformans in the area of the carotid bifurcation and the initial part of the internal carotid, which sites are fairly often a source of *embolism* to intracranial arteries, on the other the not uncommon occurrence at an early stage or even in isolated form of endarteritis chronica deformans in the carotid bifurcation and the initial part of the carotid artery.

Conclusions and critique

These words, written in 1905, are as valid today as they were then, with the proviso that they were written in German, that the italics are ours, and that 'endarteritis chronica deformans' is currently called 'atherosclerosis' or 'atheroma'. However, despite the advent of angiography in the 1920s, it took some six to seven decades before the essence of these observations had permeated to the rank and file of physicians and neurologists. This delay can be attributed not only to medical conservatism but also to the modest sphere of resonance of the journal in which the article appeared. Germany may have emulated France—or rather Paris—as the centre of medical progress in the second half of the nineteenth century, but the Journal of the German Pathological Society, in its ninth year, probably did not enjoy a wide and international circulation.

Cerebral infarction continued to be attributed to *in situ* thrombosis of intracranial arteries throughout the first half of the twentieth century, as attested by authoritative textbooks up to 1968 [5], despite observations that the carotid arteries were occasionally occluded by a thrombus that extended intracranially [6]. That medical attention was eventually drawn again to extracranial atherosclerosis resulted, firstly, from carotid angiography and other imaging techniques (see section 5.2) and, secondly, from the studies of Miller Fisher (1913–2012). He correlated atherosclerosis at the carotid bifurcation not only with contralateral hemiplegia but also with attacks of monocular blindness in the ipsilateral eye [7]. Fisher's observations established the notion of 'transient ischaemic attacks' and, eventually, that of artery to artery embolism as the most common cause of cerebral infarction. Chiari's observations were finally confirmed by the success of carotid endarterectomy in reducing the risk of ischaemic stroke (see section 5.3) which is only technically possible because atheroma is indeed restricted to 'the area of the carotid bifurcation and the initial part of the internal carotid', allowing the surgeon to clamp the artery above and below atheromatous plaque before removing it.

5.2 **Angiography**

Main paper: Moniz E. L'encéphalographie artérielle, son importance dans la localisation des tumeurs cérébrales. [Arterial encephalography – its importance in the localisation of cerebral tumours] *Rev Neurol* 1927; 48:72–90.

Background

After the discovery of X-rays in 1895 by Wilhelm Röntgen (1845–1923) [8], changes in the skull or calcified intracranial lesions could be detected without invasive methods, but the soft tissues of the brain remained as mysterious as ever. Walter Dandy (1886–1946) had pioneered ventriculography in 1918 [9], but many tumours, cysts, or abscesses did not impinge on—and so distort the images of air in—the cerebral ventricles.

Methods

Moniz (1874–1955), whose full name was António Caetano de Abreu Freire Egas Moniz, started by searching for a contrast agent that could be mixed with circulating blood. The only opacifying substances in use at the time were lipiodol, an oily substance the French neurologists Sicard and Forestier had injected into the spinal subarachnoid space to demonstrate tumours and cysts [10]; bromide; and iodine salts of phenolphthalein, injected intravenously, by which method the American surgeons Graham and Cole tried to visualize the gallbladder, but it had toxic adverse effects [11].

Moniz tested several substances in animals and human cadavers. The ideal agent had to not only be opaque but also soluble and rapidly injectable, as a bolus into the internal carotid artery. He initially settled on a solution of strontium bromide, which he then tried in a few patients. The first patient had syphilitic general paralysis; most of the others had postencephalitic parkinsonism. (The first experiments in the latter category of patients were to test systemic tolerance through intravenous injections; remarkably, their symptoms seemed to improve somewhat afterwards.) However, the sixth patient undergoing carotid injection with strontium bromide died eight hours after the procedure and Moniz changed to strontium iodine. Another adjustment in his technique was the approach to the artery: percutaneous puncture was successful in the first three patients (and much later became standard practice before catheterization from the femoral artery), but in the fourth, the needle slipped out and the contrast fluid ended up in subcutaneous tissue. (Luckily, the damage was limited to a 'Claude Bernard-Horner syndrome' but, from then on, the carotid artery was dissected by a helpful surgeon, who also applied a temporary ligature to the vessel and then performed the injection more distally.) The greatest practical difficulty, however, according to Moniz, was the long exposure time—a quarter of a second—required for the imaging by the Potter-Buckey X-ray apparatus.

Results

Eventually, Moniz managed to catch a picture of the contrast fluid during its passage through the intracerebral arteries, in the sixth and last patient of the bromide series. It was in the third patient of the new series, with iodine, that he first found evidence of a tumour. This patient was a 20-year-old man, in whom a hypophyseal tumour had been suspected on clinical grounds (syndrome of Frölich-Babinski, blindness with gradual onset, severe headaches, and vomiting). For the first time, the needle had been placed in the artery before the ligature was applied. The X-ray showed displacement of the intracranial arteries, consistent with a tumour in the sellar region (Fig. 5.1).

This first of Moniz's papers about angiography was, in fact, a transcript of a lecture that he had given on 7 July 1927, for which he had travelled from Lisbon to Paris. Interestingly, the first discussant was Joseph Babinski (1857–1932), who found the pictures 'remarkable'.

Conclusion and critique

Neuroimaging had taken off, and we now take it for granted—indeed, we could not do without it. Unlike ventriculography, cerebral angiography is still carried out today, although in a different way. Even more importantly, Moniz's diagnostic technique has, in our professional lifetime, spawned therapeutic endovascular procedures that Moniz could not have dreamed of.

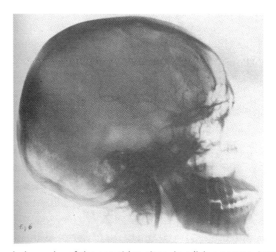

Fig. 5.1 Arterial encephalography of the carotid territory in a living person. Large tumour of the hypophysis. The carotid artery is displaced forwards, as well as the origin of the middle cerebral artery higher up. The anterior cerebral artery, of very small calibre, has an abnormal direction. (Translation of original text in French from Moniz, 1927.)

5.3 **Carotid endarterectomy**

Main paper: Eastcott HHG, Pickering GW, Robb CG. Reconstruction of internal carotid artery in a patient with intermittent attacks of hemiplegia. *Lancet* 1954; 264:994–6.

Background

Felix Eastcott, a vascular surgeon at St Mary's Hospital in London, was not the first to report operating on the carotid artery. There had been a few earlier reports from Argentina and China but because this paper was published in *The Lancet* it was so highly visible that it had a major effect on practice.

Methods and results

Eastcott's operation was in fact not an endarterectomy but a resection and reconstruction of a severely stenosed internal carotid artery to improve blood flow—so he and his co-authors thought—to the brain, in a single patient whose 33 focal neurological episodes were almost certainly caused by a cardiac arrhythmia leading to a brief fall in cardiac output and, so, cerebral blood flow, not by embolism. Along with the fairly new technique of carotid angiography (see section 5.2), this report ushered in what became an epidemic of carotid endarterectomies for patients with transient ischaemic attacks, and often quite serious strokes too, whose main cause became established as being embolism, not low flow, originating from atheromatous stenosis at the origin of the internal carotid artery (see section 5.1). At one point, surgery was also even being offered to patients with not a lot of carotid stenosis and no symptoms at all.

Conclusions and critique

In the early days, neurologists were seldom involved to help get the diagnosis right and a lot of 'dizzy' and other people with vague symptoms had unnecessary surgery. There was no computer tomography (CT) scanning to avoid operating on patients with intracerebral haemorrhage or even the occasional brain tumour, who also happened to have carotid stenosis, and there was no non-invasive imaging. The result was that thousands of patients, with and without cerebrovascular symptoms, were subjected to the risk of stroke and other complications of intra-arterial angiography, most of whom would not have had carotid stenosis. Despite the best attempts of Bill Fields, a Canadian neurologist working in the USA, who organized a randomized trial in the 1960s that was too small to assess the benefits and harms of surgery [12], the epidemic continued apace, at least in the USA if not in the UK (where, typically, there was much more caution, and some would say too much nihilism and not enough health care funding). The literature was dominated by surgical case series with no controls at all.

And so matters might have rested were it not for the publication, in the November–December edition of *Stroke* in 1984, of a series of papers criticizing the operation and pointing out that it carried higher risks than many surgeons were prepared to admit, and that it might not actually prevent strokes at all. It was no coincidence that the editor was

Henry Barnett, a hugely respected and influential Canadian neurologist working in London, Ontario. These papers captured the increasing alarm being expressed by neurologists all over the world and were probably responsible for the eventual success of the two major randomized trials of carotid endarterectomy in symptomatic patients—the European Carotid Surgery Trial (ECST) and the North American Symptomatic Carotid Endarterectomy Trial (NASCET)—and subsequent trials in asymptomatic patients. The initial results of ECST and NASCET were published almost simultaneously in 1991 and came to the same conclusion; yes, the operation carried an immediate risk of stroke, but, on average, there was also a benefit—it reduced the long-term risk of ipsilateral ischaemic strokes [13, 14]. Crucially, the *balance* of risk and benefit was favourable in the long term, if there was severe carotid stenosis. Much to the surprise of many neurologists, and to the relief of all vascular surgeons, the operation 'worked', at least on average, in the right sort of patients. Moreover, these trials also proved that carotid stenosis was indeed a cause of ipsilateral ischaemic stroke.

However, this was by no means the end of the story because it very soon became clear that several—maybe 10 or so—patients had to be operated on to prevent one stroke. This was because not all patients were destined to have a stroke, even without surgery, and because sometimes surgery caused stroke. Put another way, patients having the operation had roughly a 10% chance of personally benefiting, but no one knew before surgery who this 10% were and who the 90% were who might be spared unnecessary surgery.

Luckily, by this time people had begun to construct prognostic mathematical models based on various baseline characteristics to predict the outcome in a wide variety of conditions, and the technique of individual patient data meta-analysis was available. Peter Rothwell, a neurologist trained in Edinburgh but by then working in Oxford, exploited both these opportunities by combining the data from ECST, NASCET, and some smaller trials, to not only construct a prognostic model but also to validate it [15]. The number of operations needed to prevent a stroke could be as low as three if male patients were operated on very quickly after symptom onset (perhaps when the atheromatous plaque was still 'active' and shedding emboli), and as safely as the surgeon knew how, if the stenosis was particularly severe and irregular, and if the symptoms were in the brain rather than in the eye. The opportunities to increase the benefit to harm ratio in asymptomatic stenosis patients are far less, simply as they have a much lower longer term risk of stroke, maybe because their atheromatous plaques are not embolizing and are, therefore, somehow 'safe' [16].

And there the story stops for now, until someone can show that endovascular techniques are safer than carotid surgery, or until early medical treatment can quickly stop a stenotic plaque from embolizing and even reduce it in size. Eastcott and his colleagues were right when they wrote surprisingly modestly that 'it should, by careful clinical examination and selection, be possible to improve or cure an occasional patient by surgery'. The rise and fall, but not collapse, of carotid surgery all stemmed from a single case report in a very visible journal. But it did take half a century to sort out the place of the operation in routine clinical practice.

5.4 **Embolism from the heart, atrial fibrillation**

Main paper: European Atrial Fibrillation Trial (EAFT) Study Group. Secondary prevention in non-rheumatic atrial fibrillation after transient ischaemic attack or minor stroke. *The Lancet* 1993; 342:1255–62.

Background

The concept of embolism from the heart to the brain and other organs was promulgated by Virchow in the mid nineteenth century, although it had been suggested even earlier by Gerard van Swieten [17]. At that time, the underlying cause was probably mostly rheumatic heart disease, because this was then such a prevalent problem, and also because people rarely reached an age at which they were likely to develop atrial fibrillation (AF) in the absence of rheumatic heart disease (i.e. non-rheumatic AF). Indeed, the term 'cerebral embolism' was generally taken to mean embolism from the heart until the last half of the twentieth century, when it was realized that artery to artery embolism was a far more likely cause of ischaemic stroke than *in situ* intracranial arterial thrombosis (see section 5.1).

Concurrently with this change of emphasis came the discovery of the anticoagulant drugs—heparin and warfarin—and of the increasing importance of non-rheumatic AF as the major cause of thrombus in the heart and then embolism to the brain, probably first appreciated in the Framingham Study [18]. Up to a quarter of stroke patients are in AF, increasingly so in the elderly. Not surprisingly, anticoagulation became, largely from the 1950s, a widely used strategy for preventing ischaemic stroke in fibrillating patients, both before the event (primary prevention) and afterwards (secondary prevention). As ever, the cardiologists were more therapeutically aggressive than the neurologists. However, at the time there was no formal evidence that the potential harm from bleeding—particularly into the brain to cause haemorrhagic stroke—was less than the theoretical benefit of reducing ischaemic stroke risk. (On top of that, in the early days there was no CT scanning to distinguish primary brain haemorrhage from ischaemia as the cause of a stroke before anticoagulation was started.) The strategy of anticoagulation ought to work, but did it? And were the evident risks worth taking? Non-randomized comparisons, of which there were many, and case series, of which there were even more, were never going to satisfactorily answer those questions, even in those days, well before so-called evidence-based medicine became such a driver for guidelines.

Methods

While several randomized controlled trials were set up by cardiologists for primary prevention, neurologists were far more cautions, probably because we saw—and so feared—the adverse and sometimes fatal effect of intracranial haemorrhage. Indeed, a previous stroke was sometimes said to be a contraindication to anticoagulation when we were medical students in the 1960s. Moreover, there was a view, shared by one of us, that it would be extraordinarily difficult—at least in the UK—to set up a trial of secondary stroke prevention of patients with non-rheumatic AF, even though by then CT had become available

[19]. Maybe this paper acted as a provocation, it was probably meant to, because the Dutch took up the challenge to prove, once and for all, that the treatment worked, or did not, with their European Atrial Fibrillation Trial (EAFT). Prior to this, there had been just one trial, with less than 50 patients [20].

Results

The EAFT randomized 1007 recent transient ischaemic attack or minor ischaemic stroke patients to open anticoagulation with a target international normalized ratio of 3.0, or to placebo, or to aspirin. The result was clear-cut. Well-controlled long-term anticoagulation reduced the risk of ischaemic stroke by about two-thirds, with a remarkably low risk of bleeding. Aspirin was not as effective, a fact confirmed in many other trials and in meta-analysis.

Conclusions and critique

This trial result was so conclusive that not only did it change practice more or less overnight, but it also did away with the need for any further major secondary prevention trials with a no-treatment control group. These days, the questions have become 'What is safer than, and as effective as, warfarin, and easier to use?' and 'What to do about intermittent AF?' which is picked up more and more the longer the heart rate is monitored. When to start anticoagulation after a stroke was answered by the first International Stroke Trial (IST)—not immediately [21]. How long to anticoagulate for remains unanswered.

5.5 **Ruptured intracranial aneurysms recognized during life**

Main paper: Symonds CP. Contributions to the clinical study of intracranial aneurysms. *Guy's Hosp Rep* 1923; 73:139–58.

Background

Before 1923, the diagnosis of a ruptured cerebral aneurysm was not considered during life, but made only in the post-mortem room. There were two reasons for this. First, most patients with subarachnoid haemorrhage from a ruptured aneurysm had sudden headache, but usually no neurological deficits. There was no loss of elementary brain functions, and so no 'stroke'. Second, a ruptured aneurysm was regarded as invariably fatal because it was found only in the dead. Of course, that is a *non sequitur*, but such erroneous logic continued and probably still continues. For example, intraventricular haemorrhage was generally considered a lethal condition (because it was only seen at post-mortem) until CT scanners became available in the 1970s and detected it in patients who were definitely alive, complaining of headache, focal deficits, or both.

Charles (Putnam) Symonds (1890–1978) received his clinical training at Guy's Hospital in London, with an interruption during the First World War. In preparation for an appointment as physician at a planned new department for nervous diseases at Guy's, he spent some time as an intern in the USA, with Adolf Meyer at the Johns Hopkins Hospital in Baltimore and with Harvey Cushing at the Brigham Hospital in Boston [22].

Methods

It was during his stay with Cushing that Symonds ventured the diagnosis of a ruptured aneurysm in a 52-year-old woman who had been admitted with a sudden severe headache and a complete third nerve palsy on the right. After a sudden exacerbation of her headache, along with a decreased level of consciousness, Cushing performed a right subtemporal craniotomy but found only clotted blood, apparently coming from the base of the brain. The patient died a day later and the post-mortem showed a ruptured aneurysm at the junction of the internal carotid and posterior communicating arteries on the right (Fig. 5.2).

Cushing is reported to have said: 'Symonds, you made the correct diagnosis; either it was a fluke or there was reason in it. If so you will prove it. You will cease your ward duties as from now, and spend all your time in the library. Anything you want translated I will arrange for.' [22]

Results

Symonds' library work resulted in the historical section of his 1923 paper in the *Guy's Hospital Reports*. In this, he described the Boston patient and four further patients from England; in two, the diagnosis had been confirmed at post-mortem; in the two surviving patients, the diagnosis came from the clinical features and a lumbar puncture. Cushing wrote an addendum with five case histories of patients who had aneurysms at the anterior communicating artery, diagnosed at operation or post-mortem; in two of them, the

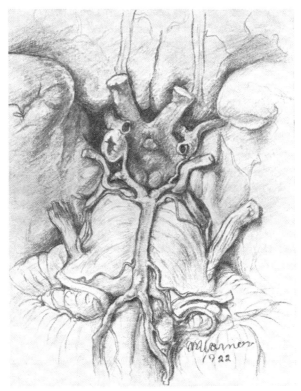

Fig. 5.2 Drawing of the base of the brain, showing the aneurysm at the junction of right internal carotid and posterior communicating arteries.
From Symonds, 1923.

aneurysm had not ruptured but compressed the optic chiasm [23]. A year later, Symonds published a full review, with an elaborate historical account and three more patients [24].

Conclusion and critique

The history of the diagnosis of aneurysmal subarachnoid haemorrhage can be briefly summarized in four phases:

1 the recognition of a ruptured aneurysm at post-mortem, more or less incidentally, by Blackall in 1813 [25];

2 the first recognition of subarachnoid haemorrhage (not its source) during life, by Froin in 1904 [26];

3 the first diagnosis of a ruptured aneurysm during life, actually not by Symonds but by Hutchinson in 1875—apparently by then medical minds were not prepared [27]; and

4 demonstration of the aneurysm during life with angiography, by Moniz in 1933 [28].

As for treatment, operative intervention for ruptured aneurysms was pioneered in the 1930s by Dott [29], became feasible by Dandy's mechanical clips [30], and was followed by many subsequent refinements in technique. The latest development is endovascular occlusion of the aneurysm by insertion of platinum coils, introduced by Guglielmi [31]. If occlusion of a ruptured aneurysm is practicable with either method, clipping or coiling, the chance of a good early outcome is definitely better with the endovascular method, also with better long-term prospects, according to a large and meticulously performed clinical trial in the UK [32].

This study was remarkable in that, in effect, it pitched neurosurgeons (with their clips and hard-won technical expertise) against the upstart interventional neuroradiologists (with their coils). Unusually, it was a randomized trial of a device very soon after it had been introduced, and it changed practice almost overnight, at least in Europe, if not the USA.

5.6 **Intracranial venous thrombosis**

Main paper: Barnett HJM, Hyland HH. Non-infective intracranial venous thrombosis. *Brain* 1953; 76:36–49.

Background

Tellingly, 'non-infective' are the first words in the title of Barnett and Hyland's article. That this qualification has disappeared in current papers is not just because extensive, purulent ear infections were more common in their day, but mainly because neurological complications in patients with such infections were practically the only circumstance when clinicians suspected (lateral) sinus thrombosis [33]. Childbirth was the one exception [34, 35].

Methods

In their article, Barnett and Hyland reviewed 39 autopsied cases with thrombosis of the dural sinuses, the superficial cortical veins, or both, collected over 20 years from the Toronto General Hospital. Before then, only case reports had been published [36, 37]. Not all 39 patients died of intracranial venous thrombosis; of 10 with associated heart disease, for example, it was the main cause of death in three and a contributing factor in four others. Other categories of preceding conditions or events were cachexia and marasmus (seven patients), operations of any kind [5], head injury [5], arterial occlusion or haemorrhage [4], and the puerperium [3].

Results

In an attempt to find some common pathogenetic denominator, the authors could not venture further than to point out that half the patients had evidence of thrombosis or embolism outside the brain, which suggested a general liability to thrombosis. Given the retrospective nature of the report, there was little available information about the clinical features. Though the authors mention gradually increasing headache as a premonitory symptom, in a paragraph about prognosis they referred—without providing details—to patients they saw in the post-partum period with a transient syndrome of convulsions and 'pseudo-tumour' (headaches, papilloedema, and increased cerebrospinal fluid pressure on lumbar puncture), as Symonds and Kendall had done more explicitly in their studies [33, 34]. In another earlier report, the diagnosis was radiologically confirmed by means of sinography [36].

Barnett and Hyland found that in patients with associated cerebral lesions, there was almost invariably haemorrhagic necrosis; often, the haemorrhage had extended into the subarachnoid space. In view of these findings, the authors wanted 'to emphasize the great danger in the use of anticoagulant therapy' that had been advocated by previous writers.

Conclusions and critique

Curiously, in our own clinical lifetime, a meta-analysis of clinical trials of anticoagulant treatment for intracranial venous thrombosis concluded that it 'appeared to be safe and was associated with a potentially important reduction in the risk of death or dependency' [38]. The discrepancy between recent evidence and the caveat from 1953, admittedly with the benefit of hindsight, is not merely ironic but also an important example of a much more fundamental kind of danger in medicine—that of reliance on intuitive logic rather than on empirical observations [39].

Although the autopsy series from Toronto did not provide new insights, it served to remind the neurological community that the diagnosis of intracranial venous thrombosis should be considered in a variety of situations, as well as in ear infections and the post-partum period. A further impulse was provided in 1967 by Kalbag and Woolf (Newcastle-upon-Tyne), in their detailed monograph [40]. Yet, it was only after the advent of CT scanning in the 1970s that the condition became prominently featured in the differential diagnosis of patients with acute or subacute brain lesions. Although modern neuroimaging is often thought to have largely replaced time-honoured clinical acumen, there are many instances where imaging has sharpened clinical judgement. Intracranial venous thrombosis is one such example where the well-founded clinical suspicion of the diagnosis, initiated by the Barnett and Hyland paper, can be confirmed with CT or magnetic resonance (MR) venography.

5.7 **Measuring outcome**

Main paper: Rankin J. Cerebral vascular accidents in patients over the age of 60: II. Prognosis. *Scot Med J* 1957; 2:200–15.

Background

In the assessment of a new treatment for acute stroke, the key question is 'How badly off is the patient in the end?', or, in the context of a clinical trial, 'How badly off is the group of patients who received the new treatment, compared with controls?'. This is rather different from trials of secondary prevention of stroke, where the usual measure of outcome is a survival curve tallying the number of major vascular events.

Initially, and almost automatically, so-called 'stroke scales' were constructed for acute stroke trials, analogous to scales for other specific neurological conditions. Such scales reflected the traditional neurological examination, by which different functions of the nervous system are separately assessed: for example, power of limbs, speech, visual fields, sometimes even reflexes. Although all these tests (or signs, as they are usually known) had evolved for the purpose of localizing lesions in the nervous system, stroke scales were aimed at measuring something completely different—the severity of a whole range of separate deficits, by assigning a numerical value to each item and then adding them up to make a total score. Not surprisingly, many physicians vaguely felt that it was problematic to try and reconstruct an individual person from such disparate building blocks. But instead of abandoning stroke scales, clinicians went on to design new scales, each time with new weights for a variety of neurological deficits. The reason for this persistence was the imaginary—but deluded—exactness of a grand total to define a patient's outcome. In reality, numbers in clinical scales such as these are misleading, since they represent not true values, like inches or kilograms, but only rank orders per item [41]. By 1992, more than 20 different stroke scales had seen the light of day [42].

That numbers were not what they seemed was only part of the problem. It gradually dawned on the neurological community that severity of disease can be measured at more than one level. After all, the greater part of the brain has no 'primary' motor, sensory, or cognitive function, and serves to connect and integrate the elementary 'functions'. Similarly, everyday life consists of a multitude of tasks that are integrated and difficult to separate. The World Health Organization's *International Classification of Functioning, Disability and Health* (ICF) describes four levels of measurement [43]:

1 of body structure, for example, the size of a cerebral infarct on a brain scan;

2 of body function (originally called the converse, an impairment, which is generally a physical sign), for example, grip strength or language production;

3 of activity and participation (originally the converse, disability), for example, the degree of independence in self-care and interaction; and finally

4 accounting for environmental factors, for example, the function of a patient within the social structure in which he or she usually lives (originally the converse, handicap).

As the perspective widens, from body organ to social circle, the measurement becomes more difficult, but the answer becomes more relevant to patients.

Since quality of life and societal roles are influenced by many factors other than just the extent of any brain damage, a pragmatic solution to measuring stroke outcome is to focus on the third level—of disability, that is, on the individual as a coherent unit (the word 'individual' stems from the Latin word for 'indivisible'). The question then becomes the degree to which a patient needs help in daily activities (disability scales), sometimes with inclusion of societal roles of an individual (handicap scales).

Methods

Such a holistic approach had, in fact, been published as early as 1957 by the Glaswegian physician John Rankin (1923–1981), as an instrument for his descriptive analysis of the natural history of stroke. Rankin was in charge of the chronic sick beds at the Academic Unit at Stobhill Hospital in his native Glasgow, and established what can be regarded as a prototypic stroke unit [44], given the emphasis he put on rehabilitation and the medical aspects of stroke.

Results

The scale is hidden within a wealth of other descriptive details about Rankin's unselected series of patients with stroke (Table 5.1). He devised it in order to describe the outcome in 196 survivors from a cohort of 202 patients who had been admitted within three weeks of stroke onset.

In 1953, Rankin emigrated and obtained a position at the University of Wisconsin in Madison, where he had already spent some time thanks to a Rockefeller fellowship, and where, eventually, he was appointed to chairs in medicine, preventive medicine, and pulmonary medicine [44, 45].

Conclusions and critique

In the days before impact factors mattered so much to universities, Rankin published his scale in his own local journal, *The Scottish Medical Journal*. Given the small circulation, it was, not surprisingly, 'lost'. However, it was rediscovered in the 1970s by a group of UK neurologists planning a secondary prevention trial of aspirin in patients with transient ischaemic attacks [46]. They hit on it in their search for a measure that might help to distinguish between 'minor' and 'disabling' strokes on follow up; the group added 'grade 0' for symptom-free patients, so it became the 'modified Rankin Scale' (mRS). Starting from this initiative, the use of the scale slowly percolated to most, if not all, research groups around the world who were faced with the shortcomings of 'stroke scales' that tabulated and summed separate impairments. The popularity of the scale was further enhanced by a formal study showing satisfactory inter-observer variation [47]. In dichotomous analyses, the split has been mostly, but not invariably, between grade 2 and 3, as in the UK TIA Study Group [46], but more sophisticated analyses include the entire distribution [48] or take account of the patient's condition at baseline [49].

Table 5.1 Rankin's original scale for measuring disability from stroke

I	*No significant disability*: able to carry out all usual duties
II	*Slight disability*: unable to carry out some of previous activities but able to look after own affairs without assistance
III	*Moderate disability*: requiring some help but able to walk without assistance
IV	*Moderately severe disability*: unable to walk without assistance and unable to attend to own bodily needs without assistance
V	*Severe disability*: bedridden, incontinent and requiring constant nursing care and attention

Reproduced from *Scot Med J*, 2, Rankin J., Cerebrovascular accidents in patients over the age of 60: II Prognosis, p. 200–15, Copyright (1957), with permission from SAGE publications.

Because the Rankin scale reflects the function of an individual person, not just that of his or her brain, it can be used to measure disability from conditions other than stroke, such as polyneuropathy or ischaemic heart disease. Yet the tradition—perhaps we should say parochialism—within research communities has largely prevented such cross-border fertilization. This is an oddity, rather than a problem, as long as the chosen measure of outcome reflects disability or handicap, as with the Karnofsky Scale for brain tumours [50], or the Glasgow (again!) Outcome Scale for head injury [51]. But, sadly enough, such provincialism is stifling if diseases continue to be assessed in the way the discarded stroke scales were, with a hotchpotch of iatrocentric measures, for example in multiple sclerosis and Parkinson's disease.

5.8 **Thrombolysis in acute ischaemic stroke**

Main paper: The National Institute of Neurological Disorders and Stroke rt-PA Stroke Study Group. Tissue plasminogen activator for acute ischaemic stroke. *New England Journal of Medicine* 1995; 333:1581–8.

Background

For centuries, strokes were regarded as untreatable. Dead brain was dead brain. Stroke was incurable. This pessimistic view began to change in the 1950s when Dyken and White, among others, suggested that ischaemic stroke—cerebral infarction—was not necessarily an all or nothing event [52]. An area of necrotic brain would not survive but it might be surrounded by 'an area of tissue reaction characterized by ischaemia and oedema'. In other words, surrounded by what is now known as the ischaemic penumbra—brain which is poorly perfused and so not functioning, but which might either recover or die. Dyken and White then went further to propose that 'If the blood flow to the ischaemic area could be increased or the surrounding tissue reaction decreased, ultimate recovery of the area might be possible'. This thought was the direct precursor of what have become the two main strands of research into the treatment of acute ischaemic stroke—the so far unsuccessful and very expensive efforts of the pharmaceutical industry to develop compounds to protect ischaemic brain from dying, and the more simple-minded plumbing approach of clearing the blocked blood vessel as quickly as possible.

The plumbing approach has, itself, two strands—dissolve the embolus or *in situ* thrombus (in other words, pharmaceutical thrombolysis), or mechanically dislodge it with some kind of arterial catheter device. Both approaches might work, although the former would be more practical. Both require speed, partly because the ischaemic penumbra is likely to die if the ischaemia lasts too long, and there is much debate about how long 'too long' is, and partly because the arterial obstruction often clears itself spontaneously, which is one reason why stroke patients can get better (and presumably why transient ischaemic attacks exist). In the background to this debate, neurologists were well aware that thrombolysis was becoming the standard treatment for acute myocardial infarction by the late 1980s, followed, more recently, by stenting of occluded coronary vessels—interventions that were well supported by randomized controlled trials (RCTs). It was therefore recognized that RCTs were needed for acute ischaemic stroke, which was a difficult task since, unlike acute myocardial infarction patients looked after in coronary care units, stroke patients were not, at the time, gathered into specialized stroke units. Furthermore, strokes had to become a medical emergency—neurologists would have to get out of bed at night—and so 'brain attacks' would have to be treated rather like 'heart attacks'. The slogan 'time is brain' was coined to encourage this necessary change of emphasis.

The early RCTs of pharmaceutical thrombolysis from the 1960s failed because the trials were far too small to show even quite a large therapeutic effect, and some were conducted before the advent of CT scanning allowed the recognition of stroke caused by intracerebral haemorrhage.

Methods and results

The thrombolysis idea dwindled, until it was reignited in 1995 when the National Institute of Neurological Disorders (NINDS) published its trial of tissue plasminogen activator. The trial had flaws, like any trial, in particular with the potential breakdown of the randomization process which took place in each hospital, rather than it being organized and recorded centrally. However, the trial demonstrated that by putting in a serious effort, strokes could be assessed, scanned, and treated very quickly—within 90 minutes of symptom onset sometimes—and that thrombolysis might well reduce both mortality and dependency, even though, not surprisingly, it increased the chance of intracranial bleeding.

Conclusions and critique

This was the seminal trial which preceded several others, culminating in the much larger third International Stroke Trial (IST3) published in 2012 [53]. Guidelines began to recommend thrombolysis within 3 hours of symptom onset, and then 4.5 hours, which is where we are now. Exactly which types of acute ischaemic stroke patients fare best, and which patients are at lowest risk of iatrogenic intracranial haemorrhage, will have to await the planned individual patient data meta-analysis of all the available trials.

Stroke is not as incurable as we thought. It might even be more successfully treated with mechanical 'clot busters'. The ongoing trials will tell us. However, whether such a labour-intensive intervention can be delivered in routine clinical practice remains to be seen. This still leaves the problem of the acute ischaemic strokes whose time of onset we do not know; in particular, those patients who awake with symptoms and strokes caused by intracerebral haemorrhage. Some strokes are still, it seems, incurable.

5.9 **Stroke units**

Main paper: Langhorne P, Williams OB, Gilchrist W, Howie K. Do stroke units save lives? *Lancet* 1993; 342:395–8.

Background

Coronary care units emerged in the late 1960s, at first just as a gathering of acute myocardial infarction patients wired up to electrocardiogram (ECG) monitors down one end of a medical ward, while the staff were poised with antiarrhythmic drugs and defibrillators. Despite some attempts, there was no RCT evidence of their effectiveness, a fact that should not suggest that they were necessarily ineffective. In those days, managers did not demand 'evidence' to be convinced that coronary care units were a 'good thing'. Intensive care units emerged in the 1970s, again without any RCT evidence of effectiveness. It just made sense to concentrate very sick patients with appropriate 24/7 expertise, even though the units were memorably criticized, but not in writing, as 'more intense than careful' by the late Tony Dornhorst, Professor of Medicine at St George's Hospital Medical School in London.

Meanwhile, stroke patients were left behind, not just in the acute phase but also for rehabilitation. They were admitted to general medical wards or to less appropriate wards if there were no beds. Often, they were regarded as 'bed blockers', and the appropriate expertise to treat them was widely scattered over the hospital (doctors, nurses, physiotherapists, occupational therapists, speech therapists, and others). Many quite severe stroke patients were not even admitted to hospital. It was no good arguing that the appropriate resources needed to be reorganized into one place; as one manager remarked, 'sometimes resources don't like being reorganized'. Although it made sense to set up stroke units to coordinate and concentrate care, by the 1980s, formal 'evidence' was required to effect any such major change in practice. Not surprisingly, the King's Fund Consensus Conference on treatment of stroke concluded, in 1988, that 'the services that are provided in hospital, primary care, and the community seem haphazard, fragmented, and poorly tailored to patients' needs' [54]. But nothing happened.

In fact, by the 1980s, there had been a few RCTs of various styles of stroke unit, all of which had a multidisciplinary team as their core, as opposed to 'ordinary' medical ward care. However, none were convincingly 'positive', so still nothing changed. By the 1990s though, systematic reviews and meta-analysis had been introduced by Richard Peto in Oxford, who applied it to aspirin; by Iain Chalmers, independently in Oxford, who applied it to perinatal medicine; by Tom Chalmers (no relation) in Boston, who applied it to anticoagulants; and by Jan Stjernsward in Stockholm, who applied it to breast cancer radiotherapy. As Richard Peto wrote to one of us: 'I don't think any of us deserve any great credit for introducing these methods in the 1970s: as soon as the need for such methods arose, they were bound to be invented independently by several groups of people (indeed there may also be others that I don't know about).'

In essence, this is a methodology to collate all the appropriate evidence from RCTs and then synthesize it into a 'bottom line'. If several trials are mostly pointing in the same sort of direction, and yet none are necessarily so-called statistically significant, then putting them together can deliver a much more compelling message (largely by increasing the effective sample size and, therefore, the precision of the estimated treatment effect). This is analogous to asking several people the way and finding that mostly they point in roughly but not exactly the same direction, so taking a rough average is the right way to head off.

Methods and results

And so it was that a meta-analysis of the available RCTs—at the time there were 10—finally produced the required evidence that specialist stroke units provided better outcomes than admitting acute stroke patients into a general medical or neurology ward and eventually rehabilitating them in an uncoordinated way. The relative risk of dying was reduced by 28% at 17 weeks post-onset (P< 0.01) and by 21% at one year (P<0.05) (Fig. 5.3). This meta-analysis was led by Peter Langhorne, on his own initiative, who at the time was a trainee geriatrician in Edinburgh. He was not even in a research post. Indeed, one of us (CPW) can remember exactly where he was standing when Peter Langhorne told him the results, and how astonished he was.

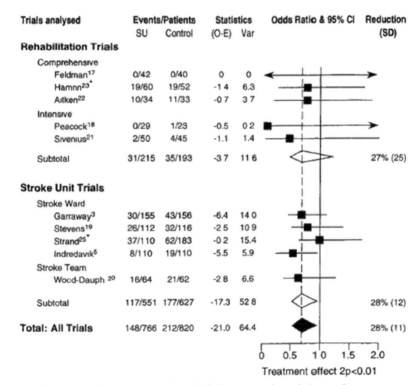

Fig. 5.3 Initial mortality after stroke: stroke unit (SU) vs general wards (control).

Reproduced from *Lancet*, 342, Langhorne P, Williams OB, Gilchrist W et al., Do stroke units save lives?, p. 395–8, Copyright (1993), with permission from Elsevier.

Conclusions and critique

In retrospect, the analysis was not as robust as one would like these days, but it did the trick, probably because it was pushing at an open door of clinical common sense. Stroke units quickly became fashionable and then demanded by clinical guidelines, as they are now. It not only makes sense to concentrate patients with the appropriate resources to treat them, but the strategy also works. Of course, one has to guard against staff 'burn out' (seeing a lot of the same sort of patients with the same sort of problems all the time can be debilitating), over-diagnosing stroke, and disadvantaging patients who might have had, but turn out not to have had, a stroke.

As time has gone on, more trials have been done and the meta-analysis enshrined in the Cochrane Library has become a little less convincing. Why less convincing? Although there are now 31 RCTs, the relative reduction of the odds of death at one year is down to 14%, albeit still statistically significant [55]. This is partly because more unpublished trials were found, and maybe partly because stroke care in general medical wards has improved. Many of the trials were not blinded, in the sense that non-fatal patient outcomes were evaluated by people who knew the treatment allocation, and many of these same people were stroke unit enthusiasts. In some of the trials, patients in stroke units received more therapy of various sorts than the control group. The stroke units were a very mixed bag, ranging from acute care units to rehabilitation units. Not all the trials were properly randomized. Nonetheless, taken in the round and with appropriate sensitivity analyses, and accounting for these criticisms, the results are still convincing. Stroke units are here to stay.

Clinical common sense, backed up by meta-analysis, has had an extraordinary impact on how stroke patients are now managed, and also made it easier to study them at all stages of their illness.

5.10 **Transient ischaemic attacks as an emergency**

Main: Rothwell PM, Giles MF, Flossmann E, et al. A simple score (ABCD) to identify individuals at high early risk after transient ischaemic attack. *Lancet* 2005; 366:29–36.

Background

Although there had been a few earlier descriptions of what we now call transient ischaemic attacks (TIAs)—for example by Osler in 1911 [56]—their widespread recognition, and the term, only evolved in the 1950s [57]. This was probably prompted by a series of papers from the Mayo Clinic by Clarke Millikan, Jack Whisnant, and others, along with papers by Miller Fisher in Boston and by Ralph Ross Russell in London. Even in those early days, it was appreciated that TIAs could herald a stroke, and so the patients were often anticoagulated on the basis of theory and hope rather than evidence. But, with the rise of RCTs from the 1970s, a more evidence-based approach led to the current widespread use of antiplatelet drugs (mainly aspirin), blood pressure lowering drugs, and statins to reduce blood cholesterol, along with carotid surgery for a few suitable patients (see section 5.3).

However, there was no sense of urgency about treating TIA patients to reduce their risk of stroke, at least not in the UK, where they would be seen—if at all—in a neurology or general medicine out-patient clinic some days, if not weeks, after the event. Months might pass before a patient had a carotid endarterectomy. In a sense, we have ourselves to blame. We criticized the Mayo Clinic workers for their observation that strokes could quickly follow TIAs because they were mostly looking backwards—in retrospect—at stroke patients, some of whom had indeed had a TIA the day before [58]. But what about the TIA patients who had never had a stroke and had not come to medical attention, or the patient with a forgotten or unrecorded TIA from years ago, as well as the recent one? Better, we thought, to look forwards—prospectively—at TIA patients as a whole. How many of them have a stroke in the next day or two? Not many we thought, but that was because in the available prospective studies, and indeed in our own clinical experience and in the big clinical trials, everyone tended to recruit TIA patients several days or even weeks after their attack, so completely missing their early natural history. In mitigation, no one in the early 1980s regarded even strokes as a medical emergency. There were other pressures on neurologists' time, and we deliberately excluded patients from TIA prognosis studies if they had had a stroke before we could see them (and stated that very clearly). Anyway, it was very difficult to get patients who might have had TIAs seen quickly.

Methods and results

All that changed when Peter Rothwell in Oxford did what he then did best—exploited data that had been collected (and fortunately stored) by other people, including us. By re-analysing data from the Oxfordshire Community Stroke Project (OCSP), and other cohort studies and randomized trials, he found that we had almost certainly missed the early natural history of TIAs [59]—something which had been suspected in the 1980s but which we had not thought was important.

Conclusions and critique

So now, in the early 2000s, everyone who might have had a TIA is very quickly referred for assessment (within hours or maybe a day), investigated quickly, and treated quickly. One difficulty, however, is that something like 50% of people who might have had TIAs, have not had them. However, the correct diagnoses (migraine, epilepsy, and other common conditions mimicking TIAs) can usually soon be sorted out by a competent physician who is readily prepared to diagnose something other than cerebrovascular disease in a stroke/TIA clinic. (Regrettably, disease-specific clinics do tend to over-diagnose their own diseases.)

More problematic is one of the paradoxes of preventive medicine—not everyone who *might* have an event, goes on to have it. So, treating everyone 'just in case' might be very expensive, cause more adverse events than could be justified by the benefit for a few, and generally lead to over-medicalizing the patients. The practical question then became how to spot the real TIAs and the real TIA patients likely to have a stroke in the next few days.

The answer was to develop a predictive score which picked out the TIA patients from the OCSP who had an early stroke, validate that score on an independent group of patients (The Oxford Vascular Study), and facilitate the adoption of the score by making it memorable and easy to use. This Peter Rothwell did, and his 'ABCD' score is now well embedded in the emergency departments of most, if not all, hospitals in the UK. It is simple, being based merely on patient age, blood pressure, straightforward clinical features, and duration of symptoms. And, reassuringly, the score has been validated in many other datasets.

Whisnant and his colleagues were right. TIA patients do need to be treated quickly to reduce their early—as well as their later—risk of stroke, but in their day, there was no reliable way of reducing that risk. Half a century later, we have effective but not perfect treatments to offer patients, and we know who to prioritize to treat at once and who can wait a few days if resources are limited.

Competing interest: although one of us (CPW) was an author on the paper, he only provided data on the OCSP and commented on the drafts.

Key unanswered questions

1 What is the cause and treatment of spontaneous intracerebral haemorrhage (ICH)?
   We did not select any papers on this 'other cause' of stroke because it still remains a mystery both to cause(s), at least in the individual patient, and treatment.

2 How much does vascular disease contribute to dementia—even, maybe, to what we currently like to call Alzheimer's disease?

3 How do we get to grips with the problem that we can diagnose before we can treat?
   So often, indeed by definition, the ability to diagnose runs far ahead of any knowledge of natural history and treatment, particularly when the natural history extends over decades and any therapeutic intervention is not obviously beneficial and safe. This would apply to how we think about cavernous malformations, only diagnosable during life with MR brain imaging, and patent foramen ovale, in a sense far too easily diagnosable with echocardiography.

4 What other causes of stroke might there be?
   Although stroke incidence and mortality are declining, perhaps because we know much more about its risk factors and causes and can treat some of them satisfactorily, there may well be other causes to be found—not just rare ones, but common ones too.

5 How can we best target therapeutic interventions?
   In an increasingly complicated world, with so many therapeutic interventions available, it would help enormously if they could be targeted on the smaller number of patients who definitely need them rather than on the much larger number that might need them.

Acknowledgements

We would like to thank Peter Langhorne, Martin Dennis, Peter Sandercock, and Peter Rothwell for their help in producing this chapter.

References

1 **Rostan L.** *Recherches sur une Maladie encore peu connue, qui a reçu le Nom de Ramollissement du Cerveau.* Paris: Béchet, Gabon & Crevot; 1820.

2 **Abercrombie J.** *Pathological and Practical Researches on Diseases of the Brain and Spinal Cord.* Edinburgh: Waugh and Innes; 1829; 25.

3 **Virchow RLK.** Ueber die akute Entzündung der Arterien. *Archiv Pathol Anat* 1847; **1**:272–378.

4 **Tubbs RS, Cohen-Gadol AA.** Hans Chiari (1851–1916). *J Neurol* 2010; **257**:1218–20.

5 **Brain WR.** *Diseases of the Nervous System*, 6th ed. Oxford: Oxford University Press; 1968.

6 **Hunt JR.** The role of the carotid arteries in the causation of vascular lesions of the brain, with remarks on special features of the symptomatology. *Am J Med Sci* 1914; **147**:704–13.

7 **Fisher CM.** Transient monocular blindness associated with hemiplegia. *Arch Ophthalmol* 1952; **47**:167–203.

8 **Röntgen WC.** Ueber eine neue Art von Strahlen (vorläufige Mittheilung). *Sitzungsberichten der Physikalisch-medicinische Gesellschaft zu Würzburg* 1895; **29**:137–47.

9 **Dandy WE.** Ventriculography following the injection of air into the cerebral ventricles. *Ann Surg* 1918; **68**:5–11.

10 **Sicard JA, Forestier J.** Méthode générale d'exploration radiologique par l'huile iodée (lipiodol). *Bull Mém Soc Méd Hôp Paris* 1922; **46**:463–8.

11 **Graham EA, Cole WH.** Roentgenologic examination of the gallbladder: preliminary report of a new method utilizing the intravenous injection of tetrabromphenolphthalein. *JAMA* 1924; **82**:613–4.

12 **Fields WS, Maslenikov V, Meyer JS, Hass WK, Remington RD, Macdonald M.** Joint study of extracranial arterial occlusion. V. Progress report of prognosis following surgery or nonsurgical treatment for transient cerebral ischaemic attacks and cervical carotid lesions. *JAMA* 1970; **211**:1993–2003.

13 **European Carotid Surgery Trialists' Collaborative Group.** MRC European Carotid Surgery Trial. Interim results for symptomatic patients with severe (70–99%) or with mild (0–29%) carotid stenosis. *Lancet* 1991; **337**:1235–43.

14 **North American Symptomatic Carotid Endarterectomy Trial Collaborators.** Beneficial effect of carotid endarterectomy in symptomatic patients with high-grade carotid stenosis. *New Engl J Med* 1991; **325**:445–53.

15 **Rothwell PM.** With what to treat which patient with recently symptomatic carotid stenosis? *Pract Neurol* 2005; **5**:68–83.

16 **Warlow CP.** Carotid endarterectomy for asymptomatic stenosis—firming up the uncertainty *Pract Neurol* 2005; **5**:2–5.

17 **Warlow CP, van Gijn J, Dennis M, et al.** *Development of Knowledge about Cerebrovascular Disease in Stroke: Practical Management.* Oxford: Blackwell Publishing; 2008.

18 **Kannel WB, Abbott RD, Savage DI, et al.** Epidemiological features of chronic atrial fibrillation: the Framingham study. *New Engl J Med* 1982; **306**:1018–21.

19 **Sandercock P, Warlow C, Bamford J, Peto R.** Is a controlled trial of long-term oral anticoagulants in patients with stroke and non-rheumatic atrial fibrillation worthwhile? *Lancet* 1986; **ii**:788–92.

20 **Ezekowitz MD, Bridgers SL, James KE, et al.**, for the Veterans Affairs Stroke Prevention in Non-rheumatic Atrial Fibrillation Investigators. Warfarin in the prevention of stroke associated with nonrheumatic atrial fibrillation. *N Engl J Med* 1992; **327**:1406–12.

21 **International Stroke Trial Collaborative Group.** The International Stroke Trial (IST): a randomised trial of aspirin, subcutaneous heparin, both, or neither among 19435 patients with acute ischaemic stroke. *Lancet* 1997; **349**:1569–81.

22 **Symonds CP.** Autobiographical introduction. In: Symonds CP, ed. *Studies in Neurology*. London: Oxford University Press; 1970; 1–23.

23 **Cushing H.** Contributions to the clinical study of cerebral aneurysms. *Guy's Hosp Rep* 1923; **73**:159–63.

24 **Symonds CP.** Spontaneous subarachnoid haemorrhage. *Quart J Med* 1924; **18**:93–122.

25 **Blackall J.** *Observations on the Nature and Cure of Dropsies*. London: Longman & Co; 1813.

26 **Froin G.** *Les Hémorrhagies sous-arachnoidiennes et le Méchanisme de L'Hématolyse en Général*. Paris: G.Steinheil; 1904.

27 **Hutchinson J.** Aneurism of the internal carotid artery within the skull diagnosed eleven years before the patient's death: spontaneous cure. *Trans Clin Soc London* 1875; **8**:127–31.

28 **Moniz E.** Anévrysme intra-cranien de la carotide interne droite rendu visible par l'artériographie cérébrale. *Rev Oto-Neuro-Ophthal* 1933; **11**:198–203.

29 **Dott N.** Intracranial aneurysms: cerebral arterio-radiography: surgical treatment. *Trans Med Chir Soc Edinb* 1932; **47**:219–40.

30 **Dandy WE.** Intracranial aneurysm of internal carotid artery, cured by operation. *Ann Surg* 1938; **107**:654–7.

31 **Guglielmi G, Vinuela F, Dion J, Duckwiler G.** Electrothrombosis of saccular aneurysms via endovascular approach. Part 2: Preliminary clinical experience. *J Neurosurg* 1991; **75**: 8–14.

32 **Molyneux AJ, Kerr RS, Birks J, et al.** Risk of recurrent subarachnoid haemorrhage, death, or dependence and standardised mortality ratios after clipping or coiling of an intracranial aneurysm in the International Subarachnoid Aneurysm Trial (ISAT): long-term follow-up. *Lancet Neurol* 2009; **8**:427–33.

33 **Symonds CP.** Hydrocephalic and focal cerebral symptoms in relation to thrombophlebitis of the dural sinuses and cerebral veins. *Brain* 1937; **60**:531–50.

34 **Kendall D.** Thrombosis of intracranial veins. *Brain* 1948; **71**:386–402.

35 **Purdon Martin JSHL.** Primary thrombosis of cerebral veins (following childbirth). *BMJ* 1941; **i**:349–53.

36 **Ray BS, Dunbar HS.** Thrombosis of the superior sagittal sinus as a cause of pseudotumor cerebri; methods of diagnosis and treatment. *Trans Am Neurol Assoc* 1950; **51**:12–7.

37 **Silbermann M, Fishman RA.** Primary (idiopathic) thrombosis of the superior longitudinal sinus. *Trans Am Neurol Assoc* 1951; **56**:164–7.

38 **Coutinho J, de Bruijn SF, DeVeber G, Stam J.** Anticoagulation for cerebral venous sinus thrombosis. *Cochrane Database Syst Rev* CD002005; **10**–8–2011.

39 **Bousser M-G.** A patient that changed my practice: in a worsening situation, treatment can do more good than harm. *Pract Neurol* 2003; **3**:112–5.

40 **Kalbag RM, Woolf AL.** *Cerebral Venous Thrombosis*. Oxford: Oxford University Press; 1967.

41 **van Gijn J, Warlow CP.** Down with stroke scales! *Cerebrovasc Dis* 1992; **2**:244–6.

42 **van Gijn J.** Measurement of outcome in stroke prevention trials. *Cerebrovasc Dis* 1992; **2** (suppl. 1):23–34.

43 **World Health Organization.** *International Classification of Functioning, Disability and Health* (ICF). WHO; 2012.

44 **Quinn TJ, Dawson J, Walters M.** Dr John Rankin: his life, legacy and the 50th Anniversary of the Rankin Stroke Scale. *Scot Med J* 2008; **53**:44–7.

45 **Lindley RI.** John Rankin (1923–81). *J Neurol* 2001; **248**: 1007–8.

46 **UK-TIA Study Group.** The United Kingdom transient ischaemic attack (UK-TIA) aspirin trial: final results. *J Neurol Neurosurg Psychiatry* 1991; **54**:1044–54.

47 van Swieten JC, Koudstaal PJ, Visser MC, Schouten HJ, van Gijn J. Interobserver agreement for the assessment of handicap in stroke patients. *Stroke* 1988; **19**:604–7.

48 **The National Institute of Neurological Disorders and Stroke rt-PA Stroke Study Group.** Tissue plasminogen activator for acute ischemic stroke. *N Engl J Med* 1995; **333**:1581–7.

49 Mendelow AD, Gregson BA, Fernandes HM, et al. Early surgery versus initial conservative treatment in patients with spontaneous supratentorial intracerebral haematomas in the International Surgical Trial in Intracerebral Haemorrhage (STICH): a randomised trial. *Lancet* 2005; **365**:387–97.

50 Karnofsky DA, Burchenal JH. The clinical evaluation of chemotherapeutic agents in cancer. In: Macleod CM, ed. *Evaluation of Chemotherapeutic Agents*. New York: Columbia University Press; 1949:191–205.

51 Jennett B, Bond M. Assessment of outcome after severe brain damage: a practical scale. *Lancet* 1975; **1**:480–4.

52 Dyken M, White P. Evaluation of cortisone in the treatment of cerebral infarction. *JAMA* 1956; **162**:1531–4.

53 The IST-3 Collaborative Group. The benefits and harms of intravenous thrombolysis with recombinant tissue plasminogen activator within 6 h of acute ischaemic stroke (the third international stroke trial [IST-3]): a randomised controlled trial. *Lancet* 2012; **379**: 2352–63.

54 King's Fund. Consensus Conference on Treatment of Stroke. *BMJ* 1988; **297**:126–8.

55 Stroke Unit Trialists' Collaboration Editorial Group: Cochrane Stroke Group. Organised inpatient (stroke unit) care for stroke. Published online: 11 September 2013. http://onlinelibrary.wiley.com/doi/10.1002/14651858.CD000197.pub3/pdf.

56 Osler W. Transient attacks of aphasia and paralysis in states of high blood pressure and arteriosclerosis. *Can Med Assoc J* 1911; **1**:919–26.

57 Hutchinson EC, Acheson EJ. *Strokes: Natural History, Pathology and Surgical Treatment*. London: Saunders; 1975.

58 Cartlidge NEF, Whisnant JP, Elveback LR. Carotid and vertebro-basilar transient cerebral ischemic attacks. A community study, Rochester, Minnesota. *Proceedings Mayo Clinic* 1977; **52**:117–20.

59 Coull AJ, Rothwell PM. Under-estimation of the early risk of recurrence after first stroke by the use of restricted definitions. *Stroke* 2004; **35**:1925–9.

Chapter 6

Epilepsy

Gregory L. Holmes

6.0 **Introduction**

Epilepsy was recognized as early as *c*.1050 BCE in Babylon, and Hippocratic writings describe epilepsy as a disorder of the brain as early as *c*.400 BCE [1]. Despite being a disorder of recognized antiquity, our understanding of this common and deadly condition remains quite limited. Epilepsy is a common and, far too often, deadly neurological disorder that affects people of all ages. Epilepsy is a spectrum of disorders—the epilepsies—with a range of severities, widely differing seizure types and causes, and varying impacts on patients and their families. Epilepsy imposes an immense burden on individuals, families, and society, affecting more than 65 million people worldwide.

Singling out ten landmark publications in epilepsy from the past century is no easy task. There have been many publications that could legitimately compete for such an honour. There is a great temptation to pick high-profile papers that describe new technologies that have aided in the evaluation of patients with epilepsy, such as magnetic resonance imaging, positron emission tomography, and magnetoencephalography. Rather, I have chosen to select papers that changed concepts about epilepsy, or in the case of more recent papers, have the potential of changing how we care for individuals with epilepsy. Even with this goal in mind, I found selecting the top 10 to be a difficult assignment. It is very likely that other colleagues involved in epilepsy research and patient care would have chosen a different set of manuscripts. Indeed, when I presented my 'top 10' to my colleagues, I received many incredulous looks. What may be considered a seminal paper to one clinician may be a minor contribution to another. Nevertheless, I hope my reasoning for including this group of articles is clear to the reader. Having been engaged in the care of individuals with epilepsy for well over three decades, I would relish feedback from readers, be it agreement or disagreement with my selection.

6.1 **First description of an epileptic syndrome**

Main paper: West WJ. On a peculiar form of infantile convulsions. *Lancet* 1841; 1:724–5.

Background and methods

In 1841, a physician in England wrote a letter to the editor of the *Lancet* titled 'On a peculiar form of infantile convulsions' [2]. Dr West's goal was to draw the attention of his colleagues to 'a very rare and singular species of convulsions peculiar to young children.' In the letter, Dr West described his son's symptoms in remarkable detail, conveying both the objectivity of the physician and the concerns of a father with a severely ill child. This description includes all of the features of the entity currently called infantile spasms or West syndrome.

Results

Dr West noted:

> The child is now near a year old; was a remarkably fine, healthy child when born, and continued to thrive till he was four months old. It was at this time that I first observed slight bobbings of the head forward, which I then regarded as a trick, but were, in fact, the first indications of disease; for these bobbings increased in frequency, and at length became so frequent and powerful, as to cause a complete heaving of the head forward towards his knees, and then immediately relaxing into the upright position, something similar to the attacks of emprosthotonos; these bowings and relaxings would be repeated alternately at intervals of a few seconds, and repeated from 10 to 20 or more times at each attack, which attack would not continue more than two or three minutes; he sometimes has two, three, or more attacks in the day; they come on whether sitting or lying; just before they come on he is all alive and in motion, making a strange noise, and then all of a sudden down goes his head and upwards his knees; he then appears frightened and screams out; at one time, he lost flesh, looked pale and exhausted, but latterly he has regained his good looks, and, independent of this affection, is a fine grown child, but he neither possesses the intellectual vivacity or the power of moving his limbs, of a child of his age; he never cries at the time of the attacks, or smiles or takes any notice, but looks placid and pitiful, yet his hearing and vision are good; he has no power of holding himself upright or using his limbs, and his head falls without support. [2]

Conclusions

Dr West described the core features of what was to become the entity of West Syndrome: flexor spasm which occurred in flurries and developmental regression.

Critique

In West's poignant report of 150 years ago, he provided the first ever description of an epilepsy syndrome. It was characterized, by spasms, as a particular seizure type not reported earlier, and also by occurrence in infancy and mental deterioration. However, the condition did not become widely recognized as an epilepsy syndrome until 100 years later, when the particular electroencephalograph (EEG) pattern associated with infantile spasms, hypsarrhythmia, was defined [3]. West syndrome is now an established condition consisting of infantile spams, developmental regression, and an EEG showing hypsarrhythmia.

West syndrome is one of the most recognized types of encephalopathic epilepsies. It constitutes a catastrophic form of epilepsy of early infancy. The disorder presents with seizures characterized by an initial contraction phase followed by a sustained tonic phase in one of three types of spasms—flexor, extensor, and mixed flexor-extensor spasms—a distinct EEG pattern of hypsarrhythmia, and psychomotor delay/arrest. Infantile spasms, a form of epileptic spasms, refers to the behavioural features of West Syndrome, with flurries of spasms occurring during infancy. Typically, the spasms involve brief symmetrical contractions of musculature of the neck, trunk, and extremities, lasting up to 5 seconds, and frequently occur in clusters. It is estimated that 60–90% of children with West syndrome have an associated underlying disorder that is evident; whereas, in other cases, there is no identifiable underlying condition.

Although West Syndrome was first described in 1841, its diagnosis, evaluation, and management continue to pose many challenges to the treating physician. The spasms spontaneously resolve, but they are often replaced by other types of refractory seizures. For many, developmental outcome is poor and a majority of children with West Syndrome have intellectual disabilities. A number of genetic causes of West Syndrome have been identified, although the pathophysiology of the syndrome remains quite limited.

Currently, adrenocorticotropic hormone (ACTH) and vigabatrin are the two first-line therapies available in the United States [4]; however, these agents are not effective in all cases and there is an urgent need for the development of additional therapeutic options for West syndrome.

Identifying epileptic syndromes is defined as the association of several clinically recognizable features, signs, symptoms, phenomena, or characteristics that occur together more commonly than chance. Identifying an epileptic syndrome such as infantile spasms affects treatment, provides prognostic information, offers insight into pathophysiological mechanisms, and is very helpful in the delineation of genetic defects.

Dr West's eloquent clinical description of his son set the stage for further investigations into the pathophysiology (see section 6.7) and genetic basis of infantile spasms and remains an exemplary example of how important clinical observations are in the diagnosis and treatment of epileptic conditions.

6.2 **Discovery of a revolutionary diagnostic test in epilepsy**

Main paper: Berger H. Uber das elektrenkephalogramm des menschen. *Arch Psychiatr Nervenkrankh* 1929; 87:527–70.

Background

Since the era of Hippocrates, epilepsy has been diagnosed by behavioural observation of seizures. The lack of any physiological markers of the condition hindered investigators for centuries. This all changed when a German psychiatrist named Hans Berger discovered a way to record electrical activity of the human brain [5], eventually known as electroencephalography (EEG).

Methods and results

Hans Berger was aware of the electrical activity of the brain from the work of Richard Caton who had recorded action potentials from rabbits and monkeys [6]. With the goal of discovering the physiological basis of psychic energy, Berger, in 1924, made the first EEG recording in man. He initially used subcutaneous silver wires placed in the front and back of the head and later switched to silver foil electrodes secured to the head by a rubber band. After using several recording devices, he settled on the Siemens recording galvanometer, which allowed him to record electrical voltages in the millivolt range. The resulting output was then photographed. Using the EEG, he was also the first to describe the different waves or rhythms which were present in the normal brain, such as the alpha wave rhythm and the changes to beta activity when the subject opened their eyes. Remarkably, in addition to recording brain activity from normal subjects, he also recorded activity from brain-injured patients. This early investigation of the pathological state laid the foundation of this technique in medicine.

It was not until 1929 that Dr Berger published results showing that variation in voltage could be recorded through the intact cranium [5]. Even then, the importance of Berger's discoveries in EEG was not recognized until 1934 when British electrophysiologists, Edgar Douglas Adrian and B.H.C. Matthews, confirmed his basic observations. His discoveries were presented at an international forum in 1937 [7] and, by 1938, EEG had gained widespread recognition by eminent researchers in the field, leading to its practical use in diagnosis in the United States, England, and France.

Berger's first six papers, published between 1929 and 1933, described the EEG during the awake and sleep states, as well as patterns from a number of disease states (Fig. 6.1). Interestingly, his early papers did not describe EEGs from patients with epilepsy, since he suspected that they contained artefacts. Only in 1988, after other authors had described high amplitude changes in the cortex of experiment animals, did he publish EEGs of absence and focal seizures.

Conclusions

The 1929 paper by Berger demonstrated that brain electrical activity could be reliably recorded using scalp electrodes in man. Further papers by Berger and others showed that

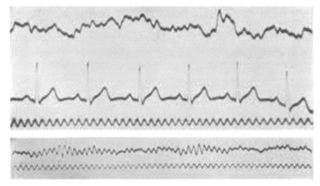

Fig. 6.1 The first reports of the human EEG from the first publication from Hans Berger in 1929. Both represent samples of EEG recorded from his son Klaus (16 years old). The bottom figure represents a sample of what he would later call the 'alpha rhythm' (a sinusoidal rhythm of approximately 10 Hz) and the figure above, what he would later call the 'beta rhythm' (or a desynchronized EEG with no obvious rhythmicity). The lowest tracing in both graphs is a generated 10 Hz sine wave, and the middle tracing from the top figure is the ECG.

Reproduced from *Arch Psychiatr Nervenkrankh*, 87, Berger H, Uber das elektrenkephalogramm des menschen, p. 527–70, Copyright (1929), with permission from Springer.

the recording of brain electrical activity could also be of enormous importance in the diagnosis of epilepsy.

Critique

Hans Berger's invention of the EEG is one of the most remarkable and momentous developments in the history of clinical neurology. The EEG remains today one of the most important and cost-effective tools in the armamentarium of a neurologist. In addition, the discovery of the EEG has had a profound effect on our understanding of the neurophysiological basis of epilepsy. At long last, the definition of epilepsy composed by John Hughlings Jackson in 1873 as a 'sudden, excessive, and rapid discharge of brain cells' could now be proven.

While modern neuroimaging such as magnetic resonance imaging (MRI) has been extremely valuable in determining the aetiology of epilepsy and providing functional information, it complements, rather than supplants, EEG which provides spatial and temporal information about the brain. The EEG has not remained a static test and, with technological advances, the research and clinical utility of the test has expanded. Long-term EEG and video monitoring, ambulatory EEG monitoring, and intracranial electrode recordings are now standard tests at tertiary epilepsy centres. Through the pioneering work of Hans Berger, the electrical activity of single cells to large networks can be sampled. The importance of Berger's early studies cannot be over-estimated.

6.3 **Discovery of the first non-sedative antiepileptic drug**

Main paper: Merritt HH, Putnam TJ. Sodium diphenylhydantoinate in the treatment of convulsive disorders. *JAMA* 1938; 111:1068–73.

Background

Prior to the discovery of phenytoin in 1938, the only two drugs available to treat epilepsy were bromides and phenobarbital. Bromides were first used in 1857 to treat women with 'hysterical epilepsy', whereas phenobarbital was first used in 1912 for both its sedative and antiepileptic properties. While phenobarbital remains widely used worldwide for treatment of epilepsy, bromides are now rarely used to treat seizures in humans, primarily because of toxicity. Based on the efficacy of phenobarbital and bromides, it was assumed that epilepsy needed to be treated by compounds that resulted in sedation. However, this assumption changed with the use of animal models in epilepsy research. By the 1930s, drugs were being studied in animal models and it is because of such animal studies that phenytoin was developed for clinical use by Tracy Putnam and H. Houston Merritt [8].

Methods

Using the maximal electroshock test in cats, Merritt and Putnam showed that phenytoin was efficacious in preventing seizures without causing sedation [8]. Because the drug was relatively non-toxic and well tolerated by laboratory animals, a clinical trial of sodium phenytoin was conducted in 200 patients with frequent convulsive seizures who had not responded to other modes of therapy.

Results

In 142 patients who received the treatment for periods varying from 2 to 11 months, generalized tonic-clonic seizures stopped in 58% and significantly decreased in frequency in an additional 27%; petit mal (absence) seizures stopped in 35% and decreased in frequency in an additional 49%; and psychic equivalent attacks (complex partial seizures) stopped in 67% and decreased in frequency in 33%. Significant skin rashes occurred in 5%; and tremors, ataxia, and dizziness occurred in 15%.

Conclusions

Phenytoin was an effective antiepileptic in a variety of seizure types and had relatively few adverse side-effects. Furthermore, the drug was effective without causing sedation.

Critique

If performed today, the study by Merritt and Putnam would not pass the scrutiny of current Food and Drug Administration (FDA) reviews due to the lack of a double-blind placebo-controlled approach. However, the efficacy of phenytoin has been proven countless times in studies comparing it with other antiepileptic drugs. The success of phenytoin as an anticonvulsant is now considered one of the most significant pharmacological advances in treating neurological disorders. Despite the introduction of more than 35 seizure medications since 1938, phenytoin remains one of the most widely used in the world [9] (Fig. 6.2). Phenytoin or fos-phenytoin (a phenytoin pro-drug) continues to be a mainstay in the treatment of status epilepticus.

While Merritt and Putnam's introduction of phenytoin as a non-sedative antiepileptic drug treatment was monumental, the application of animal studies to support its use in humans may be even more important. The work by Merritt and Putnam led to the widespread use of animal studies to investigate efficacy, pharmacokinetics, mechanism of action, toxicity, and safety of potential antiepileptic drugs. In addition to the maximal electroshock (MES) test used by Merritt and Putnam, other tests have been developed including subcutaneous pentylenetetrazol, picrotoxin, and bicuculline, among others. These tests have some specificity for seizure type. For example, the MES test identifies agents with activity against generalized tonic-clonic seizures, while the pentylenetetrazol test identifies compounds that are effective against absences and myoclonic seizures. The maximal electroshock model has served to identify antiepileptic drugs that are functionally similar to phenytoin. For example, drugs that have a mechanism of action at the voltage-gated sodium channel are effective in this model. The pentylenetetrazol model has proven to be a good predictor of clinical efficacy against generalized spike-wave epilepsies of the absence

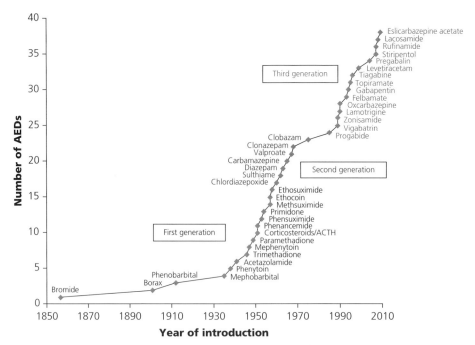

Fig. 6.2 Introduction of antiepileptic drugs (AEDs) to the market from 1853 to 2010.

Reproduced from *Epilepsia*, 52, Loscher W, Schmidt D, Modern antiepileptic drug development has failed to deliver: ways out of the current dilemma, p. 657–78, Copyright (2011), with permission from John Wiley and Sons.

type. Compounds that suppress Ca^{2+} flux across low-threshold T-type channels, such as ethosuximide or valproate, as well as compounds that enhance gamma-aminobutyric acid (GABA) receptor-mediated Cl^- currents, such as the benzodiazepines, are effective in the pentylenetetrazol model.

Animal screening of putative antiepileptic drugs (AEDs) became so useful that the National Institutes of Health funded the Anticonvulsant Screening Program in 1975. This programme relies on animal studies for preclinical discovery and evaluation for new drugs in epilepsy. Candidate compounds are compared against standard marketed antiepileptic drugs, new agents undergoing development, as well as similarly tested candidate drugs representing a specific chemical class under investigation. Such evaluations have proved invaluable to researchers, saving them years in development as well as human resource effort used in optimizing lead compounds. Multiple new AEDs have come to the market because of this programme. Most, if not all, of this progress is owed to the pioneering work of Merritt and Putnam.

6.4 **Epilepsy surgery provides insight into normal brain function**

Main paper: Scoville WB, Milner B. Loss of recent memory after bilateral hippocampal lesions. *J Neurol Neurosurg Psychiat* 1957; 20:11–20.

Background

One of the most important areas of study in neuroscience is how we learn, remember, and forget. The success or failure of our memory has profound effects on our lives, so understanding the anatomical and physiological processes involved in memory are critical. In some instances, studying disease processes can provide great insight into how the brain functions normally. Epilepsy is one of the premiere examples of how rigorous observation of phenomenology in a disease state can lead to understanding normal brain function. For example, correlating and locating EEG discharges with behavioural changes during the seizure has resulted in a better functional localization in the neocortex. In the instance of memory, studying patients with temporal lobe epilepsy has had a major impact on understanding normal memory processes.

Methods and results

In 1953, at age 27, a man referred to by his initials of H.M. underwent resection of the bilateral hippocampal structures [10]. H.M. had had epilepsy since age 16 and had both focal and generalized seizures (Fig. 6.3).

While the surgery was successful, he was left with a severe and pervasive disorder of learning and memory which persisted until his death in 2008 at age 82. He had severe impairment in the ability to acquire and retain new material (anterograde amnesia) and the ability to make use of pre-surgery resection acquired memory before the onset of the amnesia (retrograde amnesia). Although H.M. was alert and attentive and could carry on social conversation, he did not know his age, date, where he lived, or his own history since high school. H.M.'s working memory was intact and he could keep track of conversations and maintain his train of thought. However, if an individual with whom he had a conversation walked out of the room and then returned 10 minutes later, H.M. would not recognize the individual or recall the previous conversation. H.M. was described by Scoville and Milner as 'forgetting of the events of daily life as quickly as they occur'. Despite the devastating effects of the surgery on memory, no other neuropsychological deficits were ever identified.

Previous studies had provided some hints that intact bilateral mesial temporal structures were necessary for memory. However, H.M. provided clear evidence of the importance of mesial temporal structures, including the hippocampus, in memory. Removal of one hippocampus, on the medial aspect of the temporal lobe, was found to result in a grave and persistent memory disorder if the patient harboured an additional, pre-operatively unsuspected lesion in the hippocampus of the opposite side [11]. Such patients showed no loss of intelligence or previously acquired knowledge and skill and they could attend normally

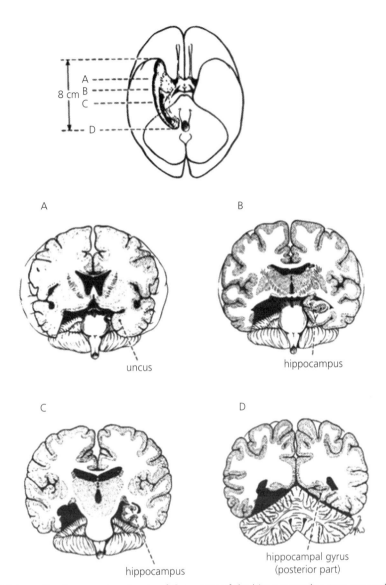

Fig. 6.3 Schematic of surgeon's estimate of the extent of the hippocampal system removal in the patient H.M. Illustrated is the extent of removal on one side of the brain at four cross-sectional levels (A, B, C, and D) along the anterior-posterior extent of the brain shown at the top. Although the surgical removal was bilateral, one side of the brain is shown intact for illustrative purposes.

Reproduced from *J Neurol Neurosurg Psychiat*, 20, Scoville WB, Milner B, Loss of recent memory after bilateral hippocampal lesions, p. 11–20, Copyright (1957), with permission from the BMJ Publishing Group Ltd.

to ongoing events. Yet, these individuals appeared to be able to add little new information to their long-term memory store, demonstrating a persistent anterograde amnesia for post-operative events. They also exhibited a retrograde amnesia that might extend back for months or even years, so that they could not recall events from this pre-operative period but were able to recount happenings from much earlier in their lives without difficulty.

Conclusions

Scoville and Milner showed that the hippocampus is a critical brain region involved in memory and that bilateral resection or injury of the hippocampi results in profound deficits in episodic memory. While memory can be preserved following resection of the mesial temporal lobe, it is critically important that the remaining hippocampus is functionally intact.

Critique

A critical part of the evaluation for patients who are being considered for temporal lobe epilepsy surgery is ascertaining whether the temporal lobe contralateral to the epileptic focus can sustain memory. The extensive studies by Milner and colleagues [11–17], in patients undergoing temporal lobe surgery, also served to spur neuroscientists to study the hippocampus in regard to the neurobiology of memory. As a result of this pioneering work, the study of hippocampal function in memory is exploding.

6.5 **The consequences of epilepsy extend beyond seizures**

Main paper: Harrison RM, Taylor DC. Childhood seizures: a 25-year follow up. Social and medical prognosis. *Lancet* 1976; 1:948–51.

Background

Since the earliest writings about epilepsy, the majority of the effort in caring for the individual has been in stopping the seizures. While it was widely recognized that individuals with epilepsy often had other issues such as intellectual disabilities and behavioural problems, this was not a focus of their care providers. The paper by Harrison and Taylor in 1976 [18] challenged the notion that epilepsy was only about seizures.

Methods

For 25 years, the authors followed 200 children who had at least one seizure, paying particular attention to the long-term prognosis in relation to medical, social, and educational problems.

Results

While two-thirds of individuals had favourable outcomes, 25% had chronic epilepsy, 10.1% had died, 11.2% were confined to institutions, and 6.6% were invalids at home. Educational problems were common, and continuing epilepsy was associated with greatly reduced educational and occupational achievement compared with the group in remission.

Conclusions

The authors dramatically noted 'there was much to fear from childhood epilepsy' since seizures in childhood can be the beginning of serious social and medical problems. The observation that occupational achievement is severely reduced in those with chronic epilepsy has been borne out by many other studies. As the authors stated, individuals with epilepsy 'are located in the most unpleasant, poorly paid jobs which offer little future or prospect of self-advancement'. The authors were well ahead of their time in noting that the cost of a seizure disorder is enormous to the community in both human and material terms.

Critique

This paper was the first to crystallize the spectrum of difficulties individuals with epilepsy face. It is now recognized that the morbidity of epilepsy involves more than seizures. Co-morbidities, defined as two supposedly separate conditions co-occurring at above chance levels, are, unfortunately, very common in epilepsy. These co-morbidities include conditions such as learning disabilities, autistic spectrum disorders, intellectual impairment, depression, and anxiety, to name just a few.

A recent Institute of Medicine report highlighted the costs of epilepsy in terms of its impact on individuals, their families, and society [19]. An estimate of the annual economic burden of epilepsy in the United States ranges from $9.6 to $12.5 billion [20, 21]. Of this total, the proportion due to direct costs (e.g. health care visits, hospitalization, medications) are dwarfed by the indirect costs to society, such as unemployment, underemployment, and premature mortality. Thirty-five years after the Harrison and Taylor paper, the Institute of Medicine committee recommended that co-morbidities be identified early and to design, implement, and evaluate interventions for individuals with epilepsy.

6.6 **Febrile seizures are usually benign**

Main paper: Nelson KB, Ellenberg JH. Predictors of epilepsy in children who have experienced febrile seizures. N Engl J Med 1976; 295:1029–1033.

Background

Febrile seizures are the most common type of seizure seen in young children, occurring in 2–5% of all children before the age of 5 years [22, 23]. While most children with febrile seizures are able to function at a normal level cognitively and socially, a higher than expected proportion have adverse outcomes, including epilepsy and cognitive deficits [24, 25]. Children with prolonged febrile seizures appear to be particularly at risk for developing mesial temporal lobe epilepsy. Epidemiological studies suggest that most children with febrile seizures have normal development and intelligence, whereas some children with prolonged febrile seizures appear to be vulnerable for long-term cognitive disturbances.

Methods

In this large epidemiological study, Nelson and Ellenberg [26] assessed the frequency of afebrile seizures in 1706 children who had experienced at least one febrile seizure. These children were followed to the age of 7 years.

Results

The authors found that epilepsy developed by 7 years of age in 2% of the participants and another 1% had at least one afebrile seizure but did not meet the definition of epilepsy, defined as two or more unprovoked seizures. The rate of epilepsy was higher in children whose neurological or developmental status was suspect or abnormal before any seizure and whose first seizure was complex (longer than 15 minutes, multiple, or focal). In this group of patients, epilepsy developed at a rate 18 times higher than in children with no febrile seizures. In children who were previously abnormal and had a non-complex first febrile seizure, epilepsy developed in only 1.1%, a percentage slightly higher than children with no history of febrile seizures. The study unambiguously demonstrated that prior neurological and developmental status and characteristics of the first febrile seizure were important predictors of epilepsy after febrile seizures.

Conclusions

This study showed that in the vast majority of children with febrile seizures, the outcome was favourable, with only a small percentage going on to develop epilepsy.

Critique

Prior to this study, many children with febrile seizures were treated with drugs such as phenobarbital to prevent the occurrence of epilepsy. Farwell et al. [27] compared IQ scores in children with at least one febrile seizure who received phenobarbital or placebo. After two years of treatment, the mean IQ was 7.03 points lower in the group assigned to phenobarbital than in the placebo group. Six months later, after the medication had been tapered and discontinued, the mean IQ was 5.2 points lower in the group assigned to phenobarbital. This study demonstrated that phenobarbital depresses cognitive performance in children treated for febrile seizures and that this impairment may outlast the administration of the drug by several months. In addition, phenobarbital did not reduce recurrence of either febrile or afebrile seizures. When the cohort of children were retested 3–5 years later, after they had entered school, the phenobarbital group scored significantly lower than the placebo group on the Wide Range Achievement Test (WRAT-R) and there was a non-significant mean difference of 3.71 IQ points on the Stanford-Binet, with the phenobarbital-treated group scoring lower (102.2 vs 105.7) [28]. Because of the short- and long-term consequences of phenobarbital, it is now rarely used to treat febrile seizures.

The low incidence of epilepsy following febrile seizures reported by Nelson and Ellenberg [26], coupled with the findings regarding the harmful effects of phenobarbital, led to a movement away from prophylactic treatment of febrile seizures. Most clinicians now agree that no preventive therapy is required for a child who has experienced a first or even a second febrile seizure. In practice parameters provided by the American Academy of Pediatrics, it was concluded that the potential adverse effects of prophylactic therapy did not justify the use of phenobarbital for febrile seizures [29]. Children who experience complex febrile seizures, characterized by partial or prolonged seizures and concomitant neurological developmental abnormality, are more likely to have recurrent seizures. These patients are frequently considered to have epilepsy initially triggered by fever and are more often treated with chronic antiepileptic drug therapy.

This study was one of the first to raise the question of whether the risks outweigh the benefits of antiepileptic drug therapy in children with seizures. The paper changed conventional thinking that all seizures should be suppressed in children, regardless of risk, and has dramatically changed the way children with febrile seizures are treated.

6.7 **Infantile spasms may have a focal onset and be amenable to surgical resection**

Main paper: Chugani HT, Shields WD, Shewmon DA, Olson DM, Phelps ME, Peacock WJ. Infantile spasms: I. PET identifies focal cortical dysgenesis in cryptogenic cases for surgical treatment. *Ann Neurol* 1990; 27:406–13.

Background

Infantile seizures are one of the most devastating epileptic syndromes to occur in children. Infantile spasms are an age-specific disorder occurring in children only during the first two years of life. The characteristic features of this syndrome are epileptic spasms, hypsarrhythmic EEG, and mental retardation—a triad sometimes referred to as West syndrome (see section 6.1). Infantile spasms frequently occur in clusters, and the intensity and frequency of the spasms in each cluster may increase to a peak before progressively decreasing. Infantile spasms are associated with markedly abnormal EEGs. The spasms typically consist of flexion of the trunk and bilateral flexion or extension of the arms and legs, although variations are often seen. The most commonly seen interictal pattern is hypsarrhythmia, which consists of very high-voltage, random, slow waves and multifocal spikes and sharp waves. The chaotic appearance of the EEG abnormality gives the impression of total disorganization of cortical voltage and rhythms. During sleep, bursts of polyspike and slow waves occur.

The poor prognosis of this syndrome has been confirmed in virtually all follow-up studies. A significant number of infants demonstrate psychomotor retardation and continue to have seizures. While it is clear that aetiology plays an important role in outcome, there is concern that the spasms themselves may cause additional harm.

The clinical and ictal EEG features of infantile spasms are highly suggestive of a generalized seizure disorder and treatment has consisted primarily of medical therapy including ACTH [30] and vigabatrin [31]. Chugani and colleagues [32] convincingly dismissed the notion that infantile spams are always a generalized seizure phenomenon.

Methods and results

Using positron emission tomography (PET) of local cerebral glucose metabolism in 13 children with infantile spasms of undetermined cause (cryptogenic spasms), the authors found unilateral hypometabolism involving the parieto-occipito-temporal region in five infants. All of the infants with abnormal PET scans had normal cranial axial tomography (CAT) scans and four of the five had normal MRI (Fig. 6.4).

Surface EEG in four infants showed hypsarrythmia at some time in the patients' courses, but at other times showed localized or lateralized abnormalities corresponding to areas of PET-detected hypometabolism. Because of poor seizure control, four infants underwent surgical removal of the cortical focus, guided by intra-operative electrocorticography, and were seizure-free post-operatively. Neuropathological examination of resected tissue in each showed microscopic cortical dysplasia.

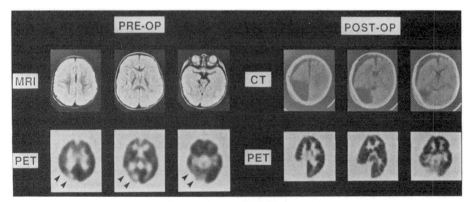

Fig. 6.4 Pre-operative MRI and PET studies using 2-deoxy-2 (¹⁸F) floro-D-glucose (FDG), and post-operative CT and PET images with FDG. MRI was normal pre-operatively, but PET revealed right parieto-occipital hypometabolism. The post-operative CT images demonstrate the extent of surgical excision, which matched the area of abnormality on intra-operative electrocorticography. Repeat PET at 1 year 3 months post-operatively revealed normal metabolic activity in remaining brain regions.

Reproduced from *Ann Neurol*, 27, Chugani HT, Shields WD, Shewmon DA, Olson DM, Phelps ME, Peacock WJ, Infantile spasms: I. PET identifies focal cortical dysgenesis in cryptogenic cases for surgical treatment, p. 406–13, Copyright (1990), with permission from John Wiley and Sons.

Conclusions

The findings showed that in infants with cryptogenic spasms, seizures can be partial, with secondary generalization, and that PET can effectively identify those due to unsuspected focal cortical dysplasia, for which resective surgery offers improved prognosis.

Critique

This paper changed the perception of infantile spasms as always being a diffuse brain disorder. Support for the concept of a 'focal pacemaker' in infantile spasms came from the observation that focal seizures might precede, accompany, or follow the cluster of spasms [33, 34]. Carrazana and colleagues [34] reported on 16 patients with infantile spasms in whom the onset of the clusters of spasms appeared to be triggered by the close temporal association with partial seizures. The authors hypothesized that while the bilateral spasms were likely generated at a subcortical level, their close temporal relation with a cortically generated partial seizure strongly suggested that the spasms were facilitated or possibly induced by the cortical event. Three of their patients had complete agenesis of the corpus callosum, which argued against interhemispheric callosal spread of focal discharges to result in the generalized spasms. Further support for the concept of an abnormality in cortical–subcortical pathways comes from the finding that children with focal cortical lesions may have total resolution of the spasms and hypsarrhythmia with focal cortical resections [32, 35, 36].

Shewmon and colleagues [37] suggested that, early in life, focal lesions may produce secondary epileptogenesis by altering the epileptic potential of other brain sites, leading to the development of multifocal seizure foci and the clinical expression of infantile spasms. The hypsarrhythmic pattern may represent the spread of the epileptic activity and recruitment of multiple brain sites which produces an age-specific seizure pattern.

The paper by Chugani and colleagues [32] dramatically changed the way clinicians view infantile spasms. Rather than limiting treatment to pharmacological agents, this study showed that a surgical approach to a disorder that, on the surface appears to be generalized, is both rational and appropriate. The paper also emphasized how the clinical and EEG features of seizures are age-dependent. Propagation patterns in young children with epilepsy clearly differ from adults and these age-related features must be considered when approaching a child with refractory epilepsy.

6.8 **A sodium channel mutation results in epilepsy**

Main paper: Wallace RH, Wang DW, Singh R, et al. Febrile seizures and generalized epilepsy associated with a mutation in the Na⁺-channel beta1 subunit gene SCN1B. *Nat Genet* 1998; 19:366–70.

Background

While it has been known for centuries that genetics play an important role in epilepsy, the first 'pure' epilepsy gene was discovered by Wallace et al. [38]. While the genetic basis for many syndromes in which epilepsy may be part of the phenotype had already been uncovered (e.g. tuberous sclerosis complex and Down syndrome), this was the first human gene discovered in which epilepsy is the primary abnormality.

The clinical observation and the presumed genetic basis of epilepsy had been first described by Scheffer and Berkovic, in 1997, as generalized seizures with febrile seizures plus (GEFS +) [39]. The authors described this as a 'genetic disorder with heterogeneous clinical phenotypes'. The description was based on the recognition that in a large extended family, febrile seizures, often of unusual duration or severity, and afebrile generalized seizures of various types appeared to be transmitted as a dominant genetic character. Simple febrile seizures constituted the most common manifestation. However, the febrile seizures often occurred beyond the usual upper limit of age 4–5 years. The afebrile seizures consisted of a variety of different types of seizures including myoclonic, absences, or even episodes of status epilepticus. These seizures are infrequent and generally respond well to pharmacological therapy. In the majority of patients, the seizures stop at puberty and those with GEFS + rarely have significant cognitive and behavioural impairments.

Due to the heterogeneity in the clinical phenotype of individuals with the condition, it was initially difficult for clinicians to recognize it as a distinct syndrome. This changed with the findings of Wallace et al. [38].

Methods and results

The authors reported linkage in a large GEFS + family to chromosome region 19q13.1 and identification of a mutation in the voltage-gated sodium Na⁺-channel beta1 subunit gene (SCN1B). It was discovered that the mutation changed a conserved cysteine residue, disrupting a putative disulfide bridge. Co-expression of the mutant beta1 subunit with a brain Na⁺-channel alpha subunit in Xenopus laevis oocytes demonstrated that the mutation interfered with the ability of the subunit to modulate channel-gating kinetics, consistent with a loss of function allele.

Conclusions

The authors' findings demonstrated that some idiopathic epilepsies are due to 'channelopathies'. Voltage-gated Na⁺ channels are important for the excitability of neurons and, in the brain, they are critical for the initiation and propagation of action potentials in neurons. The mutant beta1 Na$^+$ channel result in abnormal kinetics of Na$^+$ currents leads to an increased susceptibility to seizures.

Critique

The Wallace et al. [38] paper is very important in a number of regards. The investigators showed, for the first time, that a gene mutation could result in epilepsy, without other abnormalities. Furthermore, they demonstrated that mutations in gene coding for an ion channel can result in epilepsy. While the fact that a mutation in an ion channel would result in epilepsy makes sense to electrophysiologists, this paper provides proof of the principle that aberration in a single ion channel can result in a disorder with paroxysmal seizures. Mutations in ion channel encoding genes have subsequently been found in a variety of inherited diseases associated with hyper- or hypo-excitability of the affected tissue, the so-called 'channelopathies' [40]. GEFS + can be caused by a variety of mutations involving channels, including the Na$^+$ channel (SCN1A, SCN2A), and γ-aminobutyric acid receptor genes (GABRG2, GABRD) that can result in similar phenotypes [41]. Other epileptic syndromes may belong to this group of rare disorders: autosomal dominant nocturnal frontal lobe epilepsy is caused by mutations in a neuronal nicotinic acetylcholine receptor (CHRNA4, CHRNB2) [42]; benign familial neonatal convulsions, by mutations in K$^+$ channels constituting the M-current (KCNQ2, KCNQ3) [43]; and episodic ataxia type 1 (which is associated with epilepsy in some), by mutations within another voltage-gated K$^+$ channel (KCNA1) [44]. These disorders, albeit rare, provide information on the molecular level on the aetiology and pathophysiology of disturbed excitability.

The finding that channelopathies can result in seizures has already produced novel antiepileptic drugs specifically targeting ion channels. Recently, retigabine (international non-proprietary name) or ezogabine (US adopted name), a drug that acts as an activator of neuronally expressed KCNQ-channels, has been approved to treat partial seizures [45–47]. Developing antiepileptic drugs aimed specifically at molecular targets identified through genetic analysis is likely to be the focus of future drug development.

6.9 **Epilepsy surgery is superior to medical therapy in patients with temporal lobe epilepsy**

Main paper: Wiebe S, Blume WT, Girvin JP, Eliasziw M, Effectiveness and Efficiency of Surgery for Temporal Lobe Epilepsy Study Group. A randomized, controlled trial of surgery for temporal-lobe epilepsy. *N Engl J Med* 2001; 345:311–8.

Background

Removal of epileptic tissue was first accomplished in 1886 when Victor Horsley resected, in a 22-year-old patient with focal motor seizures, a scar of the motor cortex that had been caused 15 years earlier by a head injury [48]. This paper could certainly be considered a landmark paper since it led to Sir Victor Horsley being regarded as the father of epilepsy surgery. While most surgical resections over the next 60 years were of visible lesions in the neocortex, in the 1950s, Penfield and Flanigin, at the Montreal Neurological Institute, showed that temporal lobe resections could be very curative in temporal lobe epilepsy [49]. Like the Horsley paper, the work by Penfield and Flanigin [49] and, later, Penfield and Jasper [50], at the Montreal Neurological Institute, was monumental in propelling epilepsy surgery as an important therapy in epilepsy.

It has now been demonstrated that mesial temporal lobe epilepsy is the most common form of human epilepsy, and its pathophysiological substrate is usually hippocampal sclerosis, the most common epileptogenic lesion encountered in patients with epilepsy. The disabling seizures associated with mesial temporal lobe epilepsy are typically resistant to antiepileptic drugs but can be totally eliminated, in most patients, by surgical treatment.

Despite compelling evidence that temporal lobe epilepsy can be cured by surgery, many patients are not offered this form of treatment, or if they are referred to an epilepsy surgery centre, it is often done very late in their course of treatment. In one disturbing report, it was shown that patients were referred for temporal lobe epilepsy surgery on average 22 years after seizure onset, and often after a decade of having medically intractable epilepsy [51]. The paper by Wiebe et al. [52] demonstrated, unequivocally, that anteromesial temporal lobe resection is highly effective and shows benefits quickly after surgery.

Methods

Eighty patients with temporal lobe epilepsy were randomly assigned to surgery (40 patients) or treatment with antiepileptic drugs for one year (40 patients). The primary outcome, using an intention to treat approach, was freedom from seizures that impair awareness of self and surroundings. Secondary outcomes were the frequency and severity of seizures, the quality of life, disability, and death.

Results

Of those receiving surgery, 58% were free of disabling seizures and 10–15% were unimproved at the end of one year. Of the group randomized to continued medical therapy, 8% were free of disabling seizures in (p<0.001). There was a significant improvement in quantitative quality of life scores and a trend towards better social function at the end of one year for patients in the surgical group compared to the medical group. The surgical group had no mortality and limited morbidity, while one patient in the medical group died.

Conclusions

For medically intractable temporal lobe epilepsy, surgery is superior to persistent medical therapy.

Critique

This study provided a strong basis for the recommendation of the American Academy of Neurology that surgery be the treatment of choice for medically intractable temporal lobe epilepsy [53]. While the benefits of such surgery are now obvious, referrals to tertiary epilepsy centres still are frequently delayed [54]. There are likely multiple reasons for this including lack of awareness of the efficacy of surgery, concerns about the risk:benefit ratio, cultural biases, and economic restraints. Nevertheless, the study of Wiebe et al. [52] eliminated doubt about the superiority of surgical versus continued medical therapy in patients with medically intractable temporal lobe epilepsy. The paper is also important since it showed that randomized trials of surgery for epilepsy are feasible and appear to yield precise estimates of treatment effects.

6.10 **The signalling pathway of tuberous sclerosis complex provides a disease-specific rationale for treatment**

Main paper: Gao X, Zhang Y, Arrazola P, et al. Tsc tumour suppressor proteins antagonize amino-acid-TOR signaling. Nature Cell Biology 2002; 4:699–704.

Background

Tuberous sclerosis complex (TSC), first identified by Désiré-Magloire Bourneville in 1880, is characterized by the widespread development of hamartomas in a variety of organs. Common clinical symptoms include seizures, mental retardation, autism, kidney failure, facial angiofibromas, and cardiac rhabdomyomas [55]. The disorder is common, occurring in approximately 1 in 6000 people, and can be devastating, particularly in regard to epilepsy and cognitive impairment. One of two tumour gene proteins, Tsc1 (also known as hamartin) or Tsc2 (also known as tuberin), has been identified in the majority of patients.

While identifying the gene products responsible for TSC was an important first step, finding that hamartin and tuberin proteins form a physical and functional complex which inhibits mammalian target of rapamycin (mTOR)—a serine/threonine protein kinase that regulates cell growth, cell proliferation, cell motility, cell survival, protein synthesis, and transcription—was monumental. mTOR mediates a signalling pathway that couples amino acid availability to S6 kinase (S6K) activation, translational initiation, and cell growth.

Methods and results

Gao et al. [56] showed that loss of the proteins Tsc1 and Tsc2 were responsible for the excessive cell growth in TSC syndrome. Tsc1 and Tsc2 were shown to activate mTOR in drosophila melanogaster and mammalian cells with loss of Tsc1 and Tsc2 resulting in a TOR-dependent increase of S6 kinase activity (Fig. 6.5). In addition, although S6 kinase is normally inactivated in animal cells in response to amino acid starvation, loss of Tsc1 and Tsc2 renders cells resistant to amino acid starvation. Thus, the loss of Tsc1 and Tsc2 leads to selective activation of the mTOR cascade causing a mTOR-dependent increase of S6 kinase, p70S6-kinase, and 4E-BP1 [56, 57]. Negative modulation of this cascade by rapamycin results in suppression of growth and restriction of cell size. Therefore, these gene mutations provide a plausible mechanism to account for cytomegaly seen in patients with TSC (Fig. 6.5).

Conclusions

This paper demonstrated how Tsc1 and Tsc2 regulate the amino acid–mTOR pathway and provided a new paradigm for how proteins involved in nutrient sense function as tumour suppressors. Furthermore, the mechanism by which Tsc1 and Tsc2 lead to excessive cell growth in TSC was demonstrated.

Critique

Understanding the molecular biology of the mTOR pathway has played a monumental role in treating TSC. Everolimus, an inhibitor of mTOR, has been shown to result in a

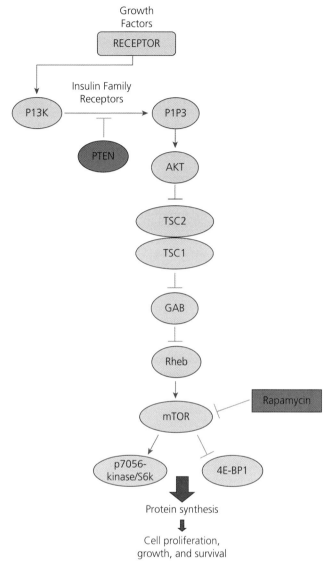

Fig. 6.5 Schematic drawing of molecular pathways involved in TSC. Protein kinase B (also known as AKT) is a potent pro-survival and pro-oncogenic protein that is activated by phosphatidylinositol triphosphate. An important negative regulator of the AKT pathway is PTEN (phosphatidylinositol triphosphate phosphatase) which decreases 3'-phosphoinositides in the cell. AKT directly phosphorylates TSC2 and inhibits its function. TSC2 inactivation by AKT may reduce GAB activity towards Rheb, subsequently leading to activation of mTOR. Both ribosomal S6 kinase (S6K) and eukaryote initiation factor 4E binding protein 1 (4E-BP1) are key regulators of protein translation. The downstream effects of the pathway would be translation, growth, survival, and cell proliferation. Rapamycin is an inhibitor of mTOR. ($\downarrow$ = activation; $\perp$ = suppression; GAP = guanosine triphosphatase activating protein; P13K = phosphatidylinositol-3 kinase; P1P3 = phosphatidylinositol triphosphate; mTOR = mammalian target of rapamycin).

marked reduction in the volume of subependymal giant-cell astrocytomas and seizure frequency in patients with TSC [58, 59]. Likewise, rapamycin treatment has been shown to induce regression of kidney angiomyolipomas [60]. While it is not known if mTOR inhibitors will be useful in treating or preventing epilepsy associated with TSC, mTOR inhibitors are effective in preventing epilepsy in a mouse model of tuberous sclerosis [61]. In addition, mTOR dysregulation has been implicated in other genetic and acquired forms of epileptogenesis and the use of mTOR inhibitors in animals can reverse some of these epileptogenic processes [62].

While Gao et al. [56] were not solely responsible for describing the signalling pathway in TSC, their work contributed dramatically to our understanding of the disorder and has helped make TSC a 'model' disease, serving as an example of how genetic disorders can be approached. In TSC, the clinical manifestations of the condition have been well established, and the genetic mutation responsible for most of the cases, as well as the aberrant signalling pathway, have been identified. This knowledge has provided a basis for medical intervention. TSC is a wonderful example of how understanding the neurogenetics of a devastating disorder can result in highly specific disease-modifying therapy.

Key unanswered questions

There are many aspects of epilepsy that must be further understood in order to aid future progression of treatment. The following questions identify key aspects that, if brought to the forefront of epilepsy research, could produce critical findings of immeasurable significance.

1 Why do such a high percentage of patients develop medically intractable epilepsy?
   For many people with epilepsy, current treatment options are effective in reducing or eliminating seizures. However, approximately 30% of people with epilepsy do not respond to medications [63]. Although surgery can be highly effective in selected patients, the number of patients who are good candidates for surgery is relatively small compared to the population with epilepsy as a whole. Further knowledge regarding patients with medically intractable epilepsy will lead to the development of novel therapeutic targets.

2 When we will ascertain the pathophysiology of sudden unexpected death in epilepsy (SUDEP)?
   Epilepsy is a life-threatening condition; SUDEP is the most common epilepsy-related cause of death. The risk of sudden death in people with epilepsy is more than 20 times greater than in the general population [64]. Research focusing on the prevention of SUDEP is of paramount importance. Ascertaining the pathophysiology of SUDEP is critical before preventive measures can be implemented.

3 Do the pathophysiological mechanisms responsible for the co-morbidities associated with epilepsy differ in individuals with epilepsy from individuals with similar co-morbidities who do not have epilepsy?
   While stopping seizures is a major goal in the treatment of epilepsy, it is not the only treatment goal. Epilepsy is associated with a range of co-morbid conditions that may also result in diminished well-being and reduced quality of life. These co-morbidities include disorders such as attention deficit disorder, depression, learning disabilities, and anxiety, to name just a few.

4 What are the mechanisms responsible for epileptogenesis?
   Among people with newly diagnosed epilepsy, the predominant known causes are cerebrovascular disease, neurodegenerative diseases, primary or metastatic brain tumours, and traumatic brain injury. However, most individuals with these conditions do not develop epilepsy. Understanding the mechanisms responsible for epileptogenesis is a critical step in developing novel therapeutics that can prevent, rather than treat epilepsy.

5 Why is it important to understand, in much more detail, the effect of recurrent seizures on immature and mature brain function?
   Cognitive impairment and behavioural disturbances are devastating co-morbidities of epilepsy and, in some patients, these co-morbidities may be of greater consequence than the epilepsy itself. There is an increasing recognition that cognitive and behavioural co-morbidities can be both chronic, primarily due to the underlying aetiology of

the epilepsy, and dynamic or evolving, because of recurrent seizures or interictal spikes. In animal models, a number of morphological changes can occur with epilepsy including cell loss, synaptic reorganization, and changes in neurogenesis. Seizures can also result in physiological changes including changes in excitatory and inhibitory currents, alterations in temporal coding of information, and impaired single-cell firing patterns.

Acknowledgements

The author wishes to thank Samantha S. Schmidt for editorial assistance. The author was supported by NIH grants NS074450 and NS073083 and the Emmory R. Shapses Research Fund.

References

1 **Temkin O.** *The Falling Sickness. A History of Epilepsy from the Greeks to the Beginning of Modern Neurology.* Baltimore: Johns Hopkins Press; 1971.

2 **West WJ.** On a particular form of infantile convulsions. *Lancet* 1841; **1**:724–5.

3 **Gibbs FA, Gibbs EL.** *Atlas of Electroencephalography. Volume 2, Epilepsy.* Cambridge, Mass.: Addison-Wesley; 1952.

4 **Ducharme G, Lowe GC, Goutagny R, Williams S.** Early alterations in hippocampal circuitry and theta rhythm generation in a mouse model of prenatal infection: implications for schizophrenia. *PLoS One* 2012; **7**:e29754.

5 **Berger H.** Uber das elektrenkephalogramm des menschen. *Arch Psychiatr Nervenkrankh* 1929; **87**:527–70.

6 **Caton R.** The electrical currents of the brain. *BMJ* 2012; **2**:278.

7 **Adrian ED, Matthews BH.** The interpretation of potential waves in the cortex. *J Physiol* 1934; **81**:440–71.

8 **Merritt HH, Putnam TJ.** A new series of anticonvulsant drugs tested by experiments on animals. *Arch Neurol Psych* 1938; **39**:1003–15.

9 **Loscher W, Schmidt D.** Modern antiepileptic drug development has failed to deliver: ways out of the current dilemma. *Epilepsia* 2011; **52**:657–78.

10 **Scoville WB, Milner B.** Loss of recent memory after bilateral hippocampal lesions. *J Neurol Neurosurg Psychiat* 1957; **20**:11–20.

11 **Milner B, Penfield W.** The effect of hippocampal lesions on recent memory. *Trans Am Neurol Assoc* 1955; 42–8.

12 **Penfield W, Milner B.** Memory deficit produced by bilateral lesions in the hippocampal zone. *AMA Arch Neurol Psychiatry* 1958; **79**:475–97.

13 **Milner B.** Psychological defects produced by temporal lobe excision. *Res Publ Assoc Res Nerv Ment Dis* 1958; **36**:244–57.

14 **Milner B.** The memory defect in bilateral hippocampal lesions. *Psychiatr Res Rep Am Psychiatr Assoc* 1959; **11**:43–58.

15 **Milner B.** Disorders of learning and memory after temporal lobe lesions in man. *Clin Neurosurg* 1972; **19**:421–46.

16 **Milner B.** Psychological aspects of focal epilepsy and its neurosurgical management. *Adv Neurol* 1975; **8**:299–321.

17 **Milner B.** The medial temporal-lobe amnesic syndrome. *Psychiatr Clin North Am* 2005; **28**:599–611, 599–611.

18 **Harrison RM, Taylor DC.** Childhood seizures: a 25-year follow-up—social and medical prognosis. *Lancet* 1976; **1**:948–51.

19 **Committee on the Public Health Dimensions of the Epilepsies, Board on Health Sciences Policy, Institute of Medicine.** *Epilepsy Across the Spectrum: Promoting Health and Understanding.* Washington, DC: The National Academies Press; 2012.

20 **Begley CE, Famulari M, Annegers JF, et al.** The cost of epilepsy in the United States: an estimate from population-based clinical and survey data. *Epilepsia* 2000; **41**:342–51.

21 **Yoon D, Frick KD, Carr DA, Austin JK.** Economic impact of epilepsy in the United States. *Epilepsia* 2009; **50**:2186–91.

22 **Nelson KB, Ellenberg JH.** Prognosis in children with febrile seizures. *Pediatrics* 1978; **61**:720–7.

23 **MacDonald BK, Johnson AL, Sander JW, Shorvon SD.** Febrile convulsions in 220 children—neurological sequelae at 12 years follow-up. *Eur Neurol* 1999; **41**:179–86.

24 **French JA, Williamson PD, Thadani VM, et al.** Characteristics of medial temporal lobe epilepsy: I. Results of history and physical examination. *Ann Neurol* 1993; **34**:774–80.

25 **Cendes F, Andermann F, Dubeau F, et al.** Early childhood prolonged febrile convulsions, atrophy and sclerosis of mesial structures, and temporal lobe epilepsy: an MRI volumetric study. *Neurology* 1993; **43**:1083–7.

26 **Nelson KB, Ellenberg JH.** Predictors of epilepsy in children who have experienced febrile seizures. *N Engl J Med* 1976; **295**:1029–33.

27 **Farwell JR, Lee YJ, Hirtz DG, Sulzbacher SI, Ellenberg JH, Nelson KB.** Phenobarbital for febrile seizures. Effects on intelligence and on seizure recurrence. *N Engl J Med* 1990; **322**:364–9.

28 **Sulzbacher S, Farwell JR, Temkin N, Lu AS, Hirtz DG.** Late cognitive effects of early treatment with phenobarbital. *Clin Pediatr (Phila)* 1999; **38**:387–94.

29 **American Academy of Pediatrics CoqISoFS.** Practice parameter: long-term treatment of the child with simple febrile seizures. *Pediatrics* 1999; **103**:1307–8.

30 **Sorel L, Dusaucy-Bauloye E.** A propos de 21 cas d'hypsarhythmia de Gibbs son traitment spectaculaire par l'ACTH. *Acta Neurol Belg* 1958; **58**:130–41.

31 **Chiron C, Dulac O, Luna D, et al.** Vigabatrin in infantile spasms. *Lancet* 1990; **335**:363–4.

32 **Chugani HT, Shields WD, Shewmon DA, Olson DM, Phelps ME, Peacock WJ.** Infantile spasms: I. PET identifies focal cortical dysgenesis in cryptogenic cases for surgical treatment. *Ann Neurol* 1990; **27**:406–13.

33 **Carrazana EJ, Barlow JK, Holmes GL.** Infantile spasms provoked by partial seizures. A case report. *J Epilepsy* 1990; **3**:97–100.

34 **Carrazana EJ, Lombroso CT, Mikati M, Helmers S, Holmes GL.** Facilitation of infantile spasms by partial seizures. *Epilepsia* 1993; **34**:97–109.

35 **Chugani HT, Shewmon DA, Peacock WJ, Shields WD, Mazziotta JC, Phelps ME.** Surgical treatment of intractable neonatal onset seizures: the role of positron emission tomography. *Neurology* 1988; **38**:1178–88.

36 **Chugani HT, Shewmon DA, Sankar R, Chen BJ, Phelps ME.** Infantile spasms: II. Lenticular nuclei and brain stem activation on positron emission tomography. *Ann Neurol* 1992; **31**:212–9.

37 **Shewmon DA, Shields WD, Chugani HT, Peacock WJ.** Contrasts between pediatric and adult epilepsy surgery: rationale and strategy for focal resection. *J Epilepsy* 1990; **3**(Suppl):1–15.

38 **Wallace RH, Wang DW, Singh R, et al.** Febrile seizures and generalized epilepsy associated with a mutation in the Na$^+$-channel beta1 subunit gene SCN1B. *Nat Genet* 1998; **19**:366–70.

39 **Scheffer IE, Berkovic SF.** Generalized epilepsy with febrile seizures plus. A genetic disorder with heterogeneous clinical phenotypes. *Brain* 1997; **120**:479–90.

40 **Lerche H, Jurkat-Rott K, Lehmann-Horn F.** Ion channels and epilepsy. *Am J Med Genet* 2001; **106**:146–59.

41 **Wallace RH, Scheffer IE, Barnett S, et al.** 2001 Neuronal sodium-channel alpha1-subunit mutations in generalized epilepsy with febrile seizures plus. *Am J Hum Genet* 2001; **68**(4):859–65.

42 **Phillips HA, Scheffer IE, Berkovic SF, Hollway GE, Sutherland GR, Mulley JC.** Localization of a gene for autosomal dominant nocturnal frontal lobe epilepsy to chromosome 20q 13.2. *Nat Genet* 1995; **10**:117–8.

43 **Singh NA, Charlier C, Stauffer D, et al.** A novel potassium channel gene, KCNQ2, is mutated in an inherited epilepsy of newborns. *Nat Genet* 1998; **18**:25–9.

44 **Zuberi SM, Eunson LH, Spauschus A, et al.** A novel mutation in the human voltage-gated potassium channel gene (Kv1.1) associates with episodic ataxia type 1 and sometimes with partial epilepsy. *Brain* 1999; **122** (Pt 5):817–25.

45 **Miceli F, Soldovieri MV, Martire M, Taglialatela M.** Molecular pharmacology and therapeutic potential of neuronal Kv7-modulating drugs. *Curr Opin Pharmacol* 2008; **8**:65–74.

46 **Schenzer A, Friedrich T, Pusch M, et al.** Molecular determinants of KCNQ (Kv7) K + channel sensitivity to the anticonvulsant retigabine. *J Neurosci* 2005; **25**:5051–60.

47 **Large CH, Sokal DM, Nehlig A, et al.** The spectrum of anticonvulsant efficacy of retigabine (ezogabine) in animal models: implications for clinical use. *Epilepsia* 2012; **53**:425–36.

48 **Horsley V.** Remarks on ten consecutive cases of operations upon the brain and cranial cavity to illustrate the details and safety of the method employed. *BM J* 1887; **1**:863–5.

49 **Penfield W, Flanigin H.** Surgical therapy of temporal lobe seizures. *Arch Neurol Psychiatry* 1950; **64**:491–500.

50 **Penfield W, Jasper HH.** *Epilepsy and Functional Anatomy of the Human Brain*. Boston: Little, Brown, & Co.; 1954.

51 **Berg AT, Langfitt J, Shinnar S, et al.** How long does it take for partial epilepsy to become intractable? *Neurology* 2003; **60**:186–90.

52 **Wiebe S, Blume WT, Girvin JP, Eliasziw M.** A randomized, controlled trial of surgery for temporal-lobe epilepsy. *N Engl J Med* 2001; **345**:311–8.

53 **Engel J, Jr.,** Wiebe S, French J, et al. Practice parameter: temporal lobe and localized neocortical resections for epilepsy: report of the Quality Standards Subcommittee of the American Academy of Neurology, in association with the American Epilepsy Society and the American Association of Neurological Surgeons. *Neurology* 2003; **60**:538–47.

54 **Haneef Z, Stern J, Dewar S, Engel Jr J.** Referral pattern for epilepsy surgery after evidence-based recommendations: a retrospective study. *Neurology* 2010; **75**:699–704.

55 **Holmes GL, Stafstrom CE.** Tuberous sclerosis complex and epilepsy: recent developments and future challenges. *Epilepsia* 2007; **48**:617–30.

56 **Gao X, Zhang Y, Arrazola P, et al.** Tsc tumour suppressor proteins antagonize amino-acid-TOR signalling. *Nat Cell Biol* 2002; **4**:699–704.

57 **Gao X, Pan D.** TSC1 and TSC2 tumor suppressors antagonize insulin signaling in cell growth. *Genes Dev* 2001; **15**:1383–92.

58 **Krueger DA, Care MM, Holland K, et al.** Everolimus for subependymal giant-cell astrocytomas in tuberous sclerosis. *N Engl J Med* 2010; **363**:1801–11.

59 **Krueger DA, Franz DN.** Current management of tuberous sclerosis complex. *Paediatr Drugs* 2008; **10**:299–313.

60 **Dabora SL, Franz DN, Ashwal S, et al.** Multicenter phase 2 trial of sirolimus for tuberous sclerosis: kidney angiomyolipomas and other tumors regress and VEGF- D levels decrease. *PLoS One* 2011; **6**:e23379.

61 **Zeng LH, Xu L, Gutmann DH, Wong M.** Rapamycin prevents epilepsy in a mouse model of tuberous sclerosis complex. *Ann Neurol* 2008; **63**:444–53.

62 **Galanopoulou AS, Gorter JA, Cepeda C.** Finding a better drug for epilepsy: the mTOR pathway as an antiepileptogenic target. *Epilepsia* 2012; **53**:1119–30.

63 **Kwan P, Brodie MJ.** Early identification of refractory epilepsy. *N Engl J Med* 2000; **342**:314–9.

64 **Ficker DM, So EL, Shen WK, et al.** Population-based study of the incidence of sudden unexplained death in epilepsy. *Neurology* 1998; **51**:1270–4.

Chapter 7

Ataxias

Elsdon Storey

7.0 **Introduction**

The cerebellum is a tantalizing enigma. The relatively simple, repetitive structure of its circuitry has been known for over 50 years, barring a few recent refinements such as Lugaro cell and unipolar brush cell interneurons, but its *modus operandi* remains elusive. Indeed, it is only a slight exaggeration to say that there are more theories of cerebellar functioning than there are workers in the field—some having proposed more than one model! A related conundrum is the differential regional susceptibility evident in various different cerebellar disorders—the basis of which is entirely unclear from its regular structure. Yet our knowledge of its structure and function continues to advance, perhaps best illustrated by the recent (and not yet universally accepted) recognition of a cognitive role for the cerebellum mediated by reciprocal connections between non-motor cortical areas such as the dorsolateral prefrontal cortex, and the lateral cerebellar hemispheres and ventral and lateral dentate, that have all expanded together in recent evolution.

Progress in anatomy and physiology has been matched or even outdone by progress in the discovery and delineation of what is now a bewildering array of genetically determined ataxias, with many more undoubtedly awaiting recognition, description, and determination of their causative genes and mutations. Yet such discoveries may pose more questions than they answer: why, for example, do some widely expressed genes such as SPTBN2 in spinocerebellar ataxia type 5 (SCA 5) manifest as neurological disorders, and predominantly cerebellar disorders at that? The non-genetically determined ataxias, too, are slowly being delineated, with isolated cerebellar toxicity from alcohol and several therapeutic agents now well described, and the potential of the cerebellum as a target of autoimmunity increasingly recognized, both in paraneoplastic syndromes and in non-cancer-related ataxias such as those due to anti-GAD and (perhaps more contentiously) (anti-)gluten ataxias.

Despite these laudable advances, however, it is a sad fact, evident to any neurologist caring for ataxic patients, that only a tiny minority of ataxias are curable or even arrestable and that even symptomatic pharmaceutical treatments are of dubious efficacy. It is clear that the next generation of neurologists will find themselves fully occupied recognizing, classifying, studying, and (it is devoutly to be hoped) effectively treating this debilitating group of disorders.

This chapter brings together 10 publications chosen by the author to represent the progress made over the last two centuries or so in understanding the cerebellum in health and disease, beginning with Flouren's 1824 report that the cerebellum was concerned with movement control rather than movement initiation. The choice of articles is necessarily somewhat arbitrary, and has been made to represent the development of ideas across the breadth of the field rather than to identify contributions of outstanding scientific merit, although most satisfy both criteria.

7.1 **The cerebellum is involved with movement control rather than movement generation**

Main paper: Flourens MJP. Recherches expérimentales sur les propriétés et les fonctions du système nerveux dans les animaux vertébrés (ed 1). *Chez Crebot* 1824; 26:20.

Background

The cerebellum was clearly distinguished from the cerebrum in the classical era, but Galen erroneously thought it an origin of motor nerves and, perhaps, the spinal cord. While Gugliemo de Saliceto, a thirteenth-century surgeon of the Bologna school, proposed that 'natural and necessary' movements were of cerebellar and voluntary movements of cerebral origin [1], most subsequent renaissance scholars, including Tulp and Vesalius, thought that the cerebellum subserved memory. The great seventeenth-century English anatomist and physician, Thomas Willis, proposed that, on the basis of comparative neuroanatomical studies and such clinical observations as were possible, the cerebellum was responsible for involuntary motor functions such as heartbeat and respiration, whereas thought and voluntary movement depended on the cerebral hemispheres [2]. Later work in the mid-eighteenth century, however, showed that animals could survive cerebellar lesions for lengthy periods of time. At the turn of the nineteenth century, debate raged as to whether brain functions were localized, as proposed by the Austrian phrenologist, Franz Joseph Gall. He thought that the cerebellum was important in sexual excitation, on the basis that sexually potent animals such as bulls and stallions had thick necks, which he equated with large cerebellums [3]. His techniques were, however, recognized to be unscientific, and the Emperor Napoleon Bonaparte asked the Academy of Sciences of Paris to resolve the issue. Flourens was eventually chosen to investigate.

Methods

Flourens improved the brain lesioning method then current (trephination followed by poorly localized destruction by trochar), instead using careful dissection under vision.

Results

Flourens showed that partial-thickness excision of the cerebellum resulted in impairment of balance and movement accuracy, but not in paresis. This was the original experimental discovery of ataxia. These findings, to some extent, contradicted those of Rolando in 1809, who described paralysis after cerebellar removal, although he did note that smaller lesions led to swaying and (ipsilateral) incoordination [4].

Conclusions and critique

Combined with Flourens's findings on partial or total cerebral hemispheric ablations (loss of voluntary initiative and intelligence) and brainstem ablations (death), these experiments provided a sound basis for locationism. They also clearly separated movement control from movement generation, which is fundamental to the concept of ataxia.

7.2 **The first recognition of a distinct spinocerebellar disorder—Friedreich's ataxia**

Main paper: Friedreich N. Über degenerative atrophie der spinalen hinterstränge. *Virkows Archiv für Pathologische Anatomie und Physiologie* 1863; (a) 26:391–419; (b) 26:433–59; (c) 27:1–26.

Background

In classical Greek (via modern Latin), 'ataxia' meant disorder or confusion (from 'taxis', meaning 'order'). In the mid-nineteenth century, locomotor ataxia was synonymous with tabes dorsalis, and was used in this sense by Duchenne. Multiple sclerosis was also recognized as a cause of ataxia, but familial ataxias had not been described until Friedreich's descriptions in 1863.

Nicholaus Friedreich was the son and grandson of Professors of Medicine at Würtzburg, where he trained under Virchow. He was appointed Professor of Pathology and Therapy at Heidelberg at age 32. He published widely in general medicine, but his major interest was in neurology. In addition to the ataxia that bears his name, he also described paramyoclonus multiplex, and wrote on progressive muscular atrophy. He died of a thoracic aortic aneurysm at age 57.

Methods

Friedreich described six siblings in two pedigrees in his three 1863 papers, adding three more from another pedigree in further papers from 1876 and 1877, which also included follow-up on the earlier cases. Post-mortem examinations were performed on four.

Results

The age of onset was typically early (about puberty). Ataxia commenced in the lower limbs, with the upper limbs affected after this. Dysarthria followed later, sometimes with scoliosis and nystagmus. (In his 1876 follow-up paper, Friedreich described absence of the knee jerks, which had been described by Erb only the year before, in 1875 [5]. Post-mortem results were described subsequently, in his 1876 paper, revealing dorsal column degeneration and fatty myocardial degeneration.)

Conclusions and critique

Other neurologists (among them Charcot) initially rejected Friedreich's conclusion that he was describing a distinct disorder, instead suggesting that his cases were due to multiple sclerosis, tabes dorsalis, or an admixture of the two. By 1880, however, William Gowers had accepted Friedreich's ataxia as a separate condition [6]. With the aid of strict diagnostic criteria formulated by Geoffroy et al. [7] and subsequently amended by Harding [8] (recessive inheritance, age of onset before age 25, progressive limb and gait ataxia, absent lower limb reflexes with extensor plantars, motor nerve conduction velocity > 40 ms^{-1} in the upper limbs with reduced/absent sensory potentials, and dysarthria within 5 years of onset), an expanded GAA intronic repeat in the gene encoding frataxin was found in 1996 [9]. There is an inverse correlation between the length of the shorter repeat and the amount of frataxin translated. There is also correlation between the length of the shorter repeat and severity, and an inverse correlation between the length of the shorter repeat and age of onset [10]. This is probably why heterozygous but *not* homozygous point mutations are occasionally seen in place of the second repeat—they typically lead to complete loss of functional frataxin, which would be fatal if homozygous.

With the advent of routine gene testing, it has become apparent that Friedreich's ataxia (FRDA) has a much wider phenotypic spectrum than initially recognized, with forms demonstrating late onset (>25 years; LOFA), very late onset (>40 years; VLOFA), and re-tained reflexes (FARR). Even patients presenting with a hereditary spastic paresis pheno-type or with chorea have been described. FRDA is common, with a prevalence rate of 1:30–40,000 in Caucasians and a carrier rate of 1 in 90 to 1 in 100. It is virtually absent in East Asian, and rare in sub-Saharan African populations.

In something of an advertisement for pure basic science, it turned out that a consider-able amount was known about the gene's yeast homologue, which plays an important role in iron-sulphur cluster assembly within mitochondria. This soon led to rationally based clinical trials, such as that of idebenone (although this was unfortunately negative) [11].

7.3 **The recognition of dominantly inherited ataxias as distinct from Friedreich's ataxia**

Main paper: Marie P. Sur l'hérédo-ataxie cérébelleuse. *Semaine Médicale (Paris)* 1893; 13:444–7.

Background

By 1893, Friedreich's ataxia was a well-accepted entity—Charcot had eventually acknowledged its existence in 1884—but a number of cases with atypical features were starting to be reported. A literature review of 165 cases, in 1890, reported that many were 'incomplete, doubtful or absolutely atypical to Friedreich' [12]. Dominant pedigrees with cerebellar ataxia plus other neurological features (such as spasticity and optic atrophy) were described by Menzel in Germany (1891) and Sanger Brown in the United States (1892).

Methods

Pierre Marie drew together and reviewed four families published in the literature in 1880, 1891, and 1892 (two families). Post-mortem information was available on a member of each of the first two families.

Results

Marie pointed out the differences between these patients and those with Friedreich's ataxia: the pedigrees Marie described exhibited (usually) dominant inheritance, older age of onset, hyperreflexia, ophthalmoplegia and/or optic atrophy, and cognitive impairment, while scoliosis and foot deformities were absent. The pathology also differed, being restricted to the cerebellum (although later pathological studies in other members of three of the families showed more variable and widespread degeneration also affecting brainstem and spinal cord [13].)

Conclusions and critique

It is clear that Marie's families were clinically and pathologically heterogeneous, and Gordon Holmes was subsequently critical of the use of 'Marie's ataxia' to refer to a nosological entity, regarding it as a 'convenient pigeon-hole in which to group together cases of obscure nature with some symptoms in common' [14]. Nevertheless, the term was soon widely accepted, and was in occasional use even as recently as the early 1990s. In retrospect, Marie's paper was important in establishing that Friedreich's was not the only form of hereditary ataxia, and in drawing attention to the range of clinical features now recognized as common manifestations of the dominantly inherited spinocerebellar ataxias. Numerous attempts were subsequently made to classify these disorders, often on pathological grounds. This led to the confusion still surrounding the term 'olivopontocerebellar atrophy' (OPCA; Fig. 7.1)—a pathological description introduced by Dejerine and Thomas in 1900, fitting some, but not all, dominant ataxias, as well as the sporadic ataxia now usually called multiple system atrophy of cerebellar type (MSA_C).

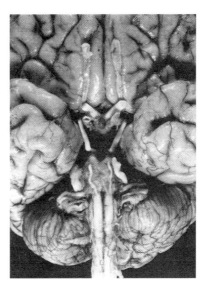

Fig. 7.1 Olivopontocerebellar degeneration: shrinkage of the pons; loss of olivary bulge; moderate atrophy of cerebellum.

Reproduced from Davis RL, Robertson DM, *Textbook of Neuropathology*, 2nd edition, Copyright (1991), with permission from John Wiley and Sons.

The dominant OPCAs were subsequently subdivided into five types by Konigsmark and Weiner [15] on the basis of clinical and pathological findings. Although their type III probably corresponds to what is now known as SCA 7, the distinctions between the other types did not readily reflect intra-familial variation of clinical features in the dominant ataxias. Yet other patients with dominantly inherited ataxias displayed cerebello-olivary degeneration or a pure parenchymatous cerebellar atrophy picture. Confusingly, the latter was sometimes termed 'Holmes ataxia' by neuropathologists, although Gordon Holmes actually described a *recessive* ataxia with hypogonadism [16]. This confusion demonstrates that, while neuropathological topography is important, it must be considered in conjunction with clinical features rather than relied on in isolation. This recognition culminated in Anita Harding's ADCA (autosomal dominant cerebellar ataxia) I–IV classification of 1982 [17], which had the virtues of simplicity and of applicability in living patients! The genetic classification (SCAs 1–37) has now largely subsumed these efforts, however [see section 7.8].

7.4 **The classic motor features of ataxia are delineated**

Main paper: Holmes G. On the clinical symptoms of cerebellar disease and their interpretation (The Croonian Lectures). *Lancet* 1922; i:1177–82, 1231–7; ii:59–65, 111–15.

Background

Rather than being a well-ordered process from the start, the neurological examination initially developed as a series of more or less disconnected signs. The organization of the neurological examination to reflect anatomical and physiological understanding is one of the triumphs of late nineteenth and early twentieth century neurology, and owes much to Gordon Holmes, especially with respect to the visual pathways and the cerebellum. While Babinski wrote about 'equilibrium' (static balance) and coined the word 'adiadococinésie' (dysdiadochokinesis) to describe difficulty with the execution of rapid patterned movements [18], a systematic study of patients with cerebellar lesions for the purpose of clarifying and classifying their motor deficits had not been undertaken, and it was universally thought that the cerebellum had a unitary, indivisible function.

Methods

In 1904, T. Granger Stewart and Holmes published on 40 patients with tumours of, or impacting on, the cerebellum [19]. Holmes subsequently studied soldiers with bullet injuries to the cerebellum, reporting the results in 1917 [20], and was the first to quantitate limb movements in ataxia, using the classical smoked drum physiology recording equipment of the time (Fig. 7.2) [21]. He drew on these studies for his Croonian lecture series on the clinical features of cerebellar disease in 1922.

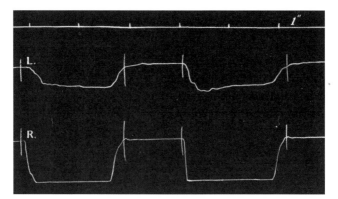

Fig. 7.2 Tracings, on a slowly rotating drum, of simultaneous depression of the right and left arms against springs of equal tension, from a man with a lesion of the left side of the cerebellum. The tracings show delay in starting and slowness in effecting the movements, reduced and irregular exertion of power, and slowness in relaxation on the affected side. Time in seconds.

Reproduced from *Brain*, 62, Holmes G, The cerebellum of man, p. 1–30, Copyright (1939), with permission from Oxford University Press.

Results

Stewart and Holmes stated that ataxia consisted of 'deficient control of the various component muscular contractions by which a complex act is executed' [19]. Holmes challenged the concept of a unitary cerebellar function, however, identifying asthenia (paresis—which he commented was frequently absent in slowly progressive cerebellar disorders), fatiguability, ataxia (including dysmetria, decomposition of movement, and intention tremor), hypotonia (causing the '(no) rebound' sign of Stewart and Holmes [19, 20] and pendular reflexes), and static (postural) tremor as separable components of the cerebellar syndrome. He thought that Babinski's 'adiadococinésie' was consequent on deficits in agonist/antagonist cooperation, at least in part, secondary to hypotonia. He addressed cerebellar localization, confirming the ipsilateral distribution of deficits in cerebellar hemisphere disease, and gait and speech abnormalities with vermal lesions. On quantitation of grasping movements in ataxic patients, he noted that reaction time was delayed by about 200 ms, phasic muscle force was reduced, and time to peak force was increased, ipsilateral to the lesion (Fig. 7.2).

Conclusions and critique

Holmes's approach to the clinical findings seen with cerebellar lesions, which he interpreted in terms of fundamental motor deficits, set the basis of the modern examination for ataxia and the analysis of ataxic motor deficits. The question as to whether ataxia is a unitary syndrome or a variable assortment of coexisting deficits based on different fundamental cerebellar functions is still debated, albeit not in the terms that Holmes employed. He did not, for example, consider motor execution in terms of feed-forward vs. feed-back control. With respect to terminology for features of the ataxic syndrome, special mention must be made of 'past pointing'. In the author's country, at least, this is often used as a synonym for dysmetria (a disturbance of limb placement/trajectory leading to inaccurate movements, as may be seen on the finger/nose test). Yet past pointing, as originally described by Barany, consists of drifting of the arm to the side of the acute cerebellar or vestibular lesion on repeated raising and lowering of the arm to an imagined target with vision abolished [22]. Dysdiadochokinesis refers to impairment of rapid alternating movements, while dyssynergia and decomposition of movement both refer to difficulty with multi-joint movements, with a tendency to move one joint at a time.

7.5 **Paraneoplastic cerebellar degeneration is formally recognized**

Main paper: Brain WR, Daniel PM, Greenfield JG. Subacute cortical cerebellar degeneration and its relation to carcinoma. *Journal of Neurology, Neurosurgery and Psychiatry* 1951; 14:59–75.

Background

Single cases of subacute cerebellar degeneration occurring in patients with cancer had been reported in 1919, 1929, 1933, and 1934, but the two diagnoses were not thought to be related. At that time, no doubt, in the absence of sophisticated neuroimaging, ataxia occurring in cancer patients was typically (and reasonably) ascribed to metastases. In 1938, Brouwer and Biemond postulated a relationship between neoplasia and cerebellar degeneration, ascribing this to 'toxicosis' [23].

Methods

The authors reported clinical details and post-mortem findings on four patients who died within 12 months of the subacute onset of cerebellar ataxia. They also reviewed the literature to that time, adding 12 further patients.

Results

One of the four had ovarian cancer (unsuspected during life), two had 'oat cell' (small cell) lung cancer (one unsuspected), and one had only a brain and spinal cord post-mortem (with no cancer known or discovered(!). All showed loss of Purkinje cells, and the three with tumours at post-mortem also had long tract degeneration (myelitis) and demonstrated a lymphocytic pleocytosis in the cerebrospinal fluid (CSF). One of the patients with an oat cell cancer had what was probably, in retrospect, limbic encephalitis, although two others also suffered cognitive decline. Eleven of the sixteen reviewed or reported cases had cancers at post-mortem—five ovarian, three lung, two uterine, and one breast.

Conclusions and critique

The authors drew attention to the much higher rate of associated carcinomas in subacute than in chronic progressive ataxias, and to the preponderance of lung and ovarian tumours. They speculated briefly on the possible pathogenesis of the cerebellar damage, but it was left to Russell, in 1961, to postulate that the central nervous system (CNS) damage was immunologically mediated [24]. The range of antibodies associated with paraneoplastic cerebellar degeneration (PCD) continues to expand, with 13 being listed in a recent monograph [25]. Most are directed against intracellular antigens (Fig. 7.3), and are thus very likely disease markers rather than directly pathogenic: anti P/Q voltage-gated calcium channel antibody-associated PCD is an exception. In most cases, cerebellar damage is accompanied by involvement of other regions of the neuraxis, and the correlations between tumour type, antibody, and paraneoplastic syndrome are not particularly tight.

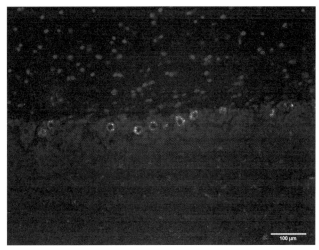

Fig. 7.3 Monkey cerebellum stained with anti-Yo antibody (FITC-white) and the nucleus with DAPI (grey). 200x magnification.

Only about 50% of patients with subacute ataxia have a paraneoplastic syndrome [25]. Subacute and more slowly evolving ataxias may also result from immunologically mediated non-paraneoplastic cerebellar damage, for example with anti-GAD antibodies [26].

In recent years, the Sheffield group have promulgated the concept of 'gluten ataxia', which can occur in the absence of coeliac enteropathy, and is claimed to be the most common definable cause of sporadic ataxia. Not all agree, however, and the dust is still settling on the argument [27], although the existence of PCD establishes beyond doubt that immunological cerebellar damage is indeed possible.

7.6 **Alcohol and truncal ataxia**

Main paper: Victor M, Adams RD, Mancall EL. A restricted form of cerebellar cortical degeneration occurring in alcoholic patients. *Archives of Neurology* 1959; 1:579–688.

Background

The effect of acute alcoholic intoxication on coordination, especially of gait, has presumably been known since alcohol was first consumed. The syndrome of cerebellar damage with more chronic alcohol intake only achieved widespread recognition, however, with the work of Victor, Adams, and Mancall; although cerebellar atrophy had been linked with chronic alcoholism by several authors following Thomas's report in 1905 [28], it was not clear that this was not just late cortical cerebellar atrophy occurring coincidentally.

Methods

The authors reviewed the literature to date and described 50 patients (personally examined in 46 cases), with clinicopathological correlations in 11.

Results

The authors described three time courses: (i) a subacutely developing ataxic syndrome that subsequently stabilized; (ii) a chronically progressive ataxic syndrome that sometimes stabilized; and (iii) more than one episode of decline with intervening stability. The ataxia was characterized by a wide-based stance and gait with truncal instability. This correlated with pathology (Purkinje cell loss) restricted to the antero-superior vermis. The lower (but not upper) limbs were often involved in more advanced cases, correlating with pathology extending to the anterior portions of the anterior lobes. Nystagmus and dysarthria were infrequent. The inferior olives were consistently involved, but the deep cerebellar nuclei (especially the dentate) usually were not.

Conclusions and critique

The restriction of pathology to the antero-superior vermis ± anterior portion of the anterior lobes, if overlaid on the cerebellar sensory homunculus mapped in monkeys by Snider and Eldred in 1952 [29], would be expected to affect the trunk, with the lower limbs involved if the atrophy extends to the anterior portions of the anterior lobes. The general features of Snider's homunculus have since been confirmed with lesion studies [30] (Fig. 7.4) and on functional magnetic resonance imaging (fMRI) [31].

Victor, Adams, and Mancall themselves thought that the syndrome they described resulted from 'malnutrition' (i.e. a form of Wernicke's encephalopathy due to thiamine deficiency), and certainly Wernicke's is under-diagnosed in life [32] and may contribute to, or indeed cause, the ataxic syndrome. However, it is now clear that Purkinje cell and granular cell damage and death can also occur with chronic alcohol ingestion in rats, independent of thiamine deficiency [e.g. 33, 34]. It seems possible that both mechanisms contribute, although if it is impossible to distinguish between them clinically or pathologically

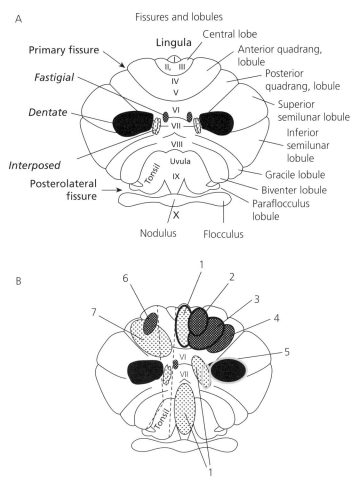

Fig. 7.4 Lesion symptom mapping. (A) Cerebellar lobules shown on an unfolded cerebellum. (B) Schematic sketch of findings in patients with focal cerebellar lesions. The figure summarizes the results of lesion symptom mapping in studies on eyeblink conditioning, cerebellar ataxia rating scores, balance in stance and gait, and upper and lower limb coordination. (1: ataxia of stance/gait; 2: lower limb ataxia; 3: upper limb ataxia; 4: dysarthria; 5: limb ataxia; 6: conditioned eyeblink response (CR) timing; 7: CR acquisition.)

Adapted from *Springer and the Cerebellum*, 7(4), Timmann D, Brandauer B, Hermsdorfer J, et al, Lesion symptom mapping of the human cerebellum, p. 602–6, Copyright (2008), with permission from Springer.

(unlike, for instance, alcohol-related and thiamine deficiency neuropathy), as seems to be the case if alcohol is indeed directly responsible in some patients, it will be very difficult to demonstrate this convincingly. It is worth noting that alcohol-related truncal ataxia may be unaccompanied by any other clinical or pathological features of Wernicke's encephalopathy, perhaps suggesting that it may, in some cases, indeed be directly alcohol-related. Furthermore, there is measurable Purkinje cell loss in moderate drinkers, more prominent in those with greater consumption [35]. On the other hand, a clinically indistinguishable picture can be seen in nutritionally compromised non-drinkers [36].

The reason for this regional susceptibility in an organ with such a uniform structure remains unexplained. There are, in fact, subtle regional differences in cerebellar architecture, with unipolar brush cells (a type of excitatory interneuron) being found particularly in inferior vermis, to a lesser extent in other vermal and intermediate regions, and, rarely, in the lateral cerebellar hemispheres. A further inhomogeneity of architecture is seen in the olivo-cerebellar projections, where there are eight major discontinuous strips orthogonal to the cerebellar folia, demonstrated in broadly congruent fashion by acetylcholinesterase, zebrin 1 and zebrin 2 distribution (Fig. 7.5). Perhaps such incompletely characterized variations on the hauntingly repetitive cerebellar microarchitecture hold the key to the regional susceptibility seen in this syndrome.

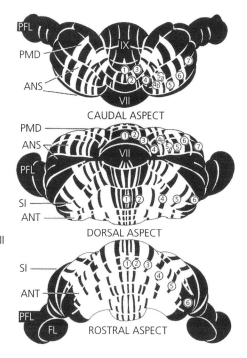

Fig. 7.5 Organization of the olivocerebellar system. Zebrin II bands 1 to 6.

Reproduced from *Trends in Neurosciences*, 21, Voogd J, Glickstein M, The anatomy of the cerebellum, p. 370–5, Copyright (1998), with permission from Elsevier.

7.7 **Long-term depression (LTD) as the substrate of motor learning in the cerebellum**

Main paper: Ito M, Kano M. Long-lasting depression of parallel fibre—Purkinje cell transmission induced by conjunctive stimulation of parallel fibres in the cerebellar cortex. *Neuroscience Letters* 1982; 33:253–8.

Background

The basic circuitry of the cerebellum had been delineated by the mid-1960s [e.g. 37], with the exception of two more recently discovered granular-cell-layer interneuron types—Lugaro cells and unipolar brush cells. The basic circuitry is shown in Fig. 7.6. On the basis

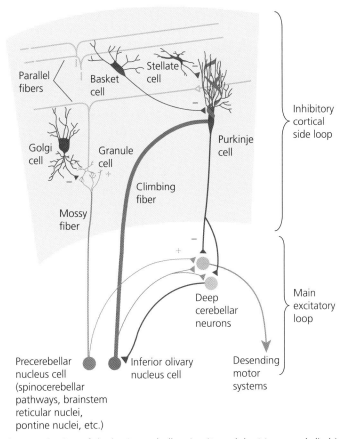

Fig. 7.6 Synaptic organization of the basic cerebellar circuit module. Mossy and climbing fibres convey output from the cerebellum, via a main excitatory loop, through the deep nuclei. This loop is modulated by an inhibitory side-loop passing through the cerebellar cortex. The excitatory (+) and inhibitory (–) connections among the cell types are shown.

Reproduced from Kandel ER, Schwartz JH, Jessell TM, *Principles of Neural Science*, 4th ed., p. 837, Copyright (2000), with permission from McGraw-Hill.

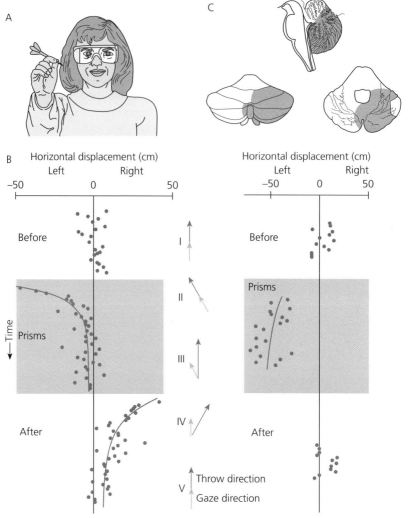

Fig. 7.7 Readjustment of eye–hand coordination during adaptation to prism glasses. (**A**) Laterally displacing prisms bend the optic path to the subject's right. The subject looks to the left along the bent light path to see the target directly in front of her. Her hand is held in position ready to throw a dart at the target in front of her. (**B**) While wearing the prisms (gaze shifted to the left), the first hit is displaced left of centre: the hand throws to where the eyes are looking, towards the target. Thereafter, hits trend to the right, away from where the eyes are looking. After removing the prisms, the gaze is centred on the target, and the first throw hits right of centre, away from where the eyes are looking. Thereafter, hits trend towards the target, where the eyes are looking. Data during and after prism use have been fitted with exponential curves. Gaze and throw directions are indicated by the *arrows* on the right. Inferred gaze (eye and head) direction assumes the subject is fixating the target. The *roman numerals* next to the arrows indicate times during the prism adaptation experiment: *I* Before donning prisms, when gaze is directed towards the target and the throw is towards the target. *II* Just after donning prisms, when gaze is directed along the bent light path away from the target and the throw is in the direction of gaze away from the target. *III* Still wearing prisms and after adapting to them, when gaze is directed along the bent light path away from the target but the throw is directed towards the target. *IV* Just after removing the prisms, when the gaze is now directed towards the target and the adapted throw is to the right of the direction of gaze and to the right of the target. *V* After disadapting

of this circuitry, Marr [38] and Albus [39] predicted that the sensitivity of Purkinje cells to parallel fibre activation might be modifiable by climbing fibre activation. This would lead to a situation whereby each cerebellar cortico-nuclear microcomplex ([40] acts as an excitatory loop (through the deep cerebellar nuclei) governed by a variable negative side-loop (through the cerebellar cortex, with variable inhibition of the deep cerebellar nuclei by the Purkinje cells). Such a process could underlie cerebellar motor learning, with the climbing fibres carrying the 'error signal' to modify subsequent inhibitory Purkinje cell output.

Methods

Decerebrate anaesthetized rabbits had cerebellar cortical field responses recorded by a glass microelectrode. Parallel fibres were stimulated 1 mm away with a second glass electrode, while the contralateral inferior olive was stimulated with a needle electrode.

Results

Conjunctive stimulation of parallel fibres and climbing fibres in rabbit cerebellar cortex led to reduction of Purkinje cell excitatory post-synaptic potential amplitudes in response to subsequent parallel fibre stimulation, lasting at least an hour. No such reduction was seen if either parallel fibres or climbing fibres were stimulated alone.

Conclusions and critique

Despite its hauntingly simple and regular circuitry, evident for half a century or so, there is still no universal agreement on what exactly the cerebellum does and how it does it. The computation is clearly the same (the 'uniform cerebellar transform' [41]), with the effects depending on the nature and location of the inputs and outputs. However, with the postulation and subsequent confirmation of LTD, a substrate for associative motor learning was revealed. LTD does, for instance, underlie the development of conditioned reflexes, which are basically examples of associative motor learning and which have been shown in both animals and humans to depend on intact paravermal cortex/interposed nuclei function. A combination of the repository for programmed motor responses concept of Marr and Albus, modified by Ito's adaptive control model (whereby LTD modifies learned motor responses both for current feed-back and subsequent feed-forward), while not explaining all features of cerebellar disease, has been the most influential model of cerebellar function since its inception.

While there remains argument as to the exact role of LTD in motor learning, it is relatively easy to demonstrate the effects of such learning on motor performance. The classic experiment (see Fig. 7.7) involves adaptation to wearing prism glasses and to their

---

the gaze–throw coordination, when gaze is now directed to the target and the throw is in the direction of gaze, towards the target, as originally. (**C**) Adaptation fails in a patient with unilateral infarctions in the territory of the posterior inferior cerebellar artery and involves inferior cerebellar peduncle (inferior olivary climbing fibres) and/or inferior lateral posterior cerebellar cortex.

subsequent removal during repeated attempts to throw at a target. Those with intact cerebellar systems rapidly adapt to the deviation in target sighting induced by the prisms, and then briefly overshoot in the opposite direction when the prisms are removed, before re-adapting to the baseline condition. Those with a cerebellar system lesion may still be accurate at baseline, but do not adapt to prism glasses and do not overshoot in the opposite direction once they are removed.

Lastly, it should be noted that, since publication of this paper, both LTD and long-term potentiation have been demonstrated at other cerebellar synapses. Clearly, the basis of cerebellar motor learning is more complex than Ito originally envisaged.

7.8 **Spinocerebellar ataxia type 1 is due to a translated expanded CAG triplet repeat**

Main paper: Orr HT, Chung M, Banfi S, et al. Expansion of an unstable trinucleotide CAG repeat in spinocerebellar ataxia type 1. *Nature Genetics* 1993; 4:221–6.

Background

Since the report of Pierre Marie in 1893 [42] (see section 7.3), it had been realized that some forms of progressive, adult-onset ataxia were dominantly inherited. The classification of these heterogeneous disorders was, for most of the twentieth century, chaotic: 'Thus, from the clinical viewpoint, it is no exaggeration to state that there are as many classifications as there are authors on the subject.' [43] Anita Harding finally brought some order to the area, outlining four types of autosomal dominant cerebellar ataxia (ADCA types I–IV) [17]. Type II was associated with retinal degeneration; Type III described those with 'pure' ataxia; Type IV separated off those rare families with myoclonus and deafness (these might actually have been mitochondrial disorders); while Type I was used for those with any other additional features (but not retinal degeneration) including optic atrophy, neuropathy, ophthalmoplegia, and dementia.

Human leukocyte antigen (HLA) linkage, implying a chromosome 6p locus, was demonstrated by Jackson et al. in 1977 [44] in some families with what would subsequently be termed ADCA I.

Methods

Orr et al. isolated a 1.2 megabase stretch of DNA (deoxyribonucleic acid) from the locus on chromosome 6p into a yeast artificial chromosome contig and subcloned this into cosmids. These were probed with triplet repeat-containing trinucleides, on the basis of observed anticipation in SCA 1 (spinocerebellar ataxia type 1) pedigrees (see 'Conclusions and critique') and variability of a CAG repeat shown on Southern blotting.

Results

A highly variable CAG triplet repeat was identified. This was expanded in individuals with SCA 1, and the repeat number was unstable, with a tendency to increase in younger generations and a strong correlation between repeat size and age of onset.

Conclusions and critique

SCA 1 was the third translated unstable triplet repeat disorder to be identified, after Huntington's disease and bulbospinal muscular atrophy (Kennedy's disease). As with Huntington's, anticipation (earlier onset in subsequent generations) had been identified in some pedigrees before the gene was found, and the unstable CAG repeat provided an explanation for this phenomenon. Subsequently, other common (SCA 2, SCA 3) and less common (SCA 7, SCA 17) SCAs, as well as dentatorubral pallidoluysian atrophy (DRPLA), were found to share the same genetic mechanism. There is some evidence that one strand in SCA 8 may also be translated as a pure polyglutamine tract [45], although its complimentary

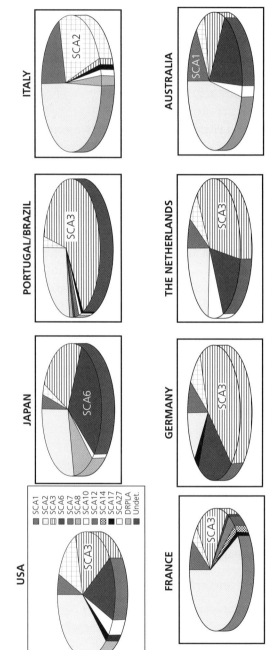

Fig. 7.8 Relative frequencies of spinocerebellar ataxias (SCAs). The SCA with highest frequency is indicated in each pie.

Reproduced from Manto MU, *Cerebellar Disorders: A Practical Approach to Diagnosis and Management*, Copyright (2010), with permission from Cambridge University Press (plate between pages 52 and 53).

strand may act as an antisense RNA (ribonucleic acid). The expanded polyglutamine tract in SCA 6 is different, however, being both much shorter than the others mentioned and stable (except in very rare pedigrees). The exact mechanisms of neurotoxicity in the expanded polyglutamine tract disorders are still unclear, although they appear to involve a gain of novel, toxic function that is at least, in part, protein context dependent (explaining different disease thresholds and pathological topographies) [46].

The SCAs now number up to 40 (as of early 2015), although several numbers are duplications or 'missing in action' [47]. These include SCA 9, SCA 16 (which turned out to be the same as SCA 15), SCA 22 (which is probably the same as SCA 19), SCA 24 (which was recessive and, therefore, should not have been numbered among the SCAs, and is now designated SCAR 4), and SCAs 33 and 39. The remainder exhibit a range of genetic mechanisms, ranging from point mutations (e.g. in SCAs 14, 27, and 28), through non-coding expansions (in SCAs 10, 12, 31, and 36), to duplications (e.g. SCA 20—probably) or deletions (e.g. SCA 15) [47]. However, the translated CAG repeat (polyglutamine tract) SCAs, plus DRPLA, together still comprise the majority of dominant pedigrees around the world, where this has been studied (Fig. 7.8). The proportion of all SCAs that are due to SCA 1 (or any other particular SCA) varies from population to population due to founder effects, and this information can be useful in deciding in what order the SCAs should be tested in a given patient. For example, although SCA 3 is the most common, worldwide, SCA 1 is the most common SCA in Australia [48], South Africa, northern Italy (with SCA 2 the most common in the south), and in parts of Siberia.

7.9 **The pathogenesis of episodic ataxia type 2—an ion channel disorder**

Main paper: Ophoff RA, Terwindt GM, Vergonne MN, et al. Familial hemiplegic migraine and episodic ataxia type 2 are caused by mutations in the Ca^{2+} channel gene CACNL1A4. *Cell* 1996; 87:543–52.

Background

Dominant episodic ataxias may have been first described in 1946 [49]. Episodic ataxia with myokymia (EA1) had been shown to be due to mutations in the KCNA1 potassium channel gene in 1994 [50]. Episodic ataxia type 2 (EA2), the most common of the episodic ataxias, is notable for attacks of nystagmus and gait ataxia lasting hours (much longer than EA1), sometimes accompanied by vertigo and vomiting, triggered by emotional stress, exercise, caffeine, alcohol, and fever. Interictal ataxia and nystagmus commonly develop over time, as does vermal atrophy on MRI. Attacks are usually prevented or diminished by acetazolamide. Onset is typically in childhood or early teenage years, but onset in a patient in their 60s has been reported. A useful summary may be found at the GeneTests website, which is conducted under the auspices of the National Institutes of Health [51].

Methods

Both EA2 and familial hemiplegic migraine (FHM; type 1) had already been mapped to chromosome 19p13, and it was suspected that they were allelic disorders. The periodic paralyses and EA1 were already known to be ion channel disorders, and it was suspected by Ophoff et al. that FHM and EA2 might be as well. They used the (now largely out-moded) technique of exon trapping to search for potential ion channel genes in the region of interest.

Results

They identified a human ion channel gene in the candidate region, homologous with a rat and rabbit P/Q type Ca^{2+} channel α-subunit, and named it CACNL1A4 (now usually known as CACNA1A). This subunit is a typical 4 x 6 transmembrane domain ion channel (see Fig. 7.9). They described missense mutations in this gene in FHM (type 1) and truncating mutations in EA2.

Conclusions and critique

Hyper- and hypokalaemic periodic paralysis, EA1, and autosomal nocturnal frontal lobe epilepsy had recently been shown to be due to mutations in voltage- or ligand-gated ion channels. The discovery that the most common form of EA, and about 50% of pedigrees with FHM, were due to mutations in an ion channel added weight to the concept that episodic neurological disorders are likely to be due to ion channel dysfunction. Subsequently, EAs 3–7 have also been described; those for which the genes are known (EAs 5 and 6) are, respectively, due to a calcium channel beta subunit mutation (CACNB4) and a glial glutamate re-uptake transporter (which doubtless disturbs glutamatergic transmission).

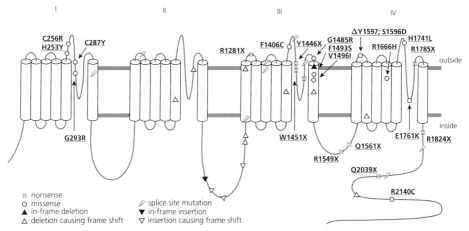

Fig. 7.9 Putative topology of Ca$_V$2.1 channel subunit and overview of the location of mutations identified to date. The complete channel complex is made up of this pore-forming and voltage-sensing subunit along with an intracytoplasmic ββ subunit, a transmembrane γ subunit, and a largely extracellular α2δ subunit.

Reproduced from Chapter 42: Episodic ataxias 1 and 2, Baloh RW, from Subramony SH, Durr A (eds), *Handbook of Clinical Neurology*, 3rd edition, p. 597, Copyright (2012), with permission from Elsevier.

Importantly, the paper also draws attention to the phenotypic heterogeneity seen with this (and other) ion channel mutations. (Another well-known example of this phenotypic heterogeneity occurs with SCN4A mutations, which can cause paramyotonia congenita, potassium-aggravated myotonia, or hyperkalaemic periodic paralysis.) Genotype–phenotype correlations are reasonably well established for CACNA1A mutations, despite some overlap in clinical presentation. Thus, SCA 6 is always due to a (CAG)$_n$ expansion, and FHM1 nearly always due to a missense mutation, while EA2 is typically due to a nonsense mutation resulting in protein truncation (although a few missense mutations have been reported as giving rise to EA2). The following year, spinocerebellar ataxia type 6 (SCA 6), one of the most common of the SCAs, was also shown to be allelic to FHM1 and EA2, being due to a small, stable translated (CAG)$_n$ repeat expansion in the CACNA1A gene [52]. It, too, overlaps with EA2 phenotypically, with a history of episodic exacerbations in the early stages not uncommon, although the onset is typically in middle age. Conversely, patients with EA2 tend to develop fixed inter-ictal signs of cerebellar dysfunction, with gaze-evoked nystagmus with rebound in most, and downbeat nystagmus in about a third. A mild truncal ataxia is often also in evidence. Despite this overlap with other CACNA1A phenotypes, it remains unclear whether the pathogenesis of SCA 6 involves Ca^{2+} channel dysfunction, or toxic gain of function due to the polyglutamine expansion, or both.

7.10 **Description of the cerebellar cognitive affective syndrome**

Main paper: Schmahmann JD, Sherman JC. The cerebellar cognitive affective syndrome. *Brain* 1998; 121(4):561–79.

Background

Gordon Holmes had not included any mention of cognition in his ultimate exposition on cerebellar function [21], but this may have reflected more on the state of development of neuropsychology in the early twentieth century than on his usually acute powers of observation and deduction. However, the advent of trans-synaptic tracer studies and of functional neuroimaging, in the last two decades of the twentieth century, prompted a re-evaluation.

Anatomically, it became clear that the cerebellum and cortex are linked in parallel, non-overlapping loops (analogous to those linking cortex and basal ganglia), and that prefrontal and other 'non-motor' cortices are reciprocally connected to posterolateral cerebellar cortex and inferior dentate nucleus [53] via non-VL thalamic nuclei (such as the medial dorsal) for cerebellar efferents, and different and non-overlapping pontine nuclei from those involved in motor circuitry for cerebellar afferents. Meanwhile, positron emission tomography (PET) and fMRI studies demonstrated posterolateral cerebellar activation with cognitive tasks, especially novel or effortful tasks, after subtraction of activation from the stimulus perception and response output portions of the task (Fig. 7.10) (reviewed by Cabeza; [54]).

Methods

Schmahmann and Sherman described 20 patients with an assortment of diseases confined to the cerebellum, including strokes, post-infectious cerebellitis, and cerebellar cortical atrophy (Fig. 7.11). Patients underwent physical and behavioural neurological examinations, an extensive neuropsychological battery, MRI, and electroencephalography (EEG).

Results

Lesions of the anterior lobe of the cerebellum resulted in the classical ataxia (motor) syndrome. Lesions in the posterior lobe and vermis caused impairment of executive ('frontal') functions, visuospatial organization and memory, and linguistic function, in addition to personality changes. Follow-up of several patients with acute lesions, over 1–9 months, showed improvement or resolution of cognitive dysfunction.

Conclusions and critique

Although there had been some earlier reports of cognitive impairment in apparently isolated cerebellar disease [e.g. 55], Schmahmann and Sherman's paper crystallized the issue and acted as a spur to other investigators. Over the last 15 years, numerous studies of patients with cerebellar infarcts or degenerations have confirmed the findings of dysexecutive function, linguistic impairment, and visuospatial compromise with cerebellar lesions,

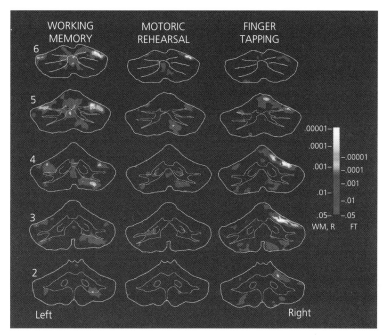

Fig. 7.10 Averaged fMRI activation in slices 2–6 for the working-memory, motoric rehearsal, and finger-tapping tasks. Sections represent oblique coronal slices taken parallel to the dorsal surface of the brain stem and slice numbers appear on the left. Slice 1, which was the most anterior slice, exhibited almost no activation and was, therefore, omitted from the figure. The maps for working memory and motoric rehearsal were averaged across eight subjects, whereas finger tapping was averaged across five subjects. Regions depicted in white represent areas that exhibited increased activation in high relative to low load conditions (in working memory and motoric rehearsal) or during finger tapping relative to rest. Decreases in activation during high load or finger tapping relative to their contrasting conditions were negligible and so are not depicted in this figure. The grey scale on the right represents the significance levels (one-tailed p values) of averaged Z scores and is scaled differently for finger tapping than for working memory and motoric rehearsal. The right side of the brain is depicted on the right. (WM, working memory; R, motoric rehearsal; FT, finger tapping.)

Reproduced from *J Neuroscience*, 17(24), Desmond JE, Lobular patterns of cerebellar activation in verbal working-memory and finger-tapping tasks as revealed by functional MRI, p. 9675–9685, Copyright (1997), with permission from Elsevier.

and the localization suggested by Schmahmann and Sherman (reviewed by O'Halloran; [56]). Behavioural and personality changes, being less readily measured, have less weight of evidence. There has also been confirmation from lesional studies of functional imaging findings demonstrating right posterolateral cerebellar dominance for effortful linguistic tasks—the 'linguistic cerebellum'. It remains unclear, however, exactly how the cerebellum plays these roles: impaired attention, impaired sequencing, or 'dysmetria of thought' have all been proposed as fundamental mechanisms. Whatever the nature of the underlying deficit, however, clinicians should remain aware of the possibility of significant cognitive

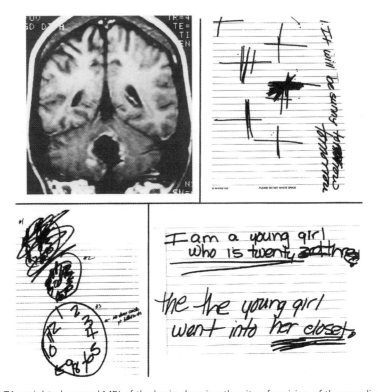

Fig. 7.11 T1-weighted coronal MRI of the brain showing the site of excision of the ganglioglioma, and subject's responses when asked to bisect a line, draw a clock, and write a sentence.

Reproduced from *Brain*, 121, Schmahmann JD, Sherman JC, The cerebellar cognitive affective syndrome, p. 561–579, Copyright (1998), with permission from Oxford University Press.

compromise in patients with even isolated cerebellar lesions involving the posterior lobe(s).

One criticism sometimes levelled against the concept of a cerebellar contribution to cognition is that cerebellar motor, visual scanning, and speech articulation difficulties artefactually impair performance on ostensibly cognitive tasks. Indeed, it is important to consider which tasks may be appropriate for testing cognition in moderately or severely ataxic patients. Tasks should either:

i) be untimed and place no premium on motor accuracy (e.g. the Wisconsin Card Sorting Test or verbal similarities), or

ii) if timed, contain an internal control for impaired visuomotor performance (e.g. the Trail-Making Test or the Stroop Test), or

iii) if timed and without an internal control, be clearly constrained by cognition rather than by loss of motor (including speech) facility (e.g. verbal fluency by initial letter—Controlled oral word association test (COWAT) or F,A,S Test).

Key unanswered questions

1 How does the cerebellum actually work?

Although cerebellar microstructure is relatively simple, and its fundamentals have been known for some 50 years, there is still no consensus as to how it does what it does. Various possibilities have been advanced, but none satisfactorily explain all experimental findings. The dominant model has been that of Albus, Marr, and Ito, but numerous others, including a non-adaptive role in movement timing, a role as an adaptive pattern generator, and various adaptive control theories have all been proposed (and criticized).

2 Is the limb motor ataxia syndrome unitary?

Many clinicians are of the view that the various clinical features of the ataxic syndrome— dysmetria, dyssynergia, dysdiadochokinesis, abnormal rebound, etc.—are consequences of a single fundamental underlying deficit. Another possibility, however, is that these manifestations are potentially separable, with the separation consequent on different afferent and efferent connections, but that they usually occur together due to proximity and the extent of the usual pathological processes. Proof of the latter would require the ability to quantify these different aspects accurately and separately, with subsequent careful study of small focal cerebellar lesions. It is conceivable that cerebellar repetitive transcranial magnetic stimulation may help in this regard.

3 What underlies differential patterns of pathological topographic involvement in a brain region with such a uniform structure?

It is well known that the superior and inferior vermis are particularly susceptible to thiamine deficiency, and perhaps less well known that the inferior vermis is relatively resistant to many of the otherwise diffuse dominantly inherited cerebellar degenerations. Yet cerebellar structure is remarkably uniform. While cholinergic projections and zebrin immunohistochemistry do define sagittally oriented cerebellar cortical modules, these are much finer-grained than the differential susceptibilities already mentioned. The relatively recently described unipolar brush cells are preferentially distributed in superior and inferior vermis—might their distribution perhaps contribute to the pattern of damage in thiamine deficiency?

4 Do all the expanded polyglutamine tract (EPGT-)-mediated SCAs (other than SCA 6) have a common pathogenesis?

While SCAs 1, 2, 3, 7, 17 and DRPLA all share a common pathological signature with Huntington's disease—intranuclear inclusions predominantly comprising EPGTs—the clinical features and pathological topographies differ despite widespread translation of the gene products in each case. This fact alone implies that the pathogeneses may differ. There is some support for this from SCA 1—not only does cerebellar damage precede, and is experimentally separable from, intranuclear inclusion formation, but SCA 1 pathogenesis is dependent on phosphorylation at a serine residue well away from the EPGT [57]. As there is no homology between the various EPGT-bearing proteins beyond the EPGTs themselves, this implies an EPGT host protein-specific contribution to pathogenesis. The importance of this is that, were the pathogenesis indeed to be unitary, advances in Huntington's disease therapy might be expected to translate to the EPGT-mediated SCAs as well.

5 What is the nature of the cerebellar contribution to cognition?
While there now remains little doubt that the cerebellum contributes to cognition, the nature of that contribution is disputed. Possibilities raised include 'dysmetria of thought' (particularly for novel cognitive tasks), impaired sequencing, and a general effect on attention. Given the uniformity of cerebellar structure and, therefore, presumably of function (the 'uniform cerebellar transform'), it may well be that further clues to this problem will actually come from further analyses of motor dysfunction in cerebellar disease.

References

1 **Giannitrapani D.** Developing concepts of lateralisation of cerebral functions. *Cortex* 1967; **3**:355–70.

2 **Willis T.** *Cerebri anatome: cui accessit nervorum descriptio et usus.* London: J. Martyn and J. Allestry. 1664 (Translation: Willis T. *The Anatomy of the Brain and Nerves.* Montreal: McGill University Press; 1965).

3 **Finger S.** *Origins of Neuroscience.* Oxford: Oxford University Press; 1994; 211.

4 **Rolando L.** 1809. Saggio sopra la Vera Struttura del Cervello del'Uomo e degli Animali e sopra la Funzione del Sistema Nervoso. (Nella Stamperia da S.S.R.M. Privilegiata, Sassari) (Translation in: McHenry LC Jnr. *Garrison's History of Neurology.* Springfield, IL: Charles C. Thomas; 1969.)

5 **Friedreich N.** Über ataxie mit besonderer berücksichtigung der hereditären formen. *Virkows Archiv für Pathologische Anatomie und Physiologie* 1876; **68**:145–245.

6 **Gowers WR.** A family affected with locomotor ataxy. *Clin Soc Transcripts* 1880; **14**:27–36.

7 **Geoffroy G, Barbeau A, Breton A, et al.** Clinical description and roentgenologic evaluation of patients with Friedreich's ataxia. *Can J Neurol Sci* 1976; **3**:279–86.

8 **Harding AE.** Friedreich's ataxia: a clinical and genetic study of 90 families with an analysis of early diagnostic criteria and intrafamilial clustering of clinical features. *Brain* 1981; **104**:589–620.

9 **Campuzano V, Montermini L, Moltó MD, et al.** Friedreich's ataxia: autosomal recessive disease caused by an intronic GAA triplet repeat expansion. *Science* 1996; **271**:1423–7.

10 **Montermini L, Richter A, Morgan K, et al.** Phenotypic variability in Friedreich ataxia: role of the associated GAA triplet repeat expansion. *Ann Neurol* 1997; **41**:675–82.

11 **Lynch DR, Perlman SL, Meier T.** A phase 3, double-blind, placebo-controlled trial of idebenone in Friedreich ataxia. *Arch Neurol* 2010; **67**:941–7.

12 **Ladame P.** Friedreich's disease. *Brain* 1890; **13**:467–537.

13 **Berciano J, Rebollo M, Coria F, Pérez JL, Leno C.** Heredotaxia de Marie. Nuevas consideraciones sobre su uso e independencia nosológica. *Med Clin (Barcelona)* 1983; **80**:506–8.

14 **Holmes G.** An attempt to classify cerebellar disease, with a note on Marie's hereditary cerebellar ataxia. *Brain* 1907; **30**:545–67.

15 **Konigsmark BW, Weiner LP.** The olivopontocerebellar atrophies: a review. *Medicine* 1970; **49**:227–41.

16 **Holmes G.** A form of familial degeneration of the cerebellum. *Brain* 1907; **30**:466–89.

17 **Harding AE.** The clinical features and classification of the late onset autosomal dominant cerebellar ataxias: a study of eleven families, including descendants of the 'Drew family of Walworth'. *Brain* 1982; **105**:1–28.

18 **Babinski J.** Sur lo rôle du cervelet dans les actes volitionnels nécessitant une succession rapide de mouvements (diadococinésie). *Rev Neurol* 1902; **10**:1013–5.

19 **Stewart TG, Holmes GM.** Symptomatology of cerebellar tumours. *Brain* 1904; **27**:522–92.

20 **Holmes GM.** The symptoms of acute cerebellar injuries due to gunshot. *Brain* 1917; **40**:461–535.

21 **Holmes G.** The cerebellum of man. *Brain* 1939; **62**:1–30.

22 **Barany R.** 1914. Nobel Prize in Physiology or Medicine lecture. Some new methods for functional testing of the vestibular apparatus and the cerebellum. In: Nobel Lectures in Physiology or Medicine 1901–1921, Elsevier Publishing Compamny, Amsterdam, 1967.

23 **Brouwer B, Biemond A.** Les affections parenchymateuses du cervelet et leur signification du point de vue de l'anatomie et la physiologie de cet organe. *J Belg Neurol Psychiatr* 1938; **38**:691–757.

24 **Russell DS.** Encephalomyelitis and carcinomatous neuropathy. In: van Bogaert L, Radermecker J, Hozay J, Lowenthal A. (eds.) *The Encephalitides.* Amsterdam: Elsevier; 1961; 131–5.

25 **De Angelis LM, Posner JB.** *Neurologic Complications of Cancer* (2nd ed.) New York: Oxford University Press; 2009; 577–617.

26 **Saiz A, Blanco Y, Sabater L, et al.** Spectrum of neurological syndromes associated with glutamic acid decarboxylase antibodies: diagnostic clues for this association. *Brain* 2008; **131**:2553–63.

27 **Grossman G.** Neurological complications of coeliac disease: what is the evidence? *Pract Neurol* 2008; **8**:77–89.

28 **Thomas A.** Atrophie lamellaire des cellules de Purkinje. *Rev Neurol* 1905; **13**:917–24.

29 **Snider RS, Eldred EJ.** Cerebro-cerebellar relationships in the monkey. *J Neurophysiology* 1952; **15**:27–40.

30 **Timmann D, Brandauer B, Hermsdörfer J, et al.** Lesion-symptom mapping of the human cerebellum. *Cerebellum* 2008; **7**:602–6.

31 **Grodd W, Hulsmann E, Lotze M, Wildgruber D, Erb M.** Sensorimotor mapping of the human cerebellum: fMRI evidence of somatotopic organisation. *Hum Brain Mapping* 2001; **13**:55–73.

33 **Harper CG.** The incidence of Wernicke's encephalopathy in Australia—a neuropathological study of 131 cases. *J Neurol Neurosurg Psychiatry* 1983; **46**:593–8.

33 **Tavares MS, Paula-Barbosa MM.** Alcohol-induced granule cell loss in the cerebellar cortex of the adult rat. *Exp Neurol* 1982; **78**:574–82.

34 **Pentney R.** Alcohol toxicity in the cerebellum: fundamental aspects. In: Manto MU, Pandolfo M (eds.). *The Cerebellum and its Disorders*. Cambridge, UK: Cambridge University Press; 2002; 327–35.

35 **Karhune PJ, Erkinjuntti T, Laippala P.** Moderate alcohol consumption and loss of Purkinje cells. *BMJ* 1994; **308**:1663–7.

36 **Mancall EL, McEntee WJ.** Alterations of the cerebellar cortex in nutritional encephalopathy. *Neurology* 1965; **15**:303–13.

37 **Eccles JC, Ito M, Szentágothai J.** *The Cerebellum as a Neuronal Machine*. Berlin: Springer Verlag; 1967.

38 **Marr D.** A theory of cerebellar cortex. *J Physiol (Lond)* 1969; **202**:437–70.

39 **Albus JS.** A theory of cerebellar function. *Math Biosci* 1971; **10**:25–61.

40 **Ito M.** *The Cerebellum and Neural Control*. New York: Raven Press; 1984.

41 **Schmahmann JD.** Disorders of the cerebellum: ataxia, dysmetria of thought, and the cerebellar cognitive affective syndrome. *J Neuropsychiat Clin Neurosci* 2004; **16**:367–78.

42 **Marie P.** Sur l'hérédoataxie cérébelleuse. *Semaines de Médicine (Paris)* 1893; **13**:444–7.

43 **Skre H, Refsum S.** Neurological approaches to the inherited ataxias. In: Kark RAP, Rosenberg RN, Schut LJ (eds.). *The Inherited Ataxias. Advances in Neurology, Vol. 21.* New York: Raven Press; 1978: 1–13.

44 **Jackson JD, Currier RD, Terasaki PI, Morton NE.** Spinocerebellar ataxia and HLA linkage: risk prediction by HLA typing. *N Engl J Med* 1977; **296**:1138–41.

45 **Moseley ML, Zu T, Ikeda Y, et al.** Bidirectional expression of CUG and CAG expansion transcripts and intranuclear polyglutamine inclusions in spinocerebellar ataxia type 8. *Nat Genet* 2006; **38**:758–69.

46 **Paulson HL, Pulst S-M.** Polyglutamine ataxias: *In vitro* and *in vivo* models. In: Brice A, Pulst S-M (eds.). *Spinocerebellar Degenerations: the Ataxias and Spastic Paraplegias*. Philadelphia: Butterworth Heinemann; 2007: 145–69.

47 **National Center for Biotechnology Information.** OMIM. Available at: <http://www.ncbi.nlm.nih.gov/omim>

48 **Storey E, du Sart D, Shaw JH, et al.** Frequency of spinocerebellar ataxia types 1, 2, 3, 6, and 7 in Australian patients with spinocerebellar ataxia. *Am J Med Genet* 2000; **95**:351–7.

49 **Parker HL.** Periodic ataxia. In: Hewlett RM, Nevling AB, Minor JR (eds). *Collected Papers of the Mayo Clinic*. Philadelphia: WB Saunders; 1946; 642–5.

50 **Browne DL, Gancher ST, Nutt JG, et al.** Episodic ataxia/myokymia syndrome is associated with point mutations in the human potassium channel gene, KCNA1. *Nat Genet* 1994; **8**:136–40.

51 **Spacey S.** Episodic ataxia type 2. *GeneReviews*®; updated 8 December 2011. Available at: <http://www.ncbi.nlm.nih.gov/books/NBK1501/>

52 **Zhuchenko O, Bailey J, Bonnen P, et al.** Autosomal dominant cerebellar ataxia (SCA 6) associated with small polyglutamine expansions in the alpha (1A)-voltage-dependent calcium channel. *Nat Genet* 1997; **15**:62–9.

53 **Middleton FA, Strick PL.** Basal ganglia and cerebellar loops: motor and cognitive circuits. *Brain Res Rev* 2000; **31**:236–50.

54 **Cabeza R, Nyberg L.** Imaging cognition II: an empirical review of 275 PET and fMRI studies. *J Cogn Neurosci* 2000; **12**:1–47.

55 **Grafman J, Litvan I, Massaquoi S, et al.** Cognitive planning deficit in patients with cerebellar atrophy. *Neurology* 1992; **42**:1493–6.

56 **O'Halloran CJ, Kinesella GJ, Storey E.** The cerebellum and neuropsychological functioning: a critical review. *J Clin Exp Neuropsychol* 2011; **34**:35–56.

57 **Emamian ES, Kaytor MD, Duvick LA, et al.** Serine 776 of ataxin-1 is critical for polyglutamine-induced disease in SCA 1 transgenic mice. *Neuron* 2003; **38**:375–87.

Chapter 8

Parkinson's disease

A. J. Lees

8.0 **Introduction**

Fragmentary literary descriptions of the shaking palsy can be found in the ancient Chinese texts, the Bible, and the Sanskrit incunabula, but the first detailed clinical descriptions from a sufferer, Wilhelm von Humboldt, and from a physician, James Parkinson, did not appear until the first half of the nineteenth century. One hundred years then went by before severe cell loss in the pars compacta of the substantia nigra was identified as the single most consistent pathological lesion and the Lewy body as an invariable marker of the disease in the brain stem. The most important landmark in this article related to the discovery of dopamine as an important brain neurotransmitter and the subsequent finding (eventually, after some unfortunate delays to the introduction of L-dopa as a highly efficacious symptomatic therapy in the late 1960s) that it was markedly deficient in the nigrostriatal bundle in individuals with Parkinson's disease. A further half century on, the pathogenesis of Parkinson's disease is still to be determined and the relative contributions of 'seed' versus 'soil' in its pathogenesis remain to be fully elucidated. Modest further advances have occurred in the symptomatic treatment of the disease but there is still no reliable biomarker or proven treatment that prevents the neurodegenerative process.

The early landmarks chose themselves, but it was less straightforward to choose the most important papers from the last forty years. I consulted a number of trusted colleagues actively involved in research into Parkinson's disease to make sure there were no glaring 'blind spots' before settling on my selections. I sought particular reassurances that the paper I had written with Julian Fearnley, in which we had predicted a pre-symptomatic phase of at least five years after nigral degeneration began and rigidity and bradykinesia became clinically detectable, justified its place above, say, the Braak hypothesis. After the paper was written and waiting for publication, its inclusion in *Brain's* 'Top Ten at Ten' collection, made up of the top two cited articles from each of the last five decades, seemed to add further external justification of its impact.

The most outstanding challenges that remain in the field of Parkinson's disease are to determine the chemical pathways that lead to the specific and localied neurodegeneration, the role of ageing in the causation of cognitive and balance difficulties, whether the Lewy body is a cause of cell death or an attempt to protect the neurone against toxins, and whether a physiological replacement of the nigrostriatal dopamine pathway early in the course of the disease could eliminate all its cardinal signs.

8.1 **The shaking palsy**

Main paper: Parkinson J. *An Essay on the Shaking Palsy.* London: Sherwood, Neely and Jones; 1817.

Background

It has remained something of a mystery why James Parkinson (1755–1824), an apothecary already in his sixty-second year, decided to write a 66-page treatise on an obscure nervous malady (Fig. 8.1). His only stated explanation was that the shaking palsy had not yet obtained a place in the classification of nosologists. As a young man, he had attended one of John Hunter's clinical demonstrations on tremor at the Royal College of Surgeons and may also have listened to the Croonian Lecture of 1776 where Hunter stated that 'Lord L's hands are almost perpetually in motion, and he never feels the sensation in them of being tired. When he is asleep his hands are perfectly at rest, but when he wakes in a little time they begin to move' [1]. Parkinson seems to have been one of those doctors who wrote up cases as part of a learning process with the intention of improving his clinical skills, and that may be sufficient justification. In his essay, he also expressed the hope that his clinical description would encourage the great anatomists of his day to find the underlying cause.

Methods

In the preface of his monograph, Parkinson emphasizes the need for repeated observation over a number of years and the differences between the early and late stages of the illness. Although uneven in content, the case reports have a modernity that was seldom matched by contemporary medical writers. His use of field neurology to identify affected cases and his aptitude in collating data over a protracted period of observation distinguish his description from the many piecemeal and fragmentary reports which preceded it. His review of the available historical literature is scholarly and characteristically thorough.

Results

All the cases were men, which may reflect the fact that far fewer women ventured into the dangerous squalid streets of nineteenth-century London. The first chapter begins with a review of the literature, followed by an overview of the natural history, emphasizing the insidious onset of the malady. Descriptions of six illustrative cases then follow, two of whom he had encountered and questioned in the street and another he had only seen at a distance. Parkinson considers a coarse tremor of the limbs at rest, lessened muscular power with an inability to respond to the dictate of the will, and a festinant gait as the cardinal triad. The sixth case had a 12-year history of disease and, having sustained a slight stroke, had been relieved of tremor in the weakened hand. He also notes that tremor could be interrupted by movement but could occur to a mild degree in the lighter stages of sleep. Parkinson also describes unilateral onset, the effortful nature of walking with risk of propulsion, problems of speech and swallowing, constipation, and the terminal phase of the illness with severe flexion of posture, delirium, and loss of sphincter controls.

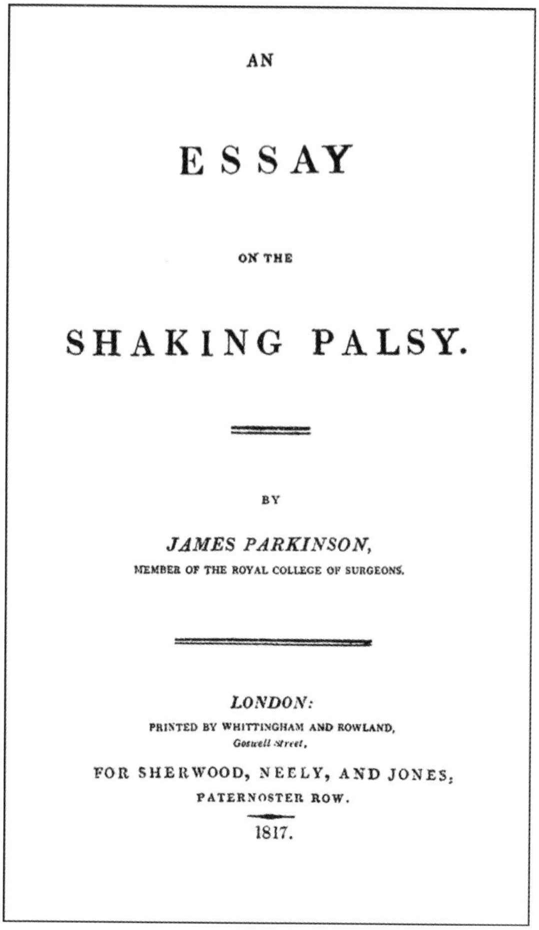

AN

ESSAY

ON THE

SHAKING PALSY.

BY

JAMES PARKINSON,

MEMBER OF THE ROYAL COLLEGE OF SURGEONS.

LONDON:

PRINTED BY WHITTINGHAM AND ROWLAND,

Goswell Street,

FOR SHERWOOD, NEELY, AND JONES,

PATERNOSTER ROW.

1817.

Fig. 8.1 The front cover of *An Essay on the Shaking Palsy* by James Parkinson, 1817.

On the grounds that all four limbs can be affected, followed by speech and swallowing difficulties, but that the senses and intellect are preserved, he speculates that trauma to the cervico-medullary junction is at fault. He concludes there is no effective treatment but is aware that early intervention is likely to be necessary for therapeutic success.

Conclusions and critique

During the eighteenth century, semiotics and nosology dominated medical thinking and diseases were classified on the grounds of clinical manifestations rather than their causation. English physician, Thomas Sydenham (1624–89), considered diseases 'as pre-existing specific entities that should be classified with the same care which we see exhibited by botanists in their phytologies' [2]. The clinico-anatomical method of Italian anatomist, Giovanni Battista Morgagni (1682–1771), linking diseases to pathology, was only beginning to be more widely accepted when Parkinson wrote *An Essay on the Shaking Palsy.*

Parkinson's monograph was acknowledged, if not widely read, in British medical circles after its publication. French neurologist, Jean-Martin Charcot (1825–1893), who experienced considerable difficulty in obtaining a copy, acknowledged the definition of the disorder now familiar to all movement disorder specialists:

> Involuntary tremulous motion, with lessened muscular power, in parts not in action and even when supported; with a propensity to bend the trunk forward, and to pass from a walking to a running pace: the senses and intellect being uninjured

Nevertheless, he considered Parkinson's description to be incomplete and added descriptions of the masked face and the notion of a variant without any tremor.

Parkinson failed to precisely distinguish paralysis from bradykinesia, but nor did anybody else for almost a century after his seminal description. He realized that field neurology based on careful observation was sufficient to make the diagnosis—a view to which Charcot would later subscribe when he wrote of paralysis agitans, 'I have seen such patients everywhere on the streets of Rome, of Amsterdam in Spain, it is always the same picture they can be identified from afar you do not need a medical history' [3].

The clinical features described by Parkinson were embellished by British neurologist. Sir William Richard Gowers (1845–1915), in his *Manual of the Diseases of the Nervous System*, the greatest single-author textbook of neurology ever to have been published, where, in over 18 pages, he describes his own findings on 50 men and 30 women. His lucid account is full of clinical pearls and augmented by his own sketches illustrating the simian posture and characteristic hand and foot deformities seen in the late stages of the disease [4]. Hoehn and Yahr, 80 years later, further emphasized the clinical heterogeneity of the malady, and provided important demographic data on the natural history and causes of death prior to the L-dopa era. They also devised a pragmatic five-point scale to describe the main stages of motor handicap [5].

8.2 **The black stuff**

Main paper: Tretiakoff KN. *Contribution a l' étude de l'anatomie pathologique du locus niger de Soemmering avec quelques déductions relatives à la pathogénie des troubles du tonus musculaire de la maladie de Parkinson.* Thèse Faculté de Médecine Paris; 1919.

Background

No consistent pathological lesion was found during the nineteenth century but, in 1893, Blocq and Marinesco published a case report describing a 38-year-old man who had died with unilateral signs of Parkinsonism and who had been found at necropsy to have an enucleated tuberculoma the size of a hazelnut in the contralateral substantia nigra. This, and one or two other similar case reports, led Édouard Brissaud (1852–1909), Charcot's successor, to speculate that ischaemia of the substantia nigra might be responsible for the disturbance of tone observed in cases of paralysis agitans [6]. Konstantin Nikolaevitch Tretiakoff (1892–1958) was born in Novvy-Margelan in Russia but, following his involvement in student demonstrations against the Czar, his father felt it better he continue his medical studies in Paris. In 1917, he was appointed Chief of the Laboratory in the Neurology Department at L'Hôpital Salpetrière—a menial, unpopular, and poorly paid post with no clinical responsibility. He had the good fortune, however, to work in the laboratory with Marinesco, and it may have been the Romanian who suggested the topic of his thesis.

Methods

Histological examination of 54 brains was undertaken, six of which had a clinical diagnosis of Parkinson's disease and three, post-encephalitic (von Economo's disease) Parkinsonism. Haematoxylin and eosin, Mann technique (methylene blue and eosin), Nissl method for formalin-fixed material, Bielschowsky method, and Alzheimer's method (aniline blue and Orange G after mordanting with phosphomolybdic acid) were some of the staining methods used.

Results

Marked loss of pigmented nerve cells with swelling of cell bodies, 'grumous degeneration', and neurofibrillary alterations was found in all six cases with Parkinson's disease. In some of the surviving nigral cells, he noted inclusion bodies which he referred to as 'corps de Lewy' in recognition of the description, by Friedrich Lewy (1885–1950), of similar inclusions in the dorsal nucleus of the vagus. In the three cases of von Economo's disease, he noted devastation of the substantia nigra with hyaline and granular degeneration. After careful consideration of his data and review of the existing contradictory literature, he concluded that the pigmented cells of the substantia nigra were invariably and severely affected in Parkinson's disease and usually associated with senile and vascular changes in other parts of the brain (Fig. 8.2). He also stated that similar findings could sometimes occur in other disorders with altered muscle tone, like torticollis and chorea.

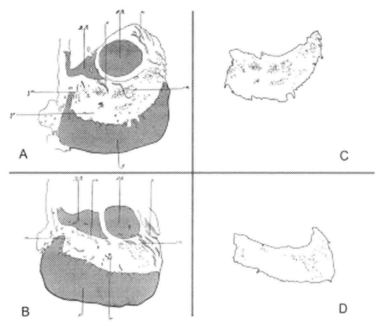

Fig. 8.2 Plates **A** and **B** are the original Figures 1 and 2 from Tretiakoff's doctoral thesis, probably drawn with the help of a camera lucida. Plates **C** and **D** are pictures drawn from A and B by selecting the neurones, in order to make the neuronal loss more easily visible. The original legends state (with modern-day terminology in brackets): Figure 1 [plate A]:— '. . . horizontal section of the cerebral peduncle [mesencephalon]. Normal aspect of the Locus Niger [substantia nigra]. . . Senile dementia, 80 years old. The numerous dots spread in the marginal zone [pas compacta] are normal pigmented neural cells. The ventral zone [pars reticulata] contains a few remaining neurones devoid of pigment and therefore, invisible with the low power view.' Figure 2 [plate B]: 'Typical Parkinson disease . . . Loss of a large number of neural cells of the Locus Niger [substantia nigra]. Those, which are spared, are in the process of degenerating.' The abbreviations are handwritten, probably by Tretiakoff himself: c.n., pigmented neural cells; N.R., red nucleus; P., pes penduculi; R.R., Reil's band [medial lemniscus]; r., roots of the third nerve; v., vessels; zm., marginal zone [pars compacta] of the Locus Niger [substantia nigra]; zv., ventral zone [pas reticulata] of the Locus Niger [substantia nigra].

Conclusions and critique

Tretiakoff could not have dreamed that his first research project would belatedly come to be accepted as the most important pathological lesion in Parkinson's disease. At the bicentenary celebrations in 1955 of James Parkinson's birth, J. Godwin Greenfield, the first neuropathologist appointed to the staff at the National Hospital, Queen Square, and whose own work had confirmed the Russian's findings, prophetically concluded:

> Paralysis agitans in its classical form is a systemic degeneration of a special type affecting a neuronal system whose nodal point is the substantia nigra. The cause of this neurodegeneration remains a problem whose solution may be found in enzyme chemistry or some other new field of investigation [7].

A year later, it was Greenfield who was responsible for finally honouring Tretiakoff at the International Congress of Neuropathology in London, a few months before the Russian's death at the age of 64.

Although much recent research has focused on alpha synuclein and Lewy bodies in sites outside the substantia nigra, greater understanding of the microarchitecture of the substantia nigra, including the significance of nigrosomes and the role of neuromelanin, remain important research goals. Severity of bradykinesia and rigidity correlate reasonably well with the degree of pars compacta nigral cell loss, and the recent progress made in the anatomical and functional neuroimaging of the nigrostriatal bundle is already aiding accurate clinical diagnosis in specific settings.

8.3 **The dopamine miracle**

Main paper: Ehringer H, Hornykiewicz O. Distribution of noradrenaline and dopamine (3-hydroxytyramine) in the human brain and their behavior in diseases of the extrapyramidal system. *Klin Wochenschr* 1960; 38:1236–9.

Background

Dopamine was first synthesized by Barger and Ewens in 1912 and was considered by Nobel Prize winning pharmacologist, Sir Henry Hallett Dale (1875–1968), to be a weak sympathomimetic adrenaline-like substance of minor interest to clinical pharmacologists. In 1956, British biochemist, Hermann Blaschko (1900–93), raised the possibility that it might be more than an inert precursor of noradrenaline and possess a physiological function of its own. On his return from a sabbatical working at the Laboratory of Chemical Pharmacology at the National Institutes of Health (NIH) Bethesda under Bernard B. Brodie, Swedish scientist, Arvid Carlsson, demonstrated that reserpine, an alkaloid extracted from the snake root plant (*Rauwolfia serpentina*) renowned in India for its sedative properties, could deplete noradrenaline in the rodent brain. Carlsson then showed that reserpine-induced catalepsy in rabbits could be reversed by L-dopa, despite its failure to restore brain noradrenaline levels. This finding led him to turn his attention to dopamine and, using a new assay procedure, he was able to show that the reversal of the behavioural effects correlated with the restoration of normal brain dopamine levels.

At a time when most of the debate centred around whether reserpine's antipsychotic properties were due to depletion of serotonin or noradrenaline, Carlsson reported, at the First Catecholamine Symposium in Bethesda in 1958, that dopamine served a function in its own right in the brain and that it was mainly concentrated in the rodent basal ganglia [8]. A year earlier, Montague, working in Weil-Malherbe's laboratory at Runwell Hospital in Wickford, UK, reported that dopamine was present in the mammalian brain, and Bertler and Rosengren [9] and Sano [10], then both independently and almost simultaneously, found that most of the dopamine was to be found in the basal ganglia where only traces of noradrenaline were present. Austrian biochemist, Oleh Hornykiewicz, who had been working with Blaschko, returned to his native Vienna and proceeded to investigate human post-mortem material for catecholamine abnormalities.

Methods

Homogenized brain material from 20 controls—two with Huntington's disease, six with extrapyramidal disease, six with Parkinson's syndrome (four, post- encephalitic; two, Parkinson's disease) was obtained from the Institute of Patho-Anatomy of the University of Vienna. The brains were dissected 3–20 hours after death and some of the tissue was fixed for histological examination. Other material was frozen immediately at –20°C and later thawed out for extraction of noradrenaline and dopamine using the method of Bertler, Carlsson, and Rosengren.

Results

Very high dopamine concentrations were found in the control basal ganglia with correspondingly low levels of noradrenaline. The six cases of Parkinson's syndrome had a marked and consistent 10-fold loss of dopamine in the putamen and caudate, whereas the Huntington's disease brains had normal levels. It was concluded that dopamine might play a significant role in the symptomatology of both Parkinson's disease and post-encephalitic Parkinsonism.

Conclusions and critique

These neurochemical findings were immediately accepted and the concept of striatal dopamine deficiency as the cause of bradykinesia, rigidity, and tremor in Parkinson's disease was soon standard textbook knowledge. The method also became a model for neurochemical study of other neurodegenerative diseases. Hornykiewicz's findings consolidated his pre-existing idea that it would be worth testing L-dopa in Parkinson's disease. He next approached Walther Birkmayer (1910–1996), a physician in charge of the neurological ward of the largest municipal home for the aged in Vienna, and, after some frustrating delays relating to difficult scientist–physician relationships, trials began with supplies of L-dopa provided by Hoffmann La Roche. Birkmayer injected 50–150 mg intravenously in saline into 20 volunteers with Parkinson's disease and post-encephalitic Parkinsonism. The results were impressive and Birkmayer later wrote:

> The effect of a single intravenous injection of l-dopa was, in short, a complete abolition or substantial relief of akinesia. Bed-ridden patients who were unable to sit up, patients who could not stand up when seated, and patients who when standing could not start walking performed after l-dopa all these activities with ease. They walked around with normal associated movements and they could even run and jump. The voiceless, aphonic speech, blurred by palilalia and unclear articulation, became forceful and clear as in a normal person. For short periods of time the people were able to perform motor activities which could not be prompted to any comparable degree by any other known drug [11].

The effects were reported to last from 3–24 hours and confined to improvement in bradykinesia, with no clear effect on tremor or rigidity. Pre-treatment with the monoamine oxidase inhibitor, isocarboxazid, increased and prolonged the anti-akinetic effect.

These findings were eventually published 11 months after the report of striatal dopamine deficiency in post-mortem brain, by which time Degkwitz [12] had reported improvement with L-dopa in reserpine-induced Parkinsonism and about the same time amelioration of rigidity for 2 hours after oral doses of 100–200 mg L-dopa (but not D-dopa) was described by Barbeau, Sourkes, and Murphy in Montreal [13].

To the sceptics, it seemed inconceivable that such efficacy could have resulted from a single dose of an amino acid for an incurable neurodegenerative disorder. Critics later attributed much of the effect to Birkmayer's charismatic personality, despite the fact that other intravenous injections with chemically related substances had not led to similar positive results.

8.4 **The magic of L-dopa**

Main paper: Cotzias GC, Van Woert MH, Schiffer LM. Aromatic amino acids and modification of parkinsonism. *New England Journal of Medicine* 1967; 276(7):374–9.

Background

The encouraging initial reports with L-dopa were not confirmed by some later placebo-controlled studies and the limited availability of the amino acid precluded longer-term studies. In 1965, anticholinergic drugs and stereotactic thalamotomy for tremor were the only available treatments for Parkinson's disease. Greek-born George Constantin Cotzias (1918–1977) had been working on manganese toxicity in Chilean miners and was interested in the possibility that a defect in melanogenesis might be the cause of Parkinson's disease. The phenothiazine anti-psychotics and manganese toxicity both caused Parkinsonism and were known to bind avidly to melanin granules. Furthermore, dopa was the amino acid precursor for both catecholamine biosynthesis and melanin formation.

Methods

Seventeen patients with Parkinson's disease and three controls were admitted to the metabolic ward at the Brookhaven National Laboratory on Long Island. Slowly increasing doses of beta melanocyte stimulating hormone (up to 40 mg/day), D-L dopa (3–16 grams/day) and D-L phenylalanine (1.6–12.6 grams/day) were given over several weeks, with some placebo control. Motor function was evaluated at baseline and then twice a day. The trial volunteers were asked to write a sentence, sit down and stand up, pick an object up from the floor, and draw a straight line. The number of steps required to walk 10 metres briskly was recorded. Rigidity, tremor, muscle strength, and mental state were also evaluated and, in some patients, sequential cinematographic records were taken.

Results

Beta melanocyte-stimulating hormone was administered to six patients and led to a reversible aggravation of tremor with transient diarrhoea and increased pigmentation of the skin. D-L dopa, on the other hand, led to complete sustained disappearance or marked amelioration of motor handicap in eight of the sixteen patients and modest benefit in a further two. Stiffness was the first symptom to improve, whereas tremor was much slower to come under control and required weeks of treatment at high dosage. Reversible choreoathetosis was a complication in some patients. Four of the responders who received the treatment for several months developed agranulocytopenia. The eight patients who had responded well to dopa were then given phenylalanine, which led to deterioration, from baseline, with exacerbation of tremor and rigidity in seven of them.

Conclusions and critique

Dopa might still be only of theoretical interest today if Cotzias and his colleagues had not had the conviction and perseverance to slowly push the dose into the therapeutic range and not be deterred by the reductions in white cell counts caused by the D-isomer. The use of pure L-dopa had been precluded by its prohibitive cost but, following the positive results, was soon made available for later studies. The fact that the paper was published in the reputable *New England Journal of Medicine* finally helped to convince the scientific world of the efficacy of dopa. Such was the Lazarus effect on severely handicapped patients of this naturally occurring amino acid, present in large quantities in broad beans, that it was hoped that the dopamine miracle would usher in a new era of scientific discovery in which neurochemical deficits would be identified in other neurodegenerative diseases with therapeutic ramifications.

The kind of meticulous observational pharmacological studies carried out by Cotzias on small groups of patients is regrettably now virtually impossible as a consequence of legal, ethical, and bureaucratic restraints, and clinical trials take three times longer than they did 25 years ago. Perhaps as a consequence of these restrictions, L-dopa is still, disappointingly, the most efficacious symptomatic therapy for Parkinson's disease, 40 years after its introduction. If it was submitted to the regulatory authorities today, critique of the trial design and fears relating to the drug's toxicity would almost certainly preclude it receiving a licence.

8.5 **The frozen addicts**

Main paper: Langston JW, Ballard P, Tetrud JW, Irwin I. Chronic Parkinsonism in humans due to a product of meperidine-analog synthesis. *Science* 1983; 219(4587): 979–80.

Background

In 1979, Davis and colleagues at the National Institutes of Mental Health, Bethesda, reported the case of a 23-year-old chemistry graduate who produced his own drugs and had been synthesizing and injecting a pethidine-like narcotic called MPPP (1-Methyl-4-phenyl-4-propionoxypiperidine). He subsequently developed irreversible Parkinsonism and died, and was found to have severe loss of neuromelanin- containing cells in the pars compacta of the substantia nigra [14].

Methods

Four heroin abusers (three men and one woman) aged between 26 and 42 years were admitted to hospital with acute severe Parkinsonism (Fig. 8.3). Two had taken a 'new heroin' sample in San José, California, and the other two, who were brothers, had obtained their batch in Watsonville. Dosages ranged between 5 g and 20 g taken over 4–8 days.

Results

Visual hallucinations, limb jerks, and stiffness were early symptoms, and severe slowness occurred within 4–14 days of the first intravenous injection. Examination revealed a complete inability to speak intelligibly, a flexed posture and shuffling gait, facial masking, and

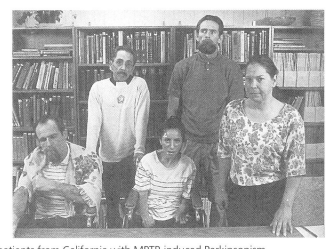

Fig. 8.3 The patients from California with MPTP-induced Parkinsonism.

severe bradykinesia and rigidity of the limbs. Three had apraxia of eyelid opening, two had a vertical gaze palsy, and one patient had a pill rolling rest tremor in the right hand. A heavy metal and toxicity screen was negative and Wilson's disease was excluded by normal caeruloplasmin levels and the absence of a Kayser-Fleischer ring. Computerized tomography of the brain was normal. All four patients responded extremely well to dopaminergic therapy but there was no spontaneous remission after five months of follow up.

Analysis of samples of the ingested white crystalline powder revealed that it contained 3% MPTP (1-methyl-4-phenyl-1,2,3,6-tetrahydropyridine) and 0.3% MPPP (by weight). After replicating the student's synthetic method reported in the paper by Davis and colleagues, it was concluded that the kitchen chemist (BK) had injected a mixture of MPPP and MPTP. Analysis of material injected by the Californian cases confirmed similar findings, and the authors concluded that MPTP was the likely culprit.

Conclusions and critique

The course of MPTP-induced Parkinsonism is static or very slowly progressive and the pathological lesion is believed to be more restrictive than occurs in sporadic Parkinson's disease. Lewy bodies have also not been conclusively demonstrated either in the patients who have died or in laboratory animals. MPTP is not, in itself, toxic but once it has entered the brain it is metabolized into the toxic cation MPP + (1-methyl-4-phenylpyridinium) by monoamine oxidase B in glial cells. MPP + interferes with complex 1 of the electron transport chain—a component of mitochondrial respiratory chain metabolism—and leads to cell death. The selectivity of MPTP toxicity is believed to be due to a high affinity uptake process involving the dopamine transporter. The MPTP-lesioned non-human primate is still the best animal model for evaluating new drug treatments in Parkinson's disease and the MPTP story fuelled an ongoing research interest in the possibility of environmental toxicity in Parkinson's disease. The mechanisms underlying MPP + mitochondrial toxicity may also have relevance to monogenetic forms of Parkinsonism like PINK1.

8.6 **The subthalamic nucleus of Luys**

Main paper: Bergman H, Wichmann T, DeLong MR. Reversal of experimental Parkinsonism by lesions of the subthalamic nucleus. *Science* 1990; 249(4975):1436–8.

Background

Unilateral lesions of the subthalamic nucleus cause contralateral hemichorea and hemiballismus but no clinical reports existed of a focal lesion of the structure alleviating Parkinsonism. Pre-clinical evidence had accumulated to indicate that loss of dopamine in Parkinson's disease causes an increased inhibitory output from the basal ganglia to the thalamus. Differential effects of dopamine occurred in the striato-pallidal pathway so that a decreased activity of striatal neurons occurred in the direct pathway to the globus pallidus interna, whereas an increased inhibitory effect was seen in the indirect pathway to the globus pallidus externa. Excessive output from the subthalamic nucleus to the internal pallidum raised the possibility that reduction could potentially improve Parkinsonism (Fig. 8.4).

Methods

Recording chambers were attached to the skull in two African green monkeys to allow access to the subthalamic region. Motor behaviour was quantified before and after treatment with the nigral neurotoxin, MPTP. Akinesia occurred after 5 days followed, a few days later, by rigidity with cogwheeling and a 5 Hz limb tremor. A combined injection and recording device was then inserted and ibotenic acid injected into the subthalamic nucleus under electrophysiological guidance.

Results

Within a minute of the chemical lesion, the animals began to move the akinetic contralateral limbs and to feed and groom themselves, and tremor was virtually abolished. Torque studies also revealed reduced stiffness in the contralateral limb. Chorea was seen in both animals in the contralateral limbs within the first 24 hours of the lesion but disappeared in one, and lessened in the other, over the 3 weeks of follow up. Although marked improvement persisted, there was also some residual akinesia and clumsiness. Histopathological examination confirmed severe loss of tyrosine hydroxylase immunoreactive pars compacta nigral cells and cresyl violet staining revealed marked gliosis and selective loss of neurons in the subthalamic nucleus.

Conclusions and critique

This study provided the scientific rationale for stereotactic deep brain stimulation [15] and lesioning [16] of the subthalamic nucleus in Parkinson's disease. It also provided evidence that abnormalities in basal ganglia circuitry were involved in the pathogenesis of rest tremor and support for the notion that akinesia resulted from excessive electrical activity

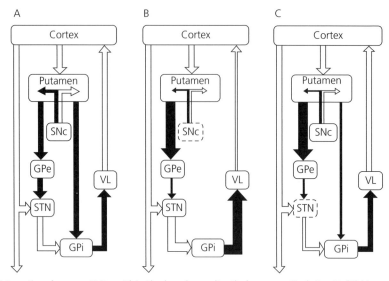

Fig. 8.4 Functional connectivity within the basal ganglia–thalamo–cortical circuit. (**A**) Normal. Open arrows, excitatory connections; filled arrows, inhibitory connections. The putamen (the 'input' stage of the circuit) is connected with GPi (the 'output' stage) by direct and indirect projections (via GPe and the STN). The postulated differential effects of dopamine on the two striatal output systems are indicated schematically. (**B**) MPTP-induced Parkinsonism. After treatment with MPTP, the SNc is damaged. Resulting changes in the overall activity in individual projection systems are indicated by changes in the width of arrows. Inactivation of the nigroputaminal projection increases GPi activity, secondary to an increase in excitatory drive from the STN and a decrease in direct inhibitory input from the striatum. The resulting over-inhibition of thalamocortical circuits may account for some of the Parkinsonian motor signs. (**C**) Effect of STN lesions in Parkinsonism. Inactivation of the STN reduces GPi output to the thalamus towards more normal levels, thus reducing Parkinsonian motor signs. (SNc, substantia nigra pars compacta; VL, ventrolateral nucleus of the thalamus.)

Reproduced from *Science*, 249(4975), Bergman, H, Wichmann, T, DeLong MR, Reversal of experimental Parkinsonism by lesions of the subthalamic nucleus, p. 1436–1438, Copyright (1990), with permission from the American Association for the Advancement of Science.

in the subthalamic nucleus and internal segment of the globus pallidus and should no longer be looked upon as a 'negative sign' of basal ganglia disease. Although not a cure for Parkinson's disease, deep brain stimulation of the subthalamic nucleus and globus pallidus can now stake a claim for being the second most efficacious symptomatic therapy behind L-dopa.

8.7 **Brain grafting**

Main paper: Lindvall O, Brundin PE, Widner H, et al. Grafts of fetal dopamine neurons survive and improve motor function in Parkinson's disease. *Science* 1990; 247(4942):574–7.

Background

Transplantation of cells and tissues of the brain has a history going back to the late nineteenth century. The idea of using cell transplants to replace damaged dopamine neurons and re-innervate the striatum occurred in the early 1980s, at a time when the shortcomings of long-term oral L-dopa therapy were increasingly apparent. Swedish neurosurgeon, Erik Olof Backlund, first carried out striatal implants at the Karolinska Institute in Stockholm, Sweden, on two patients, using their own adrenal medullas. Lars Olson, who had provided the scientific rationale for the procedures, then collaborated with the neurologist, Olle Lindvall, who devised a more rigorous protocol for assessment in future studies. Two more adrenal medullary implant operations were then carried out, in 1986, with reports of modest benefit. Lindvall reported the results at the New York Academy of Sciences and was heavily criticized on the grounds that the clinical studies were premature. One of the ethical issues relating to fetal implantation was whether the disease would damage the transplant. The authors argued that if the disease process was intrinsic to the neurons, then the grafted cells would be unaffected, but if it was extrinsic and due to a toxic mechanism, then the new cells might also be damaged.

In 1987, Ignacio Madrazo published positive results in the *New England Journal of Medicine* of caudate adrenal medullary grafts in two patients in their thirties. A glowing editorial accompanied the article and many of those who had been critical of the procedure changed their mind overnight. Eventually, however, Madrazo's claims were found to be unjustified. Nonetheless, encouraging preclinical experiments with fetal tissue transplantation in six hydroxydopamine-lesioned rodents began in Sweden in late 1985, and Lindvall and Anders Björklund then decided to go ahead with the first transplantation with fetal tissue in 1987.

Methods

A 49-year-old man with Parkinson's disease who had presented, in 1977, with unilateral tremor and rigidity in the right arm and had responded well to L-dopa but developed severe refractory motor fluctuations and dyskinesias was selected for surgery. At the time of first assessment, he continued to have an excellent response to L-dopa (700 mg/day) combined with bromocripitine and benzhexol when 'on' but had four or five refractory troughs of severe motor handicap with asymmetrical bradykinesia, rigidity, and tremor, worse on the right than left. He was assessed regularly for 11 months before surgery at the University of Lund Neurology Department. Immunosuppression with azathioprine was begun 2 days before the operation. Dissociated ventral mesencephalic tissue from four 8–9-week fetuses was implanted stereotactically with a very thin cannula into the left putamen. A protocol called the Core Assessment Programme for Intracerebral Transplantations in

Parkinson's disease (CAPIT) was used to counter the shortcomings of an open design study on small numbers of patients and was combined with the use of pre- and post-operative 18F Fluorodopa positron emission tomography (PET) to provide evidence for survival and growth of the graft.

Results

A marked reduction in 'off' period duration, nocturnal and early morning immobility, and the severity of rigidity and bradykinesia, especially on the contralateral side to the graft, started about 2 months after surgery and persisted for the following 3 months. Fluorodopa PET studies carried out at the Hammersmith Hospital in London, UK, 5 months after the operation, indicated an increased tracer uptake of 130% in the left putamen compared with baseline scanning and restored dopamine synthesis and storage on the grafted side (Fig. 8.5).

Conclusions and critique

The first two fetal implants were unsuccessful and the size of the cannula was identified as one contributory factor. The delay in the therapeutic improvement and the sustained benefit seen in the third patient described in this report who underwent surgery made it unlikely that the degree of benefit could be entirely attributed to a placebo response. Other

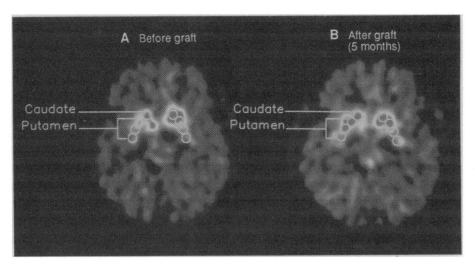

Fig. 8.5 PET scans obtained with 6-L-[18F] fluorodopa at the level of the caudate and putamen. The scan shows activity in caudate and putamen (**A**) before and (**B**) after the grafting. A clear focal increase of the tracer is seen in the anterior aspect of the left putamen. The colour code is arbitrary, with red representing the highest uptake and blue the lowest.

Reproduced from *Science*, 247(4942), Lindvall O, Brundin PE, Widner H, Rehnecrona S, Gustavii B, Frackowiak R, Leenders KL, Sawle G, Rothwell JC, Marsden CD, Björklund A, Grafts of fetal dopamine neurons survive and improve motor function in Parkinson's disease, p. 574–577, Copyright (1990), with permission from the American Association for the Advancement of Science.

open label programmes followed in a number of countries and were complemented by two controlled studies with sham surgery in the USA. It became clear that efficacy was extremely variable, even within the same centre. Furthermore, with one or two notable exceptions, overall amelioration of motor handicap did not exceed the best results with subcutaneous apomorphine pump therapy or deep brain stimulation of the subthalamic nucleus. Reports of severe graft-induced 'runaway' dyskinesias, possibly due to the creation of 'hot spots' in a supersensitive corpus striatum or to serotonergic hyperinnervation, along with continuing difficulties in harvesting fetal tissue have further slowed research progress.

Human neuroblasts for transplantation by pre-differentiation from stem cells have now been produced in several laboratories, but concerns about tumour formation have not yet been allayed and further animal studies are needed to show that these cells can reinnervate the striatum and restore dopamine release *in vivo*. To be effective, it is probable that at least 100,000 cell-derived dopamine neuroblasts with the phenotypic characteristics of human pars compacta nigral cells will need to be implanted into each putamen. The ideal candidate for future trials should be free from severe L-dopa-induced dyskinesias and have dopaminergic denervation largely restricted to the dorsal striatum.

8.8 **A pre-symptomatic phase**

Main paper: Fearnley JM, Lees AJ. Ageing and Parkinson's disease: substantia nigra regional selectivity. *Brain* 1991; 114:2283–301.

Background

Accelerated ageing was still considered to be a possible cause for Parkinson's disease at the time of publication of this paper. A second hypothesis had also recently suggested that neuronal loss due to ageing could decompensate previous subclinical damage to the substantia nigra that had occurred in the first two decades of life and result in the much later appearance of bradykinesia. About a third of patients were known to have a prodromata of non-specific symptoms prior to the onset of motor symptoms, but research into the tempo of neurodegeneration in Parkinson's disease was hampered by limited information on the speed of nigral neuronal loss.

Methods

A semi-quantitative study of the pars compacta of the substantia nigra was performed on 36 control brains with ages ranging from 21–91, 7 additional incidental Lewy body pathology controls, 20 Parkinson's disease brains, 15 MSA-P brains, and 14 PSP brains. A single 7 mu haematoxylin- and eosin-stained section of the caudal nigra was used for morphometry. In each case, the nigra was divided into ventral and dorsal tiers and split into six morphometric regions by marking the coverslip of the slide with a Rotring pen under 40x and 100x magnification. Slides were coded to blind the morphometrist from the age at death. Pigmented cells were counted twice using the cell body and then the nucleolus. Counting was carried out under 400x magnification using an eyepiece graticule. The regional counts were summated to give the total nigral count. Corrections of the counts for age were made and the pathological count expressed as a percentage of the predicted control.

Results

Using regression analysis, the pre-symptomatic phase of nigral cell loss was calculated to be 4.7 years. During this asymptomatic period, 64% of ventrolateral tier and 31% of total nigral cell loss had occurred. The loss due to ageing was calculated from the control regression equations and found to be 24–26% of the total count and 10–11% of the ventrolateral count. The average combined nigral count at the time of symptom onset was 48% total count and 68% ventrolateral count. Based on the findings in those brains with Parkinson's disease, it was predicted that two of the incidental Lewy body cases might have had subtle bradykinetic symptoms at the time of their death, both aged 78. In Parkinson's disease, there was an exponential or possibly sigmoid loss of cells, with 45% of total neuronal loss occurring in the first 10 years of disease—a figure 10 times greater than that found in normal ageing where a linear fallout of pigmented neurons at a rate of 4.8% per decade, with a predilection for the dorsal tier, was found (Fig. 8.6).

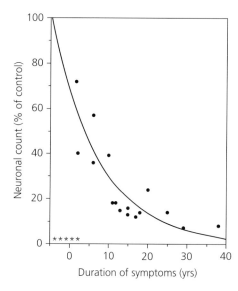

Fig. 8.6 Total age-adjusted nigral cell count vs symptom duration in cases with Parkinson's disease.

Reproduced from *Brain*, 114, JM Fearnley, AJ Lees, Ageing and Parkinson's disease: substantia nigra regional selectivity, p. 2283–2301, Copyright (1991), with permission from Oxford University Press.

Conclusions and critique

The lasting importance of this paper was that it was one of the first pathological studies to focus on the possibility of a compensatory phase before the emergence of motor symptoms in Parkinson's disease and to raise the possibility that nigral cell loss might begin only a few years prior to the onset of the presenting symptoms, a finding that was subsequently supported by functional imaging studies and two other pathological investigations. The study also provided further support for the notion that individuals with incidental Lewy body pathology in their brains might represent an at-risk group for Parkinson's disease [17] and that the ventrolateral tier of the nigra is the earliest and most severely damaged region of the pars compacta in both incidental Lewy body pathology brains and Parkinson's disease [18].

8.9 **The first cause**

Main paper: Polymeropolous M, Lavedan C, Leroy E, et al. Mutation in the alpha synuclein gene identified in families with Parkinson's disease. *Science* 1997; 276:2045–7.

Background

In the late 1980s, much research into the pathogenesis of Parkinson's disease was focused on the search for environmental risk factors and, although hereditary factors had been acknowledged in some cases, for a century, the disease was regarded as a sporadic disorder. A large family of Italian descent, with early onset Parkinson's disease, had been carefully studied by the neurologists at Robert Wood Johnson University, New Jersey, USA and more than 60 affected cases identified, but neither genetic linkage or the causative locus could be found. Directors of the then National Human Genome Research Institute (NHGRI) and National Institute of Neurological Disorders and Stroke (NINDS) intervened, and the samples were sent to the laboratory of Dr Bob Nussbaum at NIH. In 1996, his group identified genetic markers on chromosome 4q21-q23 that segregated with disease.

Methods

The region of the genome on chromosome 4, co-inheriting with disease, was first defined by running genetic markers from all across the genome through the family. The genes in this segment were then sequenced, one by one, by polymerase chain reaction amplification of each exon. Alpha synuclein was identified as a strong candidate and a variant was finally identified in all affected family members. They then tested other Italian and Greek families to see if this mutation turned up again, as well as sequencing large numbers of control samples to check it was not a normal harmless variant.

Results

A mutation of a single base pair in the presynaptic 140 amino acid protein alpha synuclein (G209A substitution resulting in an alanine 53 threonine amino acid substitution) was found in the large kindred and then in three smaller, apparently unrelated, Greek families with Parkinsonism (Fig. 8.7). The pattern of inheritance was confirmed as autosomal dominant. It was proposed that the mutation led to either an increased production of alpha synuclein or the formation of an abnormal toxic form causing beta sheets to aggregate and damage nerve cells.

Conclusions and critique

The importance of this work is that it led directly to the identification of the first precise cause of Parkinson's disease and focused attention of scientists on alpha synuclein, which was rapidly identified as an important component of Lewy bodies [19]. Prior to the discovery of the mutation, fragments of alpha synuclein had also been identified in the non-beta component of amyloid plaques, raising the possibility that Alzheimer's and Parkinson's disease may share some pathogenic mechanisms. It also proved, once and for all,

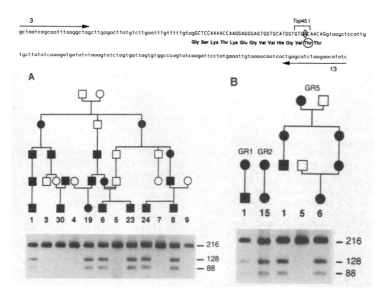

Fig. 8.7 Mutation of a single base pair in the presynpatic 140 amino acid protein, alpha synuclein. Oligonucleotide primers are shown by arrows and the numerals 3 and 13. Intron sequence is shown in lower case and exon sequence in upper case. Amino acid translation of the exon is shown below the DNA sequence. The circled base represents the G209A in the mutant allele. The resulting amino acid Ala53Thr change is represented by the circled amino acid. Mutation analysis of the G209A change is shown in a sub-pedigree of the Italian kindred (**A**) and the three Greek pedigrees (**B**). Filled symbols represent affected individuals. Numerical identifiers denote the individuals immediately above. Tsp45 I digestion of PCR products is shown at the bottom of the figure, and fragment sizes are indicated on the right, in base pairs.

Reproduced from *Science*, 276(5321), Polymeropolous M., Lavedan C., Leroy E., et al., Mutation in the alpha synuclein gene identified in families with Parkinson's disease, p. 2045–7, Copyright (1997), with permission from the American Association for the Advancement of Science.

that genetic factors were important in Parkinson's disease and presaged the identification of many other genetic loci and risk factors. Genome-wide association studies have linked SNCA (the gene coding for alpha synuclein) to sporadic Parkinson's disease. Production of toxic alpha synuclein protofibrils due to abnormal oligomeric conformations may mediate cell death in sporadic cases, and synuclein vaccines are under development to try to arrest disease progression. Although alpha synuclein deposition occurs early in the disease, it is still uncertain whether it is a primary factor in the disease process. Alpha synuclein pathology in the central nervous system is mainly deposited in neuritic processes and it is believed to be involved in neurotransmitter release. It has also been found in tissues like the gut and the olfactory bulb, not traditionally associated with Parkinson's disease.

Two other autosomally dominantly inherited gene mutations and six recessively inherited genes have now been identified, accounting for around 5% of all cases previously diagnosed as having sporadic Parkinson's disease. One of the most interesting recent genetic insights into Parkinson's disease has come from the finding that there is an increased frequency of mutations in the genes for Gaucher's disease, glucocerebrosidase (GBA), among patients with Parkinson's disease [20] which, in some Levantine and North African populations, is a risk factor in up to 20% of cases. This is the first example in genetics where heterozygosity for a recessive gene has been shown to predispose to a different late-onset disease. The finding has also directed attention to the lysosome in the pathogenesis of the disease.

8.10 **Spread of the disease process**

Main paper: Li JY, Englund E, Holton J, et al. Lewy bodies in grafted neurons in subjects with Parkinson's disease suggest host to graft propagation. *Nature Medicine* 2008; 14:501–3.

Background

Grafts of fetal ventral mesencephalic tissue can produce long-lasting functional benefits in some patients with Parkinson's disease. PET fluorodopa and raclopride studies showed that grafted neurons were functionally integrated and could release dopamine for more than 10 years after implantation. Post-mortem examination of grafted patients who died less than 5 years after transplantation showed large numbers of surviving dopaminergic neurons in the grafts.

Methods

A post-mortem examination, including neuropathological examination of the whole brain, was carried out on one patient who had died of a cardiac arrest. The brain was removed and fixed in 6% buffered formaldehyde solution and, after 2 months' fixation, the basal ganglia and midbrain was cut into 10–15 mm blocks for frozen section preparations. The remaining brain slices, including small slices of the basal ganglia, were paraffin embedded for subsequent sectioning. 5 mu sections were stained with haematoxylin and eosin for routine morphology, and with Luxol fast blue with Nissl counterstaining for myelin and intracellular structures. The second patient, with a 12-year-old graft, whose brain had been donated to the Queen Square Brain Bank (at The National Hospital for Neurology and Neurosurgery, London, UK) and who had died of aspiration pneumonia, had the left-half brain flash frozen and the other half fixed in 10% buffered formalin. Immunohistochemistry and cell counting were carried out.

Results

Both patients died from causes unrelated to Parkinson's disease and had severe nigral loss and Lewy bodies in several brain regions including the substantia nigra. Consistent with functional imaging studies performed during life, both brains contained large numbers of dopaminergic neurons in the graft. Alpha synuclein was found in 40% of tyrosine hydroxylase positive grafted cells in the 12-year-old implant and in 80% of the 16-year-old graft—similar figures to expression detected in the host nigras (Fig. 8.8). Alpha synuclein and ubiquitin immunoreactive Lewy bodies and Lewy neuritis were found in some surviving graft cells in both cases. This suggests that the alpha synuclein pathology spreads slowly over time, at a rate of about 1% per year.

Conclusions and critique

Support for these findings came in the same issue of *Nature Medicine*, from a paper published by Kordower and colleagues in which they reported similar findings in a patient

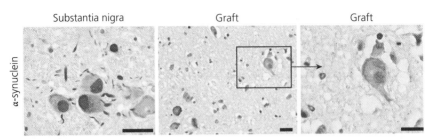

Fig. 8.8 Classical Lewy bodies and Lewy neurites in neurons of the substantia nigra (left) and in the grafts (middle and right) are immunoreactive for α-synuclein in paraffin-embedded tissue sections.

Reproduced from *Nature Medicine*, 14, Li J-Y, England E, Holton JL, Soulet D, Hagell P, et al., Lewy bodies in grafted neurons in subjects with Parkinson's disease suggest host-to-graft disease propagation, p. 501–503, Copyright (2008), with permission from Macmillan.

grafted 14 years earlier [21]. Interestingly, previous pathological studies had not revealed the presence of Lewy bodies or Lewy neurites in patients dying 18–52 months post grafting. The finding of Lewy bodies in some grafted neurons could be interpreted as supporting the notion of permissive templating, in which disease propagation can occur along neuronal pathways in Parkinson's disease and spread to the graft tissue by a prion-like mechanism triggered by misfolding of alpha synuclein in the host. Braak and Braak, based on neuroanatomical studies relating to Lewy body distribution in post-mortem brain, have also suggested that the disease may start in the gut, sympathetic ganglia, and olfactory bulb, and then spread into the medulla before ascending up the brain stem into the cerebral cortex [22]. If this is correct, then it implies that very early intervention will be required to arrest the disease process. Alternatively, it may be a reaction to inflammation at the graft–host interface, possibly mediated by cellular stress induced by reactive microglia. In a later publication on the original patient described by Lindvall and colleagues (see section 8.7) where unilateral grafting was followed, 4 years later, by a graft on the other side, both grafts contained Lewy bodies (2% of surviving neurons in the 12-year-graft and 5% in the 16-year-old-graft, in the same patient).

Although increased alpha synuclein could be detrimental to grafted neurons and limit the potential of cell-based therapies, the fact that functional imaging has confirmed that fetal grafts can still synthesize and release normal amounts of dopamine 10 years after implantation, with associated clinical benefit in some patients, is encouraging and suggests that although some of the grafted neurons may be compromised by Lewy body formation, the majority seem to function effectively.

Key unanswered questions

1   Can we improve on early accurate diagnosis?

A period of compensation in the brain seems likely before the emergence of the first detectable symptoms of Parkinson's disease. The latent interval before the onset of the pathological process is considered to be, at least, several years. Impaired olfaction and REM (rapid eye movement) sleep behaviour disorder are now considered risk factors for the development of Parkinson's disease and subtle, and sometimes intermittent, difficulties with motor function are also reported in some patients, extending back several years before the diagnosis is made. Carriers of the LRRK-2 and GBA genetic mutations are recognized genetic risk factors. An important research aim, therefore, is to identify a group of individuals with increased risk of developing Parkinson's disease, with a view to conducting trials with putative neuroprotective agents.

2   Why is Parkinson's disease asymmetrical?

Pathological studies and functional imaging have demonstrated that there is greater nigral cell loss in the side of the brain contralateral to the more severely affected limbs in patients with asymmetrical Parkinson's disease. Although there is no significant difference in the number of cases presenting with right- or left-sided symptoms, some association between dominant left-handedness and left-sided presentation has been reported. Nigral cell counts on the two sides of the brain in normal controls and in individuals dying with incidental Lewy body pathology may help to answer whether unilateral presentation reflects an intrinsic developmental difference in the number of nigral neurons on the two sides of the brain.

3   Is there a second Parkinson's disease?

Lewy body pathology and nigral cell loss have been associated with a dementing syndrome characterized by delirium, visual hallucinations, and prominent visuo-spatial difficulties (dementia with Lewy bodies) and also with a later onset Parkinsonism (usually presenting over 65 years of age) with prominent early axial and bulbar symptoms, poorer response to L-dopa, and a more rapid deterioration to the terminal milestones of falls, visual hallucinations, and dementia. Many of these patients die within 10 years of the onset of symptoms and have greater tau, beta amyloid, and cortical Lewy body burden at autopsy than the classical presentation. The respective roles of Alzheimer pathology and cerebrovascular disease in this 'senile' Parkinsonism need to be further characterized.

4   Is Parkinson's disease a dopamine deficiency disorder?

Drugs enhancing dopaminergic transmission are the most efficacious symptomatic therapy for Parkinson's disease, and the severity of dopaminergic cell loss in the pars compacta of the substantia nigra correlates reasonably well with the severity of bradykinesia. Damage to non-dopaminergic systems also occurs but its clinical relevance still remains to be clarified. Monogenic autosomal recessive Parkinsonism due to parkin mutations and MPTP-induced Parkinsonism, where the lesion is centred on the substantia nigra, has a more benign prognosis than Parkinson's disease and is not linked with dementia, whereas autosomal dominant Parkinsonism due to alpha synuclein mutations has, not uncommonly, associated memory and visuospatial cognitive impairment. Further insight into this critical question can potentially be provided by early physiological restoration of normal striatal dopaminergic transmission by cell-based or gene-therapy approaches.

5 What is the mechanism of alpha synuclein spread?

The spread of alpha synuclein pathology, as proposed by Braak and Braak, from the enteric nervous system and the olfactory bulb into the brain, would require transport of aggregated protein along long unmyelinated neurons with seeding in new nerve cells, in a process that occurs over many years. Recent experimental studies have demonstrated that alpha synuclein can transfer from cell to cell, but no study has demonstrated transport of alpha synuclein from one brain structure to another in Parkinson's disease. Identifying the precise mechanisms of cell to cell spread and transport of alpha synuclein might lead to the development of agents that could block this process and prevent disease spread in the brain.

References

1 **Hunter J.** Croonian Lecture recorded in *Hunterian Reminiscences* edited by Parkinson JWK Sherwood Gilbert and Piper, London 1833.

2 **Sydenham T.** *Observationes medicae circa morborum acutorum historiam et curationem.* London: G Kettilby; 1676.

3 **Charcot J-M.** *Lecons du Mardi: Policlinique: 1887–1888.* Paris: Bureaux du Progres Medical; 1888.

4 **Gowers W.** *A Manual of Diseases of the Nervous System.* London: Churchill; 1886.

5 **Hoehn MM, Yahr MD.** *Parkinsonism: onset, progression and mortality. Neurology* 1967; **17**(5):427–42.

6 **Brissaud E.** *Nature et pathogenie de la maladie de Parkinson (lecon 23). Lecons sur les Maladies du Systeme Nerveux. Recueiles et Publiees par Henry Meige.* Paris: Masson; 1895; 488–501.

7 **Critchley M.** *A bicentenary volume of papers dealing with Parkinson's Disease, incorporating the original 'Essay on the Shaking Palsy.'* Macmillan 1955.

8 **Carlsson A.** et al. *On the presence of 3-hydroxytyramine in brain. Science* 1958; **127**(3296):471.

9 **Bertler A, Rosengren E.** *Occurrence and distribution of dopamine in brain and other tissues. Experientia* 1959; **15**(1):10–11.

10 **Sano I, et al.** *Distribution of catechol compounds in human brain. Biochim Biophys Acta* 1959; **32**:586–7.

11 **Birkmayer W, Hornykiewicz O.** *The L-3,4-dioxyphenylalanine (DOPA)-effect in Parkinson-akinesia. Wien Klin Wochenschr* 1961; **73**: 787–8.

12 **Degkwitz R, et al.** *On the effects of L-dopa in man and their modification by reserpine, chlorpromazine, iproniazid and vitamin B6. Klin Wochenschr* 1960; **38**:120–3.

13 **Barbeau A, Murphy GF, Sourkes TL.** *Excretion of dopamine in diseases of basal ganglia. Science* 1961; **133**(3465):1706–7.

14 **Davis GC, et al.** *Chronic Parkinsonism secondary to intravenous injection of meperidine analogues. Psychiatry Res* 1979; **1**(3):249–54.

15 **Limousin P, et al.** *Effect of Parkinsonian signs and symptoms of bilateral subthalamic nucleus stimulation. Lancet* 1995; **345**(8942):91–5.

16 **Alvarez L, et al.** *Dorsal subthalamotomy for Parkinson's disease. Mov Disord* 2001; **16**(1):72–8.

17 **Forno L, Alvord E.** *The pathology of Parkinsonism: some new observations and correlations.* In: McDowell F, Markham C, ed. *Contemporary Neurology Series: Recent Advances in Parkinson's Disease.* Oxford: Blackwell Scientific; 1971; 119–30.

18 **Hassler R.** *Zur pathologie der paralysis agitans und des post-enzephalitischen Parkinsonismus. J Psychol Neurol* 1938; **48**:387–476.

19 **Spillantini MG, et al.** *Alpha-synuclein in Lewy bodies. Nature* 1997; **388**(6645):839–40.

20 **Sidransky E, et al.** *Multicenter analysis of glucocerebrosidase mutations in Parkinson's disease. N Engl J Med* 2009; **361**(17):1651–61.

21 **Kordower JH, et al.** *Lewy body-like pathology in long-term embryonic nigral transplants in Parkinson's disease. Nat Med* 2008; **14**(5):504–6.

22 **Braak H, et al.** *Staging of brain pathology related to sporadic Parkinson's disease. Neurobiol Aging* 2003; **24**(2):197–211.

Chapter 9

Motor neurone disease

Andrew Eisen

9.0 **Introduction**

Motor meurone disease (better known as amyotrophic lateral sclerosis, or Lou Gehrig's disease or Charcot's disease), is one of the major neurodegenrerations, uniquely restricted to humans. Early, comprehensive descriptions of motor neurone disease (MND), were ascribed to Jean-Martin Charcot (1825–1893), from Paris, where he established a neurological clinic at the Salpetriere Hospital. It is interesting to speculate why amytrophic lateral sclerosis (ALS) and other human neurodegenerations were not recognized before the mid-nineteenth century. Increasing longevity from that time is certainly relevant, but other, thus far unrecognized factors, possibly associated with the rise of the Industrial Revolution and a much altered human life style, must surely play a role.

Since Charcot's original descriptions of MND (1865), the literature on the subject has expanded exponentially. In 2014, the US National Library of Medicine cited approximately 32,000 papers. Sadly, despite the vast amount of research on ALS in the last decades, meaningful therapy and preventive measures remain elusive, and many important questions about the disease remain unanswered.

In this chapter, the '10 key papers' related to MND have been selected on the basis that each contributed significantly to an important, but unanswered question about the disease. Particular questions were asked, as indicated in the title of each paper. Given the huge publication record on MND and the many hundreds of very important contributions, it was a daunting task to choose 10. It is hoped that readers will view each in their correct context, namely 'a road to travel down and explore the many paths that lead from it'. Undoubtedly, there are other papers that could have equally or, maybe, even been better employed for the task at hand, and I apologize in advance to authors who would have selected their own or other works. Despite this limitation, it is believed that, taken together, the choice of papers made will introduce significant provocation and food for further thought.

9.1 **The first cases of amyotrophic lateral sclerosis**

Main paper: Veltema AN. The case of the saltimbanque Prosper Lecomte. A contribution to the study of the history of progressive muscular atrophy (Aran-Duchenne) and amyotrophic lateral sclerosis (Charcot). *Clin Neurol Neurosurg* 1975; 78:204–9.

Background

The French physician, Jean-Martin Charcot (1825–1893), coined the term 'sclérose latérale amyotrophique', emphasizing that both upper and lower motor neuron deficits characterized the disease. Charcot published a case of ALS in as early as 1865, in a female previously considered a 'hysteric'. However, prior to this, a pure lower motor neuron (LMN) syndrome termed 'progressive muscular atrophy' (now accepted as part of the spectrum of ALS/MND) was described by Cruveilhier (Fig. 9.1), Duchenne de Boulogne in France [1], and by Lockhart Clarke (1817–1880) [2] in the United Kingdom, who had made observations about the upper motor neuron (UMN) involvement well before Charcot.

Methods

In September 1848, Prosper Lecomte, a 30-year-old proprietor of a small circus, arrived in a town to prepare for some performances. Several weeks later, Lecomte noticed a certain weakness in the right hand. This inconvenience was slowly progressive. However, in January 1849, he was still able to write a letter. In July 1849, he observed a weakness in both

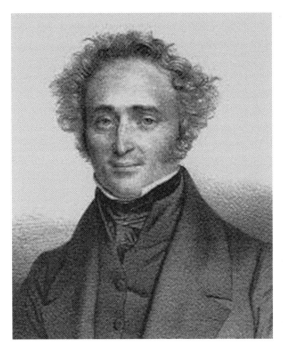

Fig. 9.1 Jean Cruveilhier, 1791–1874. In 1853, Cruveilhier described the case history of Prosper Lecomte, a French circus owner [2]. He appears to be the first patient in the historical literature in whom the diagnosis of ALS can be established with sufficient certainty.

legs. Walking became tiresome. In September 1849, weakness of the left hand developed. Sometimes, there was an indistinctness of speech. Towards the end of the year, Lecomte had to give up his work and, overcome by his illness, he decided to go to Paris. In July 1850, Lecomte was admitted to the 'Hopital de la Charite' on the service of Professor Cruveilhier, two years after symptom onset. Between July 1850 and February 1853, the paralysis together, with muscular atrophy, progressed slowly and steadily. In January 1853, one month before his death, the examination revealed a severe wasting of the arms, which were almost completely paralysed. In sharp contrast, although there was a marked weakness of the legs, there was no apparent muscle wasting. The patient could not swallow and the tongue was completely paralysed. The voice was weak; the articulation, very defective and guttural. Lecomte developed bronchitis; he was unable to cough up the secretions. On the twelfth of February he was found dead.

Results

The patient died of bronchopneumonia. The gross examination of the cerebrum, the spinal cord, and the dorsal roots of the spinal nerves revealed no pathology. On the other hand, there was a marked atrophy of the ventral roots, especially in the cervical region, while the ventral roots in the dorsal and lumbar regions were only reduced in size. After a treatment with diluted nitric acid, the motor roots were examined again, now with a strong magnifying glass. They were visible as grey filaments, often reduced to their neurilemma without a trace of nervous tissue. The gross examination of the muscular system showed a variable degree of atrophy. Several muscles had a normal aspect, others were only reduced in volume and pale in colour. The muscles in the upper extremities were extremely atrophied, very often with an accumulation of fat.

Conclusions and critique

This remarkable 'first case' of ALS described by Cruveilhier was analysed in detail by Veltema [3]. The clinical picture was that of a 30-year-old male with a slow progressive course lasting 4.5 years. Onset was in the right hand and then spread to the other arm. A bulbar syndrome developed with tongue fasciculations. There was spasticity, hyperreflexia, and cramps in the legs. There were no sensory abnormalities, cognition was normal, and there were no sphincter abnormalities. Although Cruveilhier considered that his patient had progressive muscular atrophy, the clinical picture had all the features of 'classic Charcot' ALS, with a combination of upper and lower motor neuron abnormalities. Others, too, described ALS before Charcot [1, 4]. Somewhat surprisingly, Charcot formulated the clinical characteristics of ALS on fewer than 10 cases [5, 6]. Although progressive muscle weakness without prominent sensory involvement in the context of combined upper and lower motor neuron deficits in someone, mid-life, has a limited (if any) differential diagnosis, most textbooks continue to produce an exhaustive differential diagnosis of ALS [7]. Difficulties really only arise when either upper or lower motor neuron features occur in isolation, but most authorities now accept that progressive muscular atrophy (PMA) and primary lateral sclerosis (PLS) reflect ends of a spectrum of a single disease [8].

9.2 **The first gene in amyotrophic lateral sclerosis**

Main paper: Rosen DR, Siddique T, Patterson D, et al. Mutations in Cu/Zn superoxide dismutase gene are associated with familial amyotrophic lateral sclerosis. *Nature* 1993; 362:59–62.

Background

Charcot was adamant that ALS was not genetic [5]. He clearly overlooked Aran's publication of 20 years earlier describing a 43-year-old sea captain presenting with cramps in the upper limb muscles and subsequent wasting and weakness [9]. He died two years later. One of his three sisters and two maternal uncles died of a similar disease. Current estimates indicate that less than 5% of ALS reports a family history of the disease [10]. This small proportion is similar to the familial incidence of Parkinson's disease (PD) and Alzheimer's disease (AD). However, even in sporadic disease which accounts for 95% of cases, if one member of a family has one of the neurodegenerative disorders, there is a higher than expected incidence that other family members will also develop a neurodegenerative disorder [11]. This suggests there is a genetic tendency to neurodegeneration. In 1993, the first genetic mutation was identified in ALS—the superoxide dismutase gene (*SOD1*) (see Fig. 9.2). There was great excitement at the time of this discovery, with a rather naïve expectation that 'the cause of ALS had been discovered'. Nevertheless, the finding resulted in the first useful animal models of ALS and considerable research in ALS cell death mechanisms and pathogenesis followed [8].

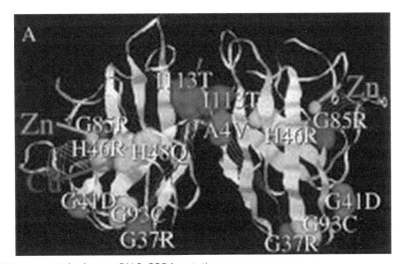

Fig. 9.2 Representative human FALS–*SOD1* mutations.

Reproduced from *PNAS*, 95 (11), Corson LB, Chaperone-facilitated copper binding is a property common to several classes of familial amyotrophic lateral sclerosis-linked superoxide dismutase mutants, p. 6361–6366, Copyright (1998), with permission from National Academy of Sciences, USA.

Methods

To determine whether familial ALS (FALS) is associated with mutations in the *SODI* gene, polymerase chain reaction (PCR) primers were designed for two of the five *SODI*. These were used for PCR amplification of *SODI* exonic deoxyribonucleic acid (DNA) from genomic DNA of normal, control individuals and of single FALS-affected individuals from families tightly linked either to *SODI* or neighbouring markers on chromosome 21q. The products of the PCR reactions were denatured and separated on a polyacrylamide gel for single-strand conformational polymorphism (SSCP) analysis, which detects mobility shifts of single-strand DNA caused by sequence variations. Autoradiograms of these gels revealed shifts in band mobility for 6 of the 15 families linked to the *SODI* region of chromosome 21q. Twelve of 135 families also revealed anomalous SSCPs; these families were too small for significant linkage analysis. Five of the FALS families were excluded from linkage to chromosome 21q; none showed abnormal SSCPs.

Results

The studies identified 11 single amino-acid changes in *SOD1* on the basis of the genomic DNA sequences of members of 13 different FALS families. These changes were not detected in more than 100 chromosomes from normal individuals and so appear not to be simply normal allelic variants. Instead, these mutations occur in association with FALS. Although it is conceivable that the mutation that causes FALS leads to the accumulation of mutations in other genes, including *SOD1*, this possibility seems unlikely. The authors stated their belief that the simplest hypothesis is that the mutations identified in the *SOD1* gene are one cause of FALS.

Conclusions and critique

It is 20 years since the first *SOD1* mutation was discovered, with over 125 mutations identified since [12, 13]. The *SOD1* gene is expressed ubiquitously and is highly conserved in evolution. Thus, it is far from clear why mutation in this gene would selectively affect the motor system, and intensive study of *SOD1* mutations has failed to answer the question of how the gene causes ALS. Several other genes have now been associated with ALS [14], and their mechanism of disease causation is equally mysterious. This is not surprising. Complex diseases, including ALS, that are caused by 'disease risk genes' form part of a molecular network. Normal control of gene–gene interactions is poorly understood and most disease-causing genes and proteins of complex diseases are scattered in gene networks without direct interactions, which renders the significance of individual genes difficult to unravel [15, 16]. In addition, the important issue of deleterious somatic (non-germ line) mutations is only now beginning to be explored [17].

Two messages follow:

1 ALS occurs as the result of the interaction of many genes (presently, we can only hazard a guess as to how many are implicated), the environment, and the epigenome [18]. As the clinical spectrum of ALS widens with gene risk discovery, the concept of 'truly sporadic ALS' will have to be re-evaluated [19].

2 Caution is required in translating animal models of ALS to the human disease, and questions remain as to how representative *SOD1* rodent models are for human sporadic and familial ALS [20]. For example, of the over 120 positive trial outcomes in the *SOD1* mouse model, none have translated to the human.

9.3 **Markers of amyotrophic lateral sclerosis progression**

Main paper: Brooks BR, Sanjak M, Ringel S, et al. The amyotrophic lateral sclerosis functional rating scale: assessment of activities of daily living in patients with amyotrophic lateral sclerosis. The ALS CNTF Treatment Study (ACTS) Phase I-II Study Group. Arch Neurol 1996; 53:141–7.

Background

ALS is uniformly fatal, and time to death is an unambiguous marker of disease progression and, as such, the best measure of the success or failure of therapeutic trials. But, as a clinical trial outcome measure, survival has limitations. Average survival of newly diagnosed patients is <3 years, so survival as an endpoint obligates a long trial duration. Survival is affected by use of non-invasive ventilation, tracheostomy and permanent-assisted ventilation, and augmented nutrition via gastrostomy tubes. Thus, although survival is an objective, easily measurable outcome, it usually reflects factors other than disease progression. Clinical rating scales that assess the activities of daily living (ADL) are useful in both natural history studies of ALS and in clinical trials. Early examples are the Norris Scale [21] and the ALS Severity Scale [22]. Presently, the ALS Functional Rating Scale (ALSFRS) and its revised version, the ALSFRS-R, are the gold standards used to measure disease progression and trial outcomes.

The ALSFRS, which was revised in 1999 to incorporate additional assessments of dyspnoea, orthopnoea, and the need for ventilator support [23], is a validated questionnaire-based scale that measures physical function in carrying out ADL of patients with ALS [24–27] (Table 9.1) It has been used in clinical trials as well as in clinical practice because of its ease of use and its correlation with both objective measures of disease status and levels of disability. The components of the scale group into four factors or domains that encompass gross motor tasks, fine motor tasks, bulbar functions, and respiratory function.

Methods

At each visit, the same evaluator administered the ALSFRS before, and without forehand knowledge of, measurement of muscle strength and pulmonary function. Maximum voluntary isometric muscle strength was measured in six muscle groups on each side of the body (shoulder extensors, elbow flexors, hip flexors, knee extensors, ankle dorsiflexors, and grip strength). The restricted set of muscles was chosen because prior natural history studies suggested that these six muscle groups adequately represented the body as a whole, and that testing these groups yielded as much information regarding rate of decline in muscle strength in ALS as testing all muscle groups.

Pulmonary function was assessed by measuring forced vital capacity (FVC) and maximum inspiratory pressure. The FVC was measured using a desktop flow spirometer, and maximum inspiratory pressure was measured by a handheld inspiratory force gauge. To measure manual dexterity, oral-labial dexterity, and walking ability, a series of timed tasks

Table 9.1 The revised ALS Functional Rating Scale (ALSFRS-R)

1. *Speech:* 4 Normal speech processes 3 Detectable speech disturbance 2 Intelligible with repeating 1 Speech combined with non-vocal communication 0 Loss of useful speech

2. *Salivation:* 4 Normal 3 Slight but definite excess of saliva in mouth; may have night-time drooling 2 Moderately excessive saliva; may have minimal drooling 1 Marked excess of saliva with some drooling 0 Marked drooling; requires constant tissue or handkerchief

3. *Swallowing:* 4 Normal eating habits 3 Early eating problems—occasional choking 2 Dietary consistency changes 1 Needs supplemental tube feeding 0 NPO (exclusively parenteral or enteral feeding)

4. *Handwriting:* 4 Normal 3 Slow or sloppy; all words are legible 2 Not all words are legible 1 Able to grip pen but unable to write 0 Unable to grip pen

5a. *Cutting food and handling utensils (patients without gastrostomy):* 4 Normal 3 Somewhat slow and clumsy, but no help needed 2 Can cut most foods, although clumsy and slow; some help needed 1 Food must be cut by someone but can still feed slowly 0 Needs to be fed

5b. *Cutting food and handling utensils (alternate scale for patients with gastrostomy):* 4 Normal 3 Clumsy but able to perform all manipulations independently 2 Some help needed with closures and fasteners 1 requires minimal assistance to caregiver 0 Unable to perform any aspect of task

6. *Dressing and hygiene:* 4 Normal function 3 Independent and complete self-care with effort or decreased efficiency 2 Intermittent assistance or substitute methods 1 Needs attendant for self-care 0 Total dependence

7. *Turning in bed and adjusting bed clothes:* 4 Normal 3 Somewhat slow and clumsy, but no help needed 2 Can turn alone or adjust sheets, but with great difficulty 1 Can initiate, but not turn or adjust sheets alone 0 Helpless

8. *Walking:* 4 Normal 3 Early ambulation difficulties 2 Walks with assistance 1 Non-ambulatory functional movement 0 No purposeful leg movement

9. *Climbing stairs:* 4 Normal 3 Slow 2 Mild unsteadiness or fatigue 1 Needs assistance 0 Cannot do

Reproduced from *Journal of the Neurological Sciences*, 169 (9), Jesse M. Cedarbaum, Nancy Stambler, et al., The ALSFRS-R: a revised ALS functional rating scale that incorporates assessments of respiratory function, Copyright (1999), with permission from Elsevier.

were used, including the Purdue Pegboard, repetition of the syllables 'pa/ta', and the time taken to walk 15 ft (approximately 4.6 m).

Results

Seventy-five patients (49 males and 26 females) were enrolled in a cross-sectional study. The mean standard deviation (±SD) patient age was 54.8 ±12.8 years, and the mean (±SD) disease duration was 3.4 ±5.5 y ears. The ALS symptoms were of bulbar onset in 18 patients, arm onset in 32, and leg onset in 25. The mean (±SD) combined megascore was 0.03 ±1.0, the mean (±SD) FVC was 2.9 ±1.1, and the mean (±SD) ALSFRS score was 28.0 ±7.0.

In a longitudinal study, the sensitivity of the ALSFRS to change in patient status over time was assessed for the 53 patients (38 males and 15 females) who had an ALSFRS score recorded at or beyond 19 weeks of follow-up. The mean (±SD) patient age was 50.4 ±11.4

years, and the mean (±SD) duration of disease was 2.6 ±2.9 years. Three of the patients had bulbar onset, 31 had arm onset, and 19 had leg onset. The mean (±SD) combined megascore was 0.17 ±0.8, the mean (±SD) FVC was 3.7 ±1.1, and the mean (±SD) ALSFRS score was 28.6 ±4.7.

Conclusions and critique

The ALSFRS remains the gold standard for determining therapeutic trial outcomes. It assesses bulbar and respiratory functions, upper extremity functions (cutting food and dressing), lower extremity functions (walking and climbing), and dressing, hygiene, and ability to turn in bed. The ALSFRS is easily administered by an allied health professional or a trained evaluator, and can be administered by phone [26]. As communication deteriorates, caregivers can provide responses, and the equivalency of caregiver and patient responses has been established, and a telephone survey system is feasible [26, 28, 29]. A revised version of the ALSFRS has added assessments of respiratory dysfunction, including dyspnoea, orthopnoea, and the need for ventilatory support. The ALSFRS-R retains the properties of the original scale and shows strong internal consistency and construct validity [23]. Measures of quality of life have now been added to the ALSFRS-R [30–32].

9.4 **Site of onset of amyotrophic lateral sclerosis**

Main paper: Mott FW. A case of amyotrophic lateral sclerosis with degeneration of the motor path from the cortex to the periphery. *Brain* 1895; 18(1):21–36.

Background

Charcot concluded that ALS was an anterograde degeneration commencing in the motor cortex with secondary demise of the anterior horn cells [5]. This was refuted by Gowers and others who argued that the upper and lower motor neurons died independently of each other [33]. The question of site of origin of ALS was largely ignored for the next 100 years but, in the last two decades, there has been considerable renewed interest and debate regarding this important question [33].

Methods

Summary of clinical phenomena: one year's duration. Commenced with weakness and numbness in right leg, gradually increasing, associated with wasting of muscles and exaggerated deep reflexes, followed by similar affection of right arm and hand, with especial wasting of thenar, hypothenar eminences, and interossei. Terminally, bulbar symptoms and paresis of diaphragm developed.

   The whole of the central nervous system and the following nerves—phrenics, vagus ulnar, median, and sciatic—were placed in Müller's fluid for hardening, after which the tissue was stained by the Marchi method and embedded in celloidin. Sections were cut and stained by Weigert- Pal carmine method and with haematoxylin and eosin.

Results

Microscopic studies showed degenerated fibres in cerebral cortex and degenerated anterior part of the posterior half of the internal capsule. The crus cerebri showed sclerosis of its middle third, as did the medulla at the level of the pyramids. There was sclerosis of the pyramidal tracts and very marked loss of anterior horn cells, especially in the lower lumbar region. It was concluded that there was simultaneous degeneration of the upper (upper motor neuron and pyramidal tracts) and lower motor pathways (anterior horn cells and exiting nerves). The appearances of degeneration and sclerosis presented by the internal capsule and the crus cerebri, in this case, were quite as advanced as the pyramidal tracts of the medulla and dorsal region of the cord.

   These findings raised the following question to Dr Mott:

> Are we to believe that the degeneration of the upper segment of the motor path begins in the terminations of the crossed pyramidal tracts in the spinal cord and spreads gradually upwards? Or is it due to degenerative changes in the cortex leading to degeneration and atrophy of the large cells of the third layer which give origin by their axis cylinder processes to the fibres of the pyramidal tract?

In other words, is the degeneration retrograde or anterograde?

Conclusions and critique

Dr Mott considered two possibilities;

> If, however, we look upon this progressive muscular atrophy as a degenerative process of the motor path, affecting in some cases the lower segment first, therefore masking the symptoms which would be produced by the subsequent affection of the upper segment, or, in some cases, in the upper segment first, producing characteristic symptoms, or affecting as in this case both segments of the motor path simultaneously, we must then conclude that there is wanting in the cells, and their processes which constitute the motor tracts.

Even meticulous pathology of ALS is unlikely to reveal whether there is 'dying forward' (cortex-anterior horn cell), 'dying back' (anterior horn cell to cortex), or if the corticomotoneurons and anterior horn cells die independently of each other. Pathological findings in ALS largely reflect late-event 'gravestones', whereas the true onset of ALS probably precedes clinical onset [34]. Recent sophisticated physiological studies and functional imaging certainly support Charcot's view that ALS is a primary disease of the brain [35]. However, it is certainly possible that once the degenerative process is advanced, focal spread of the disease occurs, although features such as diffuse fasciculation in the face of very focal muscle weakness and wasting and electromyographic evidence of disease outside the clinically affected area both indicate more diffuse disease than is clinically evident.

9.5 **Frontotemporal dementia and amyotrophic lateral sclerosis**

Main paper: Hodges J. Scientific commentary: familial frontotemporal dementia and amyotrophic lateral sclerosis associated with the C9ORF72 hexanucleotide repeat. *Brain* 2012; 135:652–65.

Background

Charcot was adamant that dementia was never associated with ALS and that the disease was never hereditary [36]. Even presently, most standard texts on ALS consider dementia to be a rare manifestation of ALS [37]. Cognitive impairment is usually ascribed to cerebral anoxia from respiratory dysfunction and/or depression [38–40]. However, genetic studies, sophisticated imaging, and neuro-psychometry clearly indicate frontotemporal dysfunction in a significant number of patients, even in the absence of overt dementia. Well-documented frontal lobe symptoms in ALS go back to Wechsler and Davison (1932) [41], who described a man aged 38 presenting with mental changes characterized by impairment of memory. 'The family noticed that he was tongue-tied, reiterated statements without being aware of it, and could not recall the names of his parents and failed to recognize the members of his family or the house and street in which he lived.' A year later, he started to develop wasting and weakness of upper extremity muscles. This became diffuse, also involving bulbar muscles. As well as typical pathological changes of ALS, there were also 'disturbances in the architecture of the cortical layers, extending from the frontal to the temporal regions'.

The March 2012 issue of *Brain* published no less than eight papers describing the clinical, radiological, and pathological characteristics of the *C9ORF72* gene-associated intronic GGGGCC hexanucelotide repeat expansion in association with frontotemporal dementia and ALS. Two previously discovered genes, the progranulin mutation (GRN) and the microtube-associated protein tau gene (MAPT), have been shown to be associated with autosomal dominantly inherited frontotemporal dementia (FTD) [42–44].

Methods

The papers reported the results of screening large cohorts of patients with FTD (almost 1200 cases), distributed fairly evenly between The Netherlands [45], Manchester [46], London [47], and the USA [48]. A study from Vancouver described the clinical and pathological findings in 30 patients from 16 unrelated families [49]. The final FTD-related paper, also from the Mayo group, contrasted the structural magnetic resonance imaging (MRI) findings in groups of patients with the various sub-forms of familial FTD compared with non-inherited FTD [50]. Two papers reported the findings in large cohorts of sporadic and familial ALS from England and from mainland Europe [51, 52].

Results

Overall, between 7% and 12% of the cohorts with FTD were found to have the mutation, but about 45% of familial ALS-FTD was associated with the *C9ORF72*-associated repeat expansion, compared to <10% of sporadic cases. Disease duration appeared shorter in those with a mutation, but otherwise, clinical features were similar to those without a mutation. Most patients had the behavioural variant of FTD, although progressive non-fluent aphasia also occurred. Semantic dementia was rarely, if ever, associated. The study from Manchester reported a very high rate of psychosis, 12 cases (38%) presenting with florid psychotic symptoms, resulting in initial diagnoses of delusional psychosis, somatoform psychosis, or paranoid schizophrenia. One patient presented complaining of 'pieces of plastic emanating from his head'. Another patient described visions of the devil and had developed behavioural strategies for keeping 'him' at bay. Autopsy findings in patients with the *C9ORF72* mutation showed classical ALS pathology with TDP-43 inclusions in spinal motor neurons and prominent neuronal cytoplasmic inclusions and glial inclusions in the hippocampus and frontal regions, in keeping with the cognitive deficits of ALS-FTD.

Conclusions and critique

In the last decade, there has been an exponential interest in ALS-FTD. FTD is an age-dependent neurodegeneration primarily associated with impairments in cognition and social behaviours, as well as personality changes. It is now recognized as the most common form of early-onset age-dependent dementia and increasing clinical, pathological, and molecular evidence indicates that FTD and ALS are closely related, and that FTD should be considered as a onset phenotype equal to bulbar, cervical, or lumbar onset ALS [53, 54]. Nevertheless, FTD remains rare, clinically, in ALS, with an incidence of about 2%. Psychometric testing and functional and positron emission tomographic (PET) imaging raises this number considerably, to 35–70%. It is more than likely that, as time goes by, genes other than the three so far identified in association with ALS-FTD will be discovered.

9.6 **Attempts to identify transmissible agents causing amyotrophic lateral sclerosis**

Main paper: Zil'ber LA, Bajdakova ZL, Gardas'jan AN, Konovalov NV, Bunina TL, Barabadze EM. Study of the etiology of amyotrophic lateral sclerosis. *Bulletin WHO* 1963; 29:449–56.

Background

Attempts to demonstrate a viral or other transmittable aetiology of ALS have surfaced in the literature, intermittently, from the 1960s onwards [55–57]. To date, there is no direct proof of a viral or other infective agent causing ALS, but viruses may be implicated in the development of ALS by means of mechanisms other than direct infection. A viral agent may act indirectly on the host cells, impairing the immune response, or may trigger and accelerate the cascade of events leading to programmed cellular death, by transactivating or altering cellular genes and transduction signals involved in this process. ALS, as other neurodegenerations, behaves in some respects akin to slow-virus disorders. The features common to slow infection include very long latency, unanimously poor prognosis, and central nervous system involvement. Bjorn Sigurdsson, in veterinary medicine, proposed slow virus as unique mode of infection in 1957 [58]. The initial concept was remodelled with the general acceptance of prion theory of sheep scrapie. Currently, the slow infections comprise subacute sclerosing panencephalitis and progressive multifocal encephalopathy in humans, visna-maedi in sheep, and prion diseases (Kuru, Creutzfeldt-Jakob disease, Gerstmann-Straussler-Scheinker syndrome in humans, and scrapie and bovine spongiform encephalopathy in animals) [59].

Methods

Pieces of the medulla oblongata and spinal cord of patients who had died of ALS were triturated in a mortar with sand and a salt solution in the ratio of 1:3. The homogenate was centrifuged at 3000–4000 revolutions per minute to clarify the liquid and precipitate the sand. The supernatant fluid, to which penicillin and streptomycin were added, was injected into the brain of the monkeys through a trephine hole. The material was administered through the dura mater into the frontal lobe of the brain to the left of the centre line and to a depth not exceeding 2–2.5 mm. To avoid deeper penetration, a sleeve was fixed on the needle. Mainly monkeys, Macaca rhesus species and some other breeds, were used for the experiments. They were of different ages but mainly under one or two years.

Results

Two Macaca rhesus monkeys (one female) were inoculated in May 1956. In May 1957, the female developed slight wasting of the muscles of the left forearm and hand, exaggeration of the tendon reflexes in the hind limbs, and weight loss. Eighteen months later (i.e. 2.5 years after infection), there was atrophy and paresis of the left hind limb, and reflexes were considerably brisker. During the next 2 months, paresis of the left hind limb was considerably intensified and a weakness of the lumbar muscles and paresis of the right hind extremity were noted.

The other monkey (male) remained in good health for the next 5 years, when it developed wasting of the left forelimb muscles, together with exaggeration of all tendon reflexes. In the subsequent 3 months, both forelimbs assumed a position of extension and pareses of the feet appeared. Reflexes were exaggerated bilaterally. The monkey ceased to bear weight on the right leg and spent most of the day on the floor and, on 20 March 1962, the monkey was sacrificed and seven monkeys, still under observation, were infected with its medullary tissue.

In another experiment in which a monkey was infected with material from an ALS patient on 14 September 1959, exaggeration of lower limb tendon reflexes and a slight wasting of the muscles in the hind limbs had developed approximately 2.5 years later. Three monkeys of other breeds were also infected from three other persons who had died of ALS. The last monkey was infected during the embryonic period in its mother's womb. By the termination of the study, the monkeys remained healthy.

Particularly marked changes were noted in the anterior horns of the spinal cord. The cells that remained were swollen and subject to chromatolysis and to Nissl's degeneration. In most cases, the cells were wrinkled and their cytoplasm had become homogeneous and hyperchromic. Some of the cells had accumulated lipoid granules. Destruction of the cells was accompanied by a marked glial reaction, and there were rounded inclusions in the cell cytoplasm. The picture of morphological changes, which was identical in all the monkeys sacrificed, pointed to a clear lesion of the central nervous system. Similar changes are observed in humans who have died of ALS, the only difference being that they are markedly more intense in human patients. This difference is probably due to the fact that the monkeys were sacrificed before they died naturally (in attempting to ensure success of the passages), whereas in study of human material, the pathologist is always dealing with fatal cases, when the intensity of the changes has reached its maximum.

Conclusions and critique

ALS has some resemblance to the transmissible spongiform encephalopathies in its dual pattern of inherited and sporadic cases, its uniform prevalence throughout the world, its late onset (suggestive of a long incubation period), and its pathological picture of neuronal degeneration without significant inflammation, although clearly marked activation of several cytokines from over-activated microglia has been demonstrated in all neurodegenerations [60]. However, to date, only the Russian group have succeeded in transmitting the human disease to primates. Gibbs and Gajdusek [61, 62] failed in their attempted to transmit ALS, ALS-PD, and PD to primates by inoculation of suspensions of tissues from patients in the United States and on Guam. Similarly, Fraser et al. [63] had negative results when inoculating mice. Nevertheless, recent research has shown a remarkable new concept of neuronal cell to cell 'propagation' of inclusions made of tau, α-synuclein, and superoxide dismutase 1. This mechanism is reminiscent of that by which prions spread through the nervous system [64].

9.7 **The first disease-modifying treatment in motor neurone disease**

Main paper: Bensimon G, Lacomblez L, Meininger V. A controlled trial of riluzole in amyotrophic lateral sclerosis. ALS/Riluzole Study Group. *N Engl J Med* 1994; 330:585–91.

Related paper: Lacomblez L, Bensimon G, Leigh PN, Guillet P, Meininger V. Dose-ranging study of riluzole in amyotrophic lateral sclerosis. ALS/Riluzole Study Group II. *Lancet* 1996; 347:1425–31.

Background

In 1956, Liversedge used a combination of glycocyamine and betaine in the therapy of MND [65]. The rationale was their involvement in the biochemical pathway of creatine production, an important component of muscle metabolism. The author recorded that, at that time, the aetiology of MND remained elusive but was attributed to 'a medley of factors, including chill, anxiety, toxicosis, injury and inevitably tobacco and alcohol'. Since then, a plethora of drugs have been tested in very variable circumstances [66], often with only small numbers of patients, and with a tenuous rationale at times. Excitotoxicity has been a lasting theme in MND pathophysiology for 20 years. It was recognized that, in culture, neuronal cell death could be induced by over-stimulation with naturally occurring excitatory amino acids such as glutamate. The findings of altered glutamate levels in the blood and cerebrospinal fluid (CSF) of ALS patients were supported by the report of reduced glutamate transport shortly afterwards [67]. This concept of over-stimulation of motor neurons as a key step in pathogenesis of MND has developed, to some extent, through inconsistent epidemiological links to physical exercise and athleticism [68], fuelled by high-profile sporting figures among the afflicted, including the legendary 1930's Yankees baseball player, Lou Gehrig, whose name continues to define ALS in the USA.

Benzothiazole riluzole found its original use as an ingredient of photographic developing solution and, later, within industrial bleach. Legend has it that two scientists, working in separate laboratories on the same floor, accidentally swapped chemicals so that riluzole was screened in an *in vitro* assay of glutamate inhibition and found to be effective. It was originally developed as a potential anticonvulsant.

Methods

Study design: A double-blind, placebo-controlled, multi-centre study to assess drug efficacy.

Number of patients: In the first study, Bensimon and colleagues reported a study of 155 patients receiving 100 mg per day. Lacomblez and colleagues then reported on 959 patients with clinically 'probable' or 'definite' ALS (by the 'El Escorial' criteria of the time [69], since modified) of less than 5 years' duration who were randomly assigned treatment with placebo or 50 mg, 100 mg, or 200 mg riluzole daily; randomization was stratified by centre and site of disease onset (bulbar or limb).

Outcome measures: The primary outcome was survival without tracheostomy. Secondary outcomes were rates of change in functional measures (muscle strength, functional status, respiratory function, patient's assessment of fasciculation, cramps, stiffness, and tiredness).

Primary analysis: This was the comparison of the 100 mg dose with placebo by intention to treat. Drug effect on survival was assessed before (log-rank test) and after adjustment for known prognostic factors (Cox's model).

Follow-up: This was at 21 months (Bensimon and colleagues) and 18 months (Lacomblez and colleagues).

Results

In the initial smaller trial, riluzole therapy was well tolerated and reduced mortality by 39% at 12 months and 19% at 21 months ($p = 0.046$). At the end of the larger dose-ranging study, 122 (50.4%) placebo-treated patients and 134 (56.8%) of those who received 100 mg/day riluzole were alive without tracheostomy (unadjusted risk 0.79, $p = 0.076$; adjusted risk 0.65, $p = 0.002$). In the groups receiving 50 mg and 200 mg riluzole daily, 131 (55.3%) and 141 (57.8%) patients were alive without tracheostomy (relative to placebo 50 mg adjusted risk 0.76, $p = 0.04$; 200 mg 0.61, $p = 0.0004$). There was a significant inverse dose response in risk of death. No functional scale discriminated between the treatment groups. (See Fig. 9.3)

Conclusions

Overall, efficacy and safety results suggest that the 100 mg dose of riluzole has the best benefit to risk ratio. This study confirmed that riluzole was well tolerated and lengthens survival of patients with ALS.

Critique

A Cochrane review of results from four eligible trials concluded that 'riluzole 100 mg daily is safe and probably prolongs median survival by about two to three months' [70]. Aside from this clearly very modest benefit, lack of subjective improvement, inability to quantify individual slowing of progression, and omission of quality of life measures from the trials, are commonly stated concerns by the significant number of neurologists who remain sceptical about the value of riluzole. The initial wave of optimism at the news, in 1994, that after decades of unsuccessful trials, one drug had at last been shown to make a difference to survival in MND, has long faded with the failure of a more effective disease-modifying drug to emerge in over 15 years. Timely implementation of a percutaneous endoscopic gastrostomy (PEG) tube, and bilevel positive airway pressure (BiPAP) have been the major two symptomatic interventions, the latter also significantly prolonging survival [71]. New approaches and a new mind-set need to be directed to drug therapy for

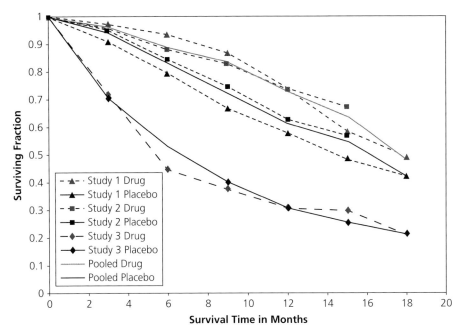

Fig. 9.3 Kaplan-Meier survival curves: pooled survival time in months. Solid lines show pooled results from the two trials that were homogeneous.

Reproduced from *Cochrane Database of Systematic Reviews*, (3), Miller RG, Mitchell JD, Moore DH., Riluzole for amyotrophic lateral sclerosis (ALS)/motor neuron disease (MND), Copyright (2012), with permission from John Wiley and Sons.

ALS since, without exception, all therapeutic trials have thus far failed. The major problems have been trying to treat a disease so late in its course, lack of appropriate animal models, and a possible need for polytherapy to tackle the many elements in the cascade of cell death.

9.8 **Inflammation in Amyotrophic lateral sclerosis akin to a smoldering fire**

Main paper: Yasojima K, Tourtellotte WW, McGeer EG, McGeer PL. Marked increase in cyclooxygenase-2 in ALS spinal cord. Implications for therapy. *Neurology* 2001; 57:952–6.

Background

Del Rio Hortega, in his classic article of 1919, identified microglia as the phagocytes of the brain and established that they were of mesenchymal origin [72]. The concepts regarding the origin and function of microglia were, until recently, regarded with considerable scepticism, but have now been confirmed through sophisticated molecular biological techniques [73]. There is considerable current interest in the roles of the innate and adaptive immune systems in diverse forms of neurodegenerative disease [74]. Microglia, a type of glial cell, are macrophages resident in the brain and spinal cord, forming a frontline defence of the innate immune system. Direct evidence for an innate inflammatory response in AD was described nearly 20 years ago and subsequent studies have also documented inflammatory components in PD. The inflammatory changes are observed in both sporadic and familial ALS and in the *SOD1* transgenic mouse model. The inflammation, considered akin to a 'smoldering fire', although not causative, may greatly influence the disease progression, and there may be potential for anti-inflammatory therapy [75]. (See Fig. 9.4)

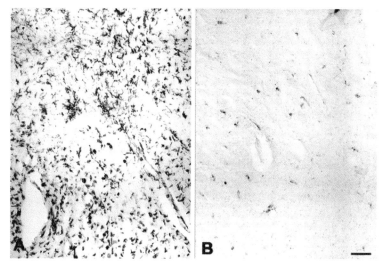

Fig. 9.4 Immunostaining of ALS and control tissue. (**A**) Anterior horn area of ALS cervical cord immunostained for HLA-DR with the antibody CR3–43 (supplied by Sigma, Oakville, Ontario, Canada). Abundant reactive microglia are seen. Most retain ramified morphology, but many in the surrounding white matter have round morphology indicative of myelin digestion. (**B**) Anterior horn area of a control case immunostained similarly to A.

Reproduced from *Muscle & Nerve*, 26 (4), McGeer PL, McGeer EG., Inflammatory processes in amyotrophic lateral sclerosis, p. 459–70, Copyright (2002), with permission from John Wiley and Sons.

Methods

ALS spinal cord (n = 11) was compared with 27 non-ALS cases (15 cases of AD, 6 cases of AD, 3 cases of cerebrovascular disease, and 3 neurologically normal individuals). Either cervical or thoracic spinal cord was studied. Extraction of total ribonucleic acid (RNA), reverse transcription of the products, and amplification of the cDNA for *COX-1*, *COX-2*, *CD11b*, and the housekeeping gene *cyclophilin* by the PCR technique were performed.

Results

In ALS compared with non-ALS spinal cord, *COX-2* mRNA was upregulated 7.09-fold ($p < 0.0001$); *COX-1*, 1.14-fold ($p < 0.05$); and *CD11b*, 1.85-fold ($p < 0.0012$). *COX-2* mRNA levels in AD, PD, cerebrovascular disease, and control cases were each significantly lower than in ALS and were not significantly different from each other. Western blots of the protein products were in general accord with the mRNA data, with *COX-2* protein levels being upregulated 3.79-fold compared with non-ALS cases ($p < 0.015$).

Conclusions and critique

Within the central nervous system (CNS), microglia are the first line of defence, responding rapidly to any type of brain injury. Microglia constantly screen their microenvironment, making them the sentinels of the CNS, and are thus active already under healthy conditions, but change their morphology and function in response to a given stimulus [76, 77]. It has been appreciated, for many decades, that there is a major inflammatory component to ALS. That is not to say that ALS is an inflammatory disorder. The inflammation is the result of the neurodegenerative process, not its cause. Astrocytes and the numerous chemical–physical inductions associated with them, represent the largest cell population in the CNS. Once regarded as merely the element that fills the space not occupied by neurons, the last 20 years of research have identified a plethora of essential functions that these cells perform in the healthy and diseased nervous system. Reactive astrocytes in ALS show increased immunoreactivity for the glial fibrillary acidic protein (GFAP) and the calcium binding protein *S100* and express inflammatory markers such as *COX-2*, inducible nitric oxide synthase (iNOS), and neuronal NOS. Increase in GFAP immunoreactive astrocytes is particularly notable in the grey matter of the spinal cord ventral horn where, normally, astrocytes express/stain for GFAP at very low levels. In addition, cytoplasmic hyaline inclusions and markers of oxidative and nitrative stress accompany astrocyte pathology.

9.9 **Environmental issues in amyotrophic lateral sclerosis—The Guam story**

Main paper: Hirano A, Kurland LT, Krooth RS, Lessell S. Parkinsonism-dementia complex, an endemic disease on the Island of Guam. I: clinical features. *Brain* 1961; 84:642–61.

Supplementary paper: Hirano A, Malamud N, Kurland LT. Parkinsonism-dementia complex, an endemic disease on the Island of Guam. II: pathological features. *Brain* 1961; 84:662–79.

Background

The first folklore account of Lytico (ALS) and Bodig (Parkinons's disease) was around 1769, originating in Umatac, a village in the south of Guam. In 1945, Dr Harry Zimmerman, a pathologist at the Guam Naval Hospital, reported that he had seen seven Chammorro patients with ALS in only one month. During the 1950s and early 1960s, it was discovered that Guam and the other Mariana Islands in the Western Pacific Ocean represented a geographic isolate with a phenomenal incidence of fatal neurological diseases. The best known of these disorders among the 38,000 indigenous Chamorro people was ALS, which accounted for about 10% of the adult deaths, or about 100 times the death ratio reported for any other population. By the end of the 1970s and 1980 onwards, the incidence of Guam-ALS was no greater than that of the rest of the world, and present cases are now clinically and pathologically typical of Western ALS [78].

Methods

The purpose of the paper was to present the clinical description of 47 selected Parkinsonism-dementia cases and to discuss their relationship to ALS and to 'presenile' dementia and Parkinsonism in other populations. The supplementary paper dealt with the pathological features of 17 autopsied cases of Parkinsonism-dementia. The cases have been divided into three groups: I. Parkinsonism-dementia complex (PDC) (30 cases); II. Parkinsonism-dementia and clinical evidence of upper MND (8 cases); and III. Parkinsonism-dementia with clinical evidence of upper and lower MND (ALS) (9 cases).

Results

The age of onset for all cases ranged from 32 to 64 years (mean, 52 years). All cases were of Chamorro descent. Seventeen of the 47 cases were familial, and there was overlap of ALS and PDC in the same families. Symptom onset was insidious and frequently first recognized by a family member. Signs and symptoms were typical of ALS, PD, and dementia of the Alzheimer type. There were no specific abnormalities in any laboratory data. The overall course of the disease was slow but progressive.

The main macroscopic neuropathological features found in the 17 cases autopsied were the presence of cortical atrophy, and depigmentation of the substantia nigra and locus caeruleus. The consistent finding on microscopic examination was widespread ganglion cell degeneration of the CNS affecting primarily the cortex of the frontal and temporal lobes, Ammon's horn, amygdaloid nucleus, hypothalamus, globus pallidus, thalamus, periaqueductal structures, substantia nigra, and tegmentum of the brain stem. There were numerous intraganglionic fibrillary changes and scattered intracytoplasmic granulovacu-olar bodies in the affected neurones of these areas. Typical senile plaques were not found in any of the cases. In addition, there was a diffuse loss of ganglion cells of variable degree, most marked in the globus pallidus and substantia nigra. Reactive glial proliferation accompanied the neuronal involvement. White matter was relatively well preserved in contrast to a severe involvement of grey matter. Degeneration of motor neurones and bilateral demyelination of the pyramidal tracts were observed in cases presenting clinically with features of ALS.

Conclusions and critique

ALS/PDC of Guam is a severe tangle-forming disorder that affects both neuronal and glial cells. The neurofibrillary tangles of the Guamanian disorder are biochemically and ultrastructurally similar to those of Western AD [79]. The striking decline in disease suggests a changing diet or decreased exposure to environmental factors. Because ALS/PDC predominates in Chamorros and their families, its cause may be influenced by the traditional, pre World War II subsistence life style of Chamorro families. Steele and McGeer reviewed the various hypotheses that have been proposed as contributing to the Guam syndrome during the past 60 years [80]. These included deficiency in calcium and magnesium, toxicity for the cycad plant, some unidentified transmissible agent, and a primary genetic defect. All of these have thus far failed to be supported by experimental evidence. An interesting observation in the Guamanian disease is the high incidence (52%) of 'linear retinal pigment epitheliopathy'. Cox et al. first reported a significant association between this eye finding and ALS/PDC of Guam, and it often predates the onset of the neurological syndrome [81]. This eye finding is unique to Guamanian ALS and further understanding of underlying biological commonality of these apparently independent aspects of the disease is important [82].

9.10 **When does amyotrophic lateral sclerosis begin?**

Main paper: Turner MR, Barnwell J, Al-Chalabi A, Eisen A. Young-onset amyotrophic lateral sclerosis: historical and other observations. *Brain* 2012; 135:2883–2891.

Background

'Juvenile ALS' refers to patients with symptom onset before age 25 years. This typically occurs in association with a positive family history and such cases characteristically are slowly progressive [83]. Early reports highlight the diagnostic difficulty in children and the distance from our current genetically defined understanding of such disorders [84, 85]. In contrast, 'Young-onset' ALS is considered to be similar to 'classic' Charcot ALS, with mixed UMN and LMN features, commencing before an arbitrary cut-off age in the region of 45 years. Such cases are apparently sporadic. In clinic-based series, younger age is then an independent predictor of longer survival [86, 87].

Methods

Approximately 200 cases of ALS that were described in the literature, from the very earliest by Cruveilhier [2] through to the early 1960s, were reviewed to determine the mean age of disease onset. The largest and most comprehensive series were those by Professor Joseph Collins (1866–1950) [88] and Professor Israel S. Wechsler (1886–1962) [89].

Results

Most (80%) of the cases were sporadic and had disease onset < 45 years (mean, 40 years; SD 9). In detailed analysis of 28 cases published between 1853 and 1931, male to female ratio was 3:1. There was bulbar onset in 18%, upper limb onset in 43%, and lower limb onset in 29%. Bulbar-onset ALS was less common in young-onset ALS. A large European, population-based analysis noted rising proportions of bulbar-onset ALS with higher age of symptom onset [90]. In the King's College London tertiary clinic database, overall, 25% of 1384 cases of sporadic ALS were bulbar-onset. Bulbar-onset frequency was independently positively correlated with higher age at symptom onset (p<0.001) and significantly under-represented among young-onset ALS cases.

Conclusions and critique

Much remains to be learned about ALS. The fact that reduced longevity in times when ALS was first recognized, may not be directly related to, or completely responsible for high numbers of young-onset ALS at that time must reflect important messages. The modifying factors, which broadly include genetic, epigenetic. and environmental influences, are poorly understood and not static. They may increase or lessen in degree, often disappearing altogether, to be replaced by new ones. If one attempts to begin to tie together a postulate for ALS, it might go something like: ALS is a perinatal disorder. Neural circuit formation and function is adversely impacted by somatic (non-germ cell) mutations during embryogenesis or in the perinatal period under the influence of epigenetic and environmental factors. The number, type, and interplay of mutations underlies ALS phenotypic variability (age of onset, site of onset, and rate of progression). The essential physiological effect of the mutations is imbalanced excitatory-inhibitory neuronal inputs resulting in chronic neuronal excitation which eventually, with the added effects of ageing, environmental factors, and epigenetic influences, culminates in the accumulation of misfolded proteins and loss of cellular homeostasis. There follows a cascade of biochemical/biophysical events that result in cell death, manifesting in clinical ALS. A similar process most likely involves all neurodegenerative disorders.

Key unanswered questions

1   What is/are the cell(s) of origin of ALS?

Conventionally, cortical and spinal motor neurons are regarded as the prime cells responsible for classic clinical UMN and LMN deficits. This may be an oversimplification. At least two other cell groups are important in ALS. One is glial cells and the other, interneurons. Important two-way conversations occur between glia and neurons and it is possible that glia are the disease-initiating cells. It is also well established that excitotoxicity (possibly longstanding and chronic in nature) is an important pathogenic mechanism in ALS. This may result from increased glutamergic activity or, more likely, from reduced GABA-ergic activity. GABA (gamma-aminobutyric acid) is the main inhibitory neurotransmitter in the adult brain and acts synaptically to inhibit neurons, primarily by binding to $GABA_A$ or $GABA_B$ receptors. In the developing nervous system, GABA is one of the earliest, and most highly evolutionarily conserved, neurotransmitters. During embryogenesis, GABA is 'excitatory' and able to depolarize progenitor cells and their progeny due to their high intracellular chloride concentration. The embryonic form of GABA signalling may provide the main excitatory drive for the immature cortical network and play a central role in regulating cortical development.

2   When does ALS begin?

The onset of ALS is commonly (and consistently, for therapeutic trials) taken as the time of first clinical manifestations. This is unlikely to reflect the onset of the degenerative process. The pathological changes that characterize both AD and PD have lengthy pre-clinical periods amounting to years, if not decades, and this is likely to be true of ALS also. During development, there are many cell divisions and, consequently, much somatic mutation must occur. Developmental mutations likely have significant risk of ALS and other neurodegenerative disorders. [Eisen A, Kiernan M, Mitsumoto H, Swash M. Amyotrophic lateral sclerosis: a long preclinical period? J Neurol Neurosurg Psychiatry 2014; 85:1232–1238.]

3   Why is it important to understand cortical–spinal interactions?

Skilled motor behaviour begins before birth but continues during a protracted postnatal period. The corticospinal system (CST) develops over a similarly protracted period. The CST is required for skilled movements in maturity and the expression of motor skills during development cannot occur until the CST achieves requisite motor milestones. Thus, motor skills are delayed until there is a structured M1 motor representation and the capacity for selective CST access to restricted spinal motor circuits. Understanding these complex interactions is essential for interpretation of what happens when they degenerate, as in ALS.

4   Why do we need to consider ALS in terms of protein–protein interactions?

For two decades, there has been a major thrust to identify 'risk' genes for ALS. The likely number will undoubtedly be large. Thus far, there is little or no knowledge on the mechanism of action of identified proteins (gene-product), but even when this occurs, a large gap in understanding would remain. Protein interactions mediate most cellular mechanisms and protein–protein interaction networks are essential in the study of cellular processes. Considering disease in terms of protein–protein interactions, rather than individual genes and proteins, will help to untangle jumbled and confusing clinical observations. For example, mutations in the same protein could lead to different diseases by disrupting different interactions. Similarly, mutations in different proteins that disrupt the same interaction could lead to the same disease. Understanding protein–protein interactions in ALS will be a major step in understanding the disorder.

5 What are the benefits of understanding neural networks in ALS?

In the healthy brain, activities in different regions are balanced for optimal overall network performance. Injuries to a specific brain (network) region can destabilize the whole network, altering activity in other brain regions that may be distant from the site of original injury, and result in unanticipated neurological deficits. Early on, this may reflect reversible dysfunction rather than loss of neurons. This would explain the striking fluctuations in patients' dysfunction from day to day. Understanding the fundamentals of disintegrating neural networks and how they result in the ultimate failure of neurological functions will open therapeutic windows in ALS.

References

1 **Clarke L, Jackson HJ.** On a case of muscular atrophy with disease of the spinal cord and medulla oblongata. *Med Chir Trans* 1867; **50**:489–98.

2 **Cruveilhier J.** Sur la paralysie musculaire progressive atrophique. *Arch Gen Med* 1853; **1**:561.

3 **Veltema AN.** The case of the saltimbanque Prosper Lecomte. A contribution to the study of the history of progressive muscular atrophy (Aran-Duchenne) and amyotrophic lateral sclerosis (Charcot). *Clin Neurol Neurosurg* 1975; **78**(3):204–9.

4 **Clarke J.** Nervous affections of the sixth and seventh decades of life. *BMJ* 1915; **2**:665–70.

5 **Charcot J-M, Joffroy A.** Deus cas d'atrophie musculaire progressive avec lesions de la substance grise et des faisceaux antéro-latérale. *Arch Physiol* 1869; **2**:354–7, 744–60.

6 **Charcot JM.** Sclérose des cordons latéraux de la moelle épinière chez une femme hystérique atteinte de contracture permanente des quatre membres. *Bull Société Méd Hôpit Paris* 1865; **10**:24–35.

7 **Eisen A.** Amyotrophic lateral sclerosis: a 40-year personal perspective. *J Clin Neurosci (Australasia)* 2009; **16**(4):505–12.

8 **Kiernan MC, Vucic S, Cheah BC, et al.** Amyotrophic lateral sclerosis. *Lancet* 2011; **377**(9769):942–55.

9 **Aran F.** Recherches sur une maladie non encore decrite du systeme musculaire (atrophie musculaire progressive). *Arch Gen Med* 1850; **3**:5–35.

10 **Byrne S, Walsh C, Lynch C, et al.** Rate of familial amyotrophic lateral sclerosis: a systematic review and meta-analysis. *J Neurol Neurosurg Psychiat* 2011; **82**(6):623–7.

11 **Fallis BA, Hardiman O.** Aggregation of neurodegenerative disease in ALS kindreds. *Amyot Lat Sclerosis* 2009; **10**(2):95–8.

12 **Hu J, Chen K, Ni B, Li L, Chen G, Shi S.** A novel SOD1 mutation in amyotrophic lateral sclerosis with a distinct clinical phenotype. *Amyot Lat Sclerosis* 2012; **13**(1):149–54.

13 **Keckarevic D, Stevic Z, Keckarevic-Markovic M, Kecmanovic M, Romac S.** A novel P66S mutation in exon 3 of the SOD1 gene with early onset and rapid progression. *Amyot Lat Sclerosis* 2012; **13**(2):237–40.

14 **Vande Velde C, Dion PA, Rouleau GA.** Amyotrophic lateral sclerosis: new genes, new models, and new mechanisms. *F1000 Biol Reps* 2011; **3**:18.

15 **Chen L, Li W, Zhang L, et al.** Disease gene interaction pathways: a potential framework for how disease genes associate by disease-risk modules. *PloS One* 2011; **6**(9):e24495.

16 **Steen KV.** Travelling the world of gene-gene interactions. *Briefings Bioinform* 2012; **13**(1):1–19.

17 **Kennedy SR, Loeb LA, Herr AJ.** Somatic mutations in aging, cancer and neurodegeneration. *Mech Ageing Develop* 2012; **133**(4):118–26.

18 **Knight J.** Resolving the variable genome and epigenome in human disease. *J Intern Med* 2012; **271**:379–391.

19 **Lattante S, Conte A, Zollino M, et al.** Contribution of major amyotrophic lateral sclerosis genes to the etiology of sporadic disease. *Neurology* 2012; **79**:66–72.

20 **Van Den Bosch L.** Genetic rodent models of amyotrophic lateral sclerosis. *J Biomed Biotechnol* 2011:11.

21 **Norris FH, Jr.** Prognosis in amyotrophic lateral sclerosis. *Trans Amer Neurol Assoc* 1971; **96**:290–1.

22 **Hillel AD, Miller RM, Yorkston K, McDonald E, Norris FH, Konikow N.** Amyotrophic lateral sclerosis severity scale. *Neuroepidemiology* 1989; **8**(3):142–50.

23 **Cedarbaum JM, Stambler N, Malta E, et al.** The ALSFRS-R: a revised ALS functional rating scale that incorporates assessments of respiratory function. BDNF ALS Study Group (Phase III). *J Neurol Sci* 1999; **169**(1–2):13–21.

24 **Castrillo-Viguera C, Grasso DL, Simpson E, Shefner J, Cudkowicz ME.** Clinical significance in the change of decline in ALSFRS-R. *Amyot Lat Sclerosis* 2010; **11**(1–2):178–80.

25 **Lechtzin N, Maragakis NJ, Kimball R, Busse A, Hoffman V, Clawson L.** Accurate ALSFRS-R scores can be generated from retrospective review of clinic notes. *Amyot Lat Sclerosis* 2009; **10**(4):244–7.

26 **Kaufmann P, Levy G, Montes J, et al.** Excellent inter-rater, intra-rater, and telephone-administered reliability of the ALSFRS-R in a multicenter clinical trial. *Amyot Lat Sclerosis* 2007; **8**(1):42–6.

27 **Gordon PH, Cheung YK.** Progression rate of ALSFRS-R at time of diagnosis predicts survival time in ALS. *Neurology* 2006; **67**(7):1314–5; author reply 5.

28 **Atsuta N, Watanabe H, Ito M, et al.** Development of a telephone survey system for patients with amyotrophic lateral sclerosis using the ALSFRS-R (Japanese version) and application of this system in a longitudinal multicenter study. *Brain Nerve* 2011; **63**(5):491–6.

29 **Kasarskis EJ, Dempsey-Hall L, Thompson MM, Luu LC, Mendiondo M, Kryscio R.** Rating the severity of ALS by caregivers over the telephone using the ALSFRS-R. *Amyot Lat Sclerosis* 2005; **6**(1):50–4.

30 **Damiano AM, Patrick DL, Guzman GI, et al.** Measurement of health-related quality of life in patients with amyotrophic lateral sclerosis in clinical trials of new therapies. *Med Care* 1999; **37**(1):15–26.

31 **Tramonti F, Bongioanni P, Di Bernardo C, Davitti S, Rossi B.** Quality of life of patients with amyotrophic lateral sclerosis. *Psychol Health Med* 2012. **17**:621–628.

32 **Montel S, Albertini L, Spitz E.** Coping strategies in relation to quality of life in amyotrophic lateral sclerosis. Muscle & Nerve 2012; **45**(1):131–4.

33 **Ravits JM, La Spada AR.** ALS motor phenotype heterogeneity, focality, and spread: deconstructing motor neuron degeneration. *Neurology* 2009; **73**(10):805–11.

34 **Eisen A.** The real onset of amyotrophic lateral sclerosis. *J Neurol Neurosurg Psychiat* 2011; **82**(6):593.

35 **Vucic S, Nicholson GA, Kiernan MC.** Cortical hyperexcitability may precede the onset of familial amyotrophic lateral sclerosis. *Brain* 2008; **131**(Pt 6):1540–50.

36 **Andersen PM.** Mutation in C9orf72 changes the boundaries of ALS and FTD. *Lancet Neurol* 2012; **11**(3):205–7.

37 **Phukan J, Pender NP, Hardiman O.** Cognitive impairment in amyotrophic lateral sclerosis. *Lancet Neurol* 2007; **6**(11):994–1003.

38 **Atassi N, Cook A, Pineda CM, Yerramilli-Rao P, Pulley D, Cudkowicz M.** Depression in amyotrophic lateral sclerosis. *Amyot Lat Sclerosis* 2011; **12**(2):109–12.

39 **Tsara V, Serasli E, Steiropoulos P, Tsorova A, Antoniadou M, Zisi P.** Respiratory function in amyotrophic lateral sclerosis patients. The role of sleep studies. *Hippokratia* 2010; **14**(1):33–6.

40 **Baumann F, Henderson RD, Morrison SC, et al.** Use of respiratory function tests to predict survival in amyotrophic lateral sclerosis. *Amyot Lat Sclerosis* 2010; **11**(1–2):194–202.

41 **Wechsler IS, Dvison C.** Amyotrophic lateral sclerosis with mental symptoms. *Arch Neurol Psychiat* 1932; **27**(4):859–80.

42 **Hutton M, Lendon CL, Rizzu P, et al.** Association of missense and 5'-splice-site mutations in tau with the inherited dementia FTDP-17. *Nature* 1998; **393**(6686):702–5.

43 **Huey ED, Grafman J, Wassermann EM, et al.** Characteristics of frontotemporal dementia patients with a Progranulin mutation. *Ann Neurol* 2006; **60**(3):374–80.

44 **Skoglund L, Brundin R, Olofsson T, et al.** Frontotemporal dementia in a large Swedish family is caused by a progranulin null mutation. *Neurogenetics* 2009; **10**(1):27–34.

45 **Simon-Sanchez J, Dopper EG, Cohn-Hokke PE, et al.** The clinical and pathological phenotype of C9ORF72 hexanucleotide repeat expansions. *Brain* 2012; **135**(Pt 3):723–35.

46 **Snowden JS, Rollinson S, Thompson JC, et al.** Distinct clinical and pathological characteristics of frontotemporal dementia associated with C9ORF72 mutations. *Brain* 2012; **135**(Pt 3):693–708.

47 **Mahoney CJ, Beck J, Rohrer JD, et al.** Frontotemporal dementia with the C9ORF72 hexanucleotide repeat expansion: clinical, neuroanatomical and neuropathological features. *Brain* 2012; **135**(Pt 3):736–50.

48 **Boeve BF, Boylan KB, Graff-Radford NR, et al.** Characterization of frontotemporal dementia and/or amyotrophic lateral sclerosis associated with the GGGGCC repeat expansion in C9ORF72. *Brain* 2012; **135**(Pt 3):765–83.

49 **Hsiung GY, DeJesus-Hernandez M, Feldman HH, et al.** Clinical and pathological features of familial frontotemporal dementia caused by C9ORF72 mutation on chromosome 9p. *Brain* 2012; **135**(Pt 3):709–22.

50 **Whitwell JL, Weigand SD, Boeve BF, et al.** Neuroimaging signatures of frontotemporal dementia genetics: C9ORF72, tau, progranulin and sporadics. *Brain* 2012; **135**(Pt 3):794–806.

51 **Chio A, Borghero G, Restagno G, et al.** Clinical characteristics of patients with familial amyotrophic lateral sclerosis carrying the pathogenic GGGGCC hexanucleotide repeat expansion of C9ORF72. *Brain* 2012; **135**(Pt 3):784–93.

52 **Cooper-Knock J, Hewitt C, Highley JR, et al.** Clinico-pathological features in amyotrophic lateral sclerosis with expansions in C9ORF72. *Brain* 2012; **135**(Pt 3):751–64.

53 **Bak TH.** Motor neuron disease and frontotemporal dementia: one, two, or three diseases? *Ann Indian Acad Neurol* 2010; **13**(Suppl 2):S81–8.

54 **Bak TH, Chandran S.** What wires together dies together: verbs, actions and neurodegeneration in motor neuron disease. *Cortex* 2011; **48**:936–944.

55 **Weiner LP, Stohlman SA, Davis RL.** Attempts to demonstrate virus in amyotrophic lateral sclerosis. *Neurology* 1980; **30**(12):1319–22.

56 **Sola P, Bedin R, Casoni F, Barozzi P, Mandrioli J, Merelli E.** New insights into the viral theory of amyotrophic lateral sclerosis: study on the possible role of Kaposi's sarcoma-associated virus/human herpesvirus 8. *Eur Neurol* 2002; **47**(2):108–12.

57 **Jubelt B.** Motor neuron diseases and viruses: poliovirus, retroviruses, and lymphomas. *Curr Opinion Neurol Neurosurg* 1992; **5**(5):655–8.

58 **Sigurdsson B.** Diagnosis of virus diseases. *Laeknabladid* 1957; **41**(4):49–53.

59 **Takasu T.** Disease concept of the slow virus infection. *Nihon Rinsho* 2007; **65**(8):1361–8.

60 **Orellana JA, von Bernhardi R, Giaume C, Saez JC.** Glial hemichannels and their involvement in aging and neurodegenerative diseases. *Revs Neurosci* 2012; **23**(2):163–77.

61 **Gibbs CJ Jr., Gajdusek DC.** Amyotrophic lateral sclerosis, Parkinson's disease, and the amyotrophic lateral sclerosis-Parkinsonism-dementia complex on Guam: a review and summary of attempts to demonstrate infection as the aetiology. *J Clin Pathol Suppl (R Coll Pathol)* 1972; **6**:132–40.

62 **Gajdusek DC, Gibbs CJ.** Attempts to demonstrate a transmissible agent in Kuru, amyotrophic lateral sclerosis, and other sub-acute and chronic nervous system degenerations of man. *Nature* 1964; **204**:257–9.

63 **Fraser H, Behan W, Chree A, Crossland G, Behan P.** Mouse inoculation studies reveal no transmissible agent in amyotrophic lateral sclerosis. *Brain Pathol* 1996; **6**(2):89–99.

64 **Kuwabara S, Yokota T.** Propagation: prion-like mechanisms can explain spreading of motor neuronal death in amyotrophic lateral sclerosis? *J Neurol Neurosurg Psychiat* 2011; **82**(11):1181–2.

65 **Liversedge LA.** Glycocyamine and betaine in motor-neurone disease. *Lancet* 1956; **271**:1136–8.

66 **Turner MR, Parton MJ, Leigh PN.** Clinical trials in ALS: an overview. *Semin Neurol* 2001; **21**(2):167–75.

67 **Rothstein JD, Martin LJ, Kuncl RW.** Decreased glutamate transport by the brain and spinal cord in amyotrophic lateral sclerosis. *N Engl J Med* 1992; **326**(22):1464–8.

68 **Harwood CA, McDermott CJ, Shaw PJ.** Physical activity as an exogenous risk factor in motor neuron disease (MND): a review of the evidence. *Amyot Lat Sclerosis* 2009; **10**(4):191–204.

69 **Brooks BR.** El Escorial World Federation of Neurology criteria for the diagnosis of amyotrophic lateral sclerosis. Subcommittee on Motor Neuron Diseases/Amyotrophic Lateral Sclerosis of the World Federation of Neurology Research Group on Neuromuscular Diseases and the El Escorial 'Clinical limits of amyotrophic lateral sclerosis' workshop contributors. *J Neurol Sci* 1994; **124** (Suppl):96–107.

70 **Miller RG, Mitchell JD, Lyon M, Moore DH.** Riluzole for amyotrophic lateral sclerosis (ALS)/motor neuron disease (MND). *Cochrane Database Syst Rev* 2007(**1**):CD001447.

71 **Miller RG, Jackson CE, Kasarskis EJ, et al.** Practice parameter update: the care of the patient with amyotrophic lateral sclerosis: multidisciplinary care, symptom management, and cognitive/behavioral impairment (an evidence-based review): report of the Quality Standards Subcommittee of the American Academy of Neurology. *Neurology* 2009; **73**(15):1227–33.

72 **Del Rio Hortega P.** El 'tercer elemento' de los centros nerviosos. Poder fagocitario y movilidad de la microglia. *Bol Soc Esp Biol Ano* 1919; **9**:154–66.

73 **Davis EJ, Foster TD, Thomas WE.** Cellular forms and functions of brain microglia. *Brain Res Bull* 1994; **34**(1):73–8.

74 **Glass CK, Saijo K, Winner B, Marchetto MC, Gage FH.** Mechanisms underlying inflammation in neurodegeneration. *Cell* 2010; **140**(6):918–34.

75 **McGeer PL, McGeer EG.** Inflammatory processes in amyotrophic lateral sclerosis. *Muscle & Nerve* 2002; **26**(4):459–70.

76 **Kreutzberg GW.** Microglia: a sensor for pathological events in the CNS. *Trends Neurosci* 1996; **19**(8):312–8.

77 **Streit WJ.** Microglia as neuroprotective, immunocompetent cells of the CNS. *Glia* 2002; **40**(2):133–9.

78 **Garruto RM, Yanagihara R, Gajdusek DC.** Disappearance of high-incidence amyotrophic lateral sclerosis and parkinsonism-dementia on Guam. *Neurology* 1985; **35**(2):193–8.

79 **Oyanagi K, Makifuchi T, Ohtoh T, et al.** Amyotrophic lateral sclerosis of Guam: the nature of the neuropathological findings. *Acta Neuropath* 1994; **88**(5):405–12.

80 **Steele JC, McGeer PL.** The ALS/PDC syndrome of Guam and the cycad hypothesis. *Neurology* 2008; **70**(21):1984–90.

81 **Cox TA, McDarby JV, Lavine L, Steele JC, Calne DB.** A retinopathy on Guam with high prevalence in Lytico-Bodig. *Ophthalmology* 1989; **96**(12):1731–5.

82 **Morris HR, Al-Sarraj S, Schwab C, et al.** A clinical and pathological study of motor neurone disease on Guam. *Brain* 2001; **124**(Pt 11):2215–22.

83 **Orban P, Devon RS, Hayden MR, Leavitt BL.** Juvenile amyotrophic lateral sclerosis. In: Eisen A, Shaw, PJ, ed. *Handbook of Clinical Neurology, Motor Neuron Disorders and Related Disorders.* Amsterdam: Elsevier B.V.; 2007; 301–12.

84 **Gordon R, Delicati JL.** The occurrence of amyotrophic lateral sclerosis in children. *J Neurol Psychopathol* 1928; **9**:30–5.

85 **Lelong J, Lereboullet J, Merklen FP.** Amyotrophic lateral sclerosis in a girl 16 years old. *Bull Soc Pediat Paris* 1932; **30**:88–93.

86 **Chio A, Logroscino G, Hardiman O, et al.** Prognostic factors in ALS: a critical review. *Amyot Lat Sclerosis* 2009; **10**(5–6):310–23.

87 **Eisen A, Schulzer M, MacNeil M, Pant B, Mak E.** Duration of amyotrophic lateral sclerosis is age dependent. *Muscle & Nerve* 1993; **16**(1):27–32.

88 **Collins J.** Amyotrophic lateral sclerosis. *Amer J Med Sci* 1903; **125**:939–66.

89 **Wechsler I, Sapirstein MR, Stein A.** Primary and symptomatic amyotrophic lateral sclerosis: a clinical study of 81 cases. *Amer J Med Sci* 1944; **208**:70–81.

90 **Chio A, Canosa A, Gallo S, et al.** Pain in amyotrophic lateral sclerosis: a population-based controlled study. Eur J Neurol 2011; **19**:551–555.

Chapter 10

Dementia

James R. Burrell and John R. Hodges

10.0 **Introduction**

Since the birth of cognitive neurology with Alzheimer's first description of the disease that now bears his name, knowledge of neurodegenerative disease has exploded. From the distinction of dementia as a pathological entity, rather than just 'normal' ageing, to more sophisticated sub-classification of dementia syndromes, much has been learned, though great challenges remain. The clinical, neuropsychological, neuroimaging, genetic, and pathological hallmarks of Alzheimer's disease, frontotemporal dementia, diffuse Lewy body disease, vascular dementia, and other dementia syndromes are now well described, but have not yet led to any effective disease-modifying treatments.

From an incredible array of worthy research studies, we have chosen 10 landmark papers in the field of dementia. In Alzheimer's disease, we discuss the initial description of the disease, both clinically and pathologically, the development of meaningful clinical assessment methods to stage and assess the severity of dementia, the description of the earliest clinical manifestations (known as mild cognitive impairment), the discovery of the first genetic causes, the precursors to symptomatic treatment, the identification of amyloid pathology *in vivo* using neuroimaging, and the staging of Alzheimer's pathology. We also discuss the clinical features and recent discovery of genetic causes of frontotemporal dementia, an important non-Alzheimer's primary dementia syndrome.

10.1 **Alzheimer's disease**

Main paper: Alzheimer A. Über eine eigenartige Erkrankung der Hirnrinde. *Allg Z Psychiat* 1907; 64:146–8.

Background

The turn of the twentieth century saw an irresistible wave of advances in neuroscience, and the clinical and research foundations of modern neurology were laid at breakneck speed. Terms such as 'neuron' [1], 'axon', 'dendrite' [2], and 'synapse' [3] were all coined in the decade leading up to 1900, as the so-called 'neuron theory' was established [1].

In cognitive neurology, the modern concept of 'senile' dementia had begun to coalesce in the latter decades of the nineteenth century [4]. Arnold Pick (1851–1924) had described, in 1892, what is now referred to as frontotemporal dementia. In neuropsychiatry, the work of Freud loomed large; his 'Interpretation of Dreams' was first published in 1900.

Alois Alzheimer (1864–1915) underwent training in psychiatry as well as neuropathology. Alzheimer—the 'psychiatrist with a microscope'—developed an interest in histopathology under the influence of Albert von Kölliker (1871–1905) as an undergraduate at the University of Würzburg. In December 1888, Alzheimer was appointed to the Municipal Asylum for the Insane and Epileptic in Frankfurt am Main, where his histopathological interests were further fostered in collaboration with Franz Nissl (1860–1919) and he first encountered the disease that would ultimately carry his name.

The case of Auguste D. (Fig. 10.1), a 51-year-old woman admitted to the Asylum in November 1901 with a multitude of cognitive symptoms, fascinated Alzheimer—so much so that he arranged to examine her brain after her death in 1906, even though by then he had left Frankfurt and was working at the Munich Medical School. Alzheimer presented the case, and the neuropathological findings, at a conference in Tübingen in November 1906, and the proceedings were published the following year. This brief report of a single case is now widely recognized as the first description of Alzheimer's disease [5].

Methods

In the traditions of nineteenth-century neuropsychiatry, Alzheimer presented a detailed description of the clinical features of the case of August D. In addition, then state of the art histopathological methods were applied to study the neuropathology. In particular, Alzheimer employed silver staining—following the technique described by Bielschowsky a few years earlier—to demonstrate the characteristic plaques and tangles of Alzheimer's disease pathology within the cerebral cortex.

Results

Modern clinicians would recognize many of the classic symptoms and signs of Alzheimer's disease in this brief case report. August D. presented with paranoid thoughts, but marked memory disturbance and disorientation soon supervened. Alzheimer described bedside testing of naming (normal) and short-term recall (impaired), using a collection of objects

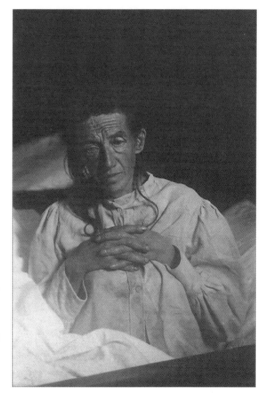

Fig. 10.1 Auguste D. The case of Auguste D. so fascinated Alzheimer that he arranged to examine her brain after death, even though he was no longer her treating doctor. Using then 'state of the art' silver staining techniques, Alzheimer discovered characteristic features of the pathology that now carries his name.

presented to the patient. In addition, he reported problems with reading—possibly due to surface dyslexia—and writing difficulties, with spelling errors. Her speech was characterized by apparent word-finding difficulties, or 'gap-fills' as Alzheimer called them, and semantic substitutions; for example, Auguste D. referred to a cup as a 'milk-pourer'. Auguste D. had obvious impairment of comprehension and trouble using tools. On physical examination, Alzheimer reported normal pupillary contraction, upper limb function, deep tendon reflexes, and gait. Auguste D. deteriorated over a period of four and a half years and by the end was bed-bound.

Alzheimer examined the brain after death. Macroscopically, he described generalized atrophy with some atherosclerotic changes in the major cerebral blood vessels. Silver staining revealed numerous 'fibrils' within neurons, often combined in thick 'bundles' or 'tangles', associated with neuronal loss.

Conclusions

Alzheimer's report links the clinical characteristics of 'pre-senile' dementia to the characteristic pathological features of Alzheimer's disease. In addition to the description of typical pathological features of Alzheimer's disease, the report emphasizes a distinction of this case, on clinical grounds, from the far more typical 'senile' dementia.

Critique

Although an obvious landmark in the cognitive neurology canon, Alzheimer's report is not without controversy; rarely has a single case report enjoyed such influence. The term 'Alzheimer's disease' was first coined in 1910 by Emil Kraeplin (1856–1926), Alzheimer's colleague and superior at the Munich Clinical School, in his textbook of psychiatry. In line with Alzheimer's original conclusions, Kraeplin presented the disease as a rapidly progressive early-onset dementia, which was clearly different to the typical 'senile' dementia. Why he applied the eponym 'Alzheimer's disease' to the condition is uncertain, but may have been, in part, due to the pressure on his academic department to 'perform' [5].

Alzheimer's distinction of this case from cases of 'senile' dementia, which he justified on the basis of several atypical and 'focal' clinical features, has had far-reaching implications, some of which are still detectable in contemporary literature. One obvious consequence was the fact that Alzheimer's disease was considered a rare disease of younger people. As such, research on Alzheimer's disease was sparse for almost 50 years following this initial report [5]. Whether early- and late-onset Alzheimer's disease represent two variations of the same disease, or separate entities, remains to be fully resolved [6]. Furthermore, the relationships of normal ageing and dementia continue to perplex, particularly as sensitive techniques for amyloid imaging become more widely available in clinical practice [7]. Alzheimer can also be credited with providing the first pathological descriptions of what became known as Pick's disease, with dense argyrophilic bodies in patients with focal frontotemporal atrophy [8, 9]. The concept of 'atypical' Alzheimer's disease phenotypes has been revived; atypical clinical presentations, in which disturbances of language, motor function, or visual function occur early and dominate the clinical presentation, may in fact be more common in younger patients [10, 11], in part validating Alzheimer's observations.

10.2 **Exploring cognitive deficits in relation to neuropathology**

Main paper: Blessed G, Tomlinson BE, Roth M. The association between quantitative measures of dementia and of senile change in the cerebral gray matter of elderly subjects. *Br J Psychiatry* 1968; 114:797–811.

Background

Sixty years after Alzheimer's landmark paper, the relationship between cognitive deficits in older people and the neuropathological changes in his original description remained uncertain. The increased incidence of Alzheimer's disease pathology with advancing age was recognized, but the presence of this pathology in the 'preserved elderly' clouded the picture. What were the pathological differences between demented patients and older control subjects? Did the pathological differences simply reflect disease burden, or was some other factor at play? Further complicating the picture, a significant proportion of elderly patients with late-onset psychiatric disease were recognized to harbour similar neuropathological changes at autopsy. Could Alzheimer's disease pathology explain such varied clinical phenotypes, or were these changes simply incidental?

In this paper, Blessed et al. addressed three main hypotheses:

1 that late-onset dementia was associated with Alzheimer's disease pathology;

2 that the severity of cognitive deficits correlated with the severity of the neuropathology identified at autopsy; and

3 that the neuropathological changes identified in demented patients differed in some critical way from the changes identified in 'preserved elderly' subjects.

Methods

Patients and controls were recruited from a psychiatric hospital, a geriatric hospital, and general hospital wards; patients with dementia and late-onset psychiatric disease were recruited. Patients were classified according to the clinical diagnosis in life. Categories included: 'senile dementia', 'depression', 'paraphrenia', and 'delirium'. Controls were recruited from 'physically ill subjects' who underwent autopsy in the general hospital. Cognition and behaviour were measured using a novel functional scale and a basic neuropsychological battery. The functional scale used an informant to grade the patient's performance on a number of everyday tasks—specifically, performance of household chores, handling money, or in finding their way around—over the preceding 6 months. A three-point grading system was used: 1 indicated inability to complete the task; 0.5 indicated variable or incomplete performance; and 0 indicated preserved ability. Tests of orientation, concentration, recent memory, and remote memory made up the neuropsychological battery. The battery was scored from 0 (complete incapacity) to 37 (flawless performance).

A standardized protocol was used to count the number of senile plaques, which were considered to be representative of Alzheimer's neuropathology. Brain specimens were sectioned in the coronal plane at 8–10 mm intervals. Brains with a large volume of ischaemic lesions (greater than 50 mL in total) were excluded from the study. Multiple 3 cm square samples of brain tissue were taken from 12 pre-defined brain regions (two from each of the frontal and occipital lobes, as well as one from each temporal lobe, and a further specimen from the opercular cortex). Hippocampal specimens were also studied, but excluded from the mean plaque count measure. Five low-power fields were randomly selected from each of the 12 brain regions so that 60 low-power fields were used to calculate the plaque count in each specimen.

Results

A total of 264 patients underwent cognitive and behavioural testing; pathological evaluation was available in 76 of these patients. Of these 76 patients, 16 had a large volume of ischaemic change and were analysed separately. Of the 60 cases in the main part of the study, 26 had dementia, 12 had functional disorders (depression or paraphrenia), 14 had delirium, and 8 were control subjects.

Patients with dementia had a significantly increased plaque count when compared to controls, whereas the plaque count was not significantly increased in patients with delirium or functional disorders. Meanwhile, patients with unequivocal vascular disease did not have a significant increase in plaque count compared to controls. The mean plaque count was significantly and strongly correlated with functional disability and poor performance on cognitive testing. When stratified according to the severity of functional and cognitive impairment, plaques and neurofibrillary tangles were distributed throughout the full thickness of the cerebral cortex, rather than limited to the superficial cortical layers, and generalized rather than limited to the hippocampus, in severely demented patients. The pathological features of Alzheimer's disease, while more frequent and widespread in demented patients, were also identified in control subjects.

Conclusions

This paper was a landmark in the history of cognitive neurology for several reasons. Firstly, an association between the severity of pathological changes of Alzheimer's disease and cognitive impairment was demonstrated unequivocally. It also pioneered a 'real world' quantitative measure of function, the Blessed-Roth Dementia Scale [12], which complemented established neuropsychological testing and became a widely used instrument in cognitive disorders clinics, setting the stage for many subsequent brief cognitive screening instruments including the Addenbrooke's Cognitive Examination [13–15]. Importantly, the lack of plaques in patients with functional or psychiatric illnesses suggested that Alzheimer's disease did not cause these illnesses. Furthermore, demented patients with extensive vascular disease, but little Alzheimer's pathology, foreshadowed the concept of vascular dementia. Finally, although this paper sought to identify differences between the neuropathological changes in dementia compared to those of 'old age', patients and controls had similar types of pathology qualitatively; the main difference was one of severity.

Critique

Senile plaques were used to quantify the degree of Alzheimer's pathology in this study, and other features such as neurofibrillary tangles were not counted or included in the correlations with clinical deficits. Neurofibrillary tangles have subsequently been shown to play a central role in Alzheimer's disease pathogenesis [16], and are important for staging of Alzheimer's pathology. Viewed in the context of the Braak and Braak staging system [17], and the more recent concept of 'pre-clinical' Alzheimer's disease [18], the observation of plaques limited to the hippocampus in controls is tantalizing.

This paper heralded a modern era of clinicopathological studies (pioneered by Alzheimer) with Blessed et al. introducing a quantitative and statistical approach. The pathological analysis of patients who have undergone systematic evaluation in life remains central to dementia research and has led to the recognition of important causes of dementia including dementia with Lewy bodies [19] and subtypes of frontotemporal dementia [20–23]. The problem of selectivity remains, in that many patients who come to autopsy are perhaps not representative of the broader populations with dementia.

10.3 **Refining pathological specificity**

Main paper: Whitehouse PJ, Price DL, Struble RG, Clark AW, Coyle JT, Delon MR. Alzheimer's disease and senile dementia: loss of neurons in the basal forebrain. *Science* 1982; 215(4537):1237–9.

Background

In the mid-1970s, the role of cholinergic systems in human memory was being explored in normal individuals using a classic experimental paradigm involving pharmacological blockade of the cholinergic system [24]. The central and peripheral effects of cholinergic blockade were studied using the pharmacokinetic differences between scopolamine, which can cross the blood-brain, with methscopolamine, which cannot. Impaired memory was detected in the individuals administered scopolamine, but individuals given methscopolamine performed as well as controls. Around the same time, a number of studies suggested a cholinergic deficit in the brains of individuals with Alzheimer's disease [25–27].

In this context, Whitehouse et al. demonstrated significant degeneration of neurons within the nucleus basalis of Meynert—a region very rich in cholinesterase activity—in a patient with familial Alzheimer's disease [28]. The authors went on to hypothesize that selective degeneration of neurons within the nucleus basalis of Meynert was a defining feature of Alzheimer's disease, not only in familial cases, but also in sporadic disease.

Methods

The brains of five demented Alzheimer's disease patients were included in the study and compared to the brains of five non-demented age-matched controls. Two raters who were blinded to the clinical diagnosis counted neurons of the nucleus basalis of Meynert independently, according to pre-defined criteria. Specifically, cells were counted if they satisfied three criteria:

1 they were larger than 30 μm in diameter;

2 abundant Nissl material was demonstrated; and

3 a nucleus was visible.

Three different methods of cell quantification were used; a seven-point grading system (with 0 indicating complete loss of neurons and 6 indicating a normal number), a mean cell count, and a total cell count.

Results

The number of neurons in the nucleus basalis of Meynert was significantly reduced in patients with Alzheimer's disease, regardless of the method used to quantify them. Specifically, the neuron density was reduced by 73% and the total number of neurons reduced by 79%. There was no overlap between the number of cells in Alzheimer's disease patients and controls.

Conclusions

This paper provided an explanation for the apparent cholinergic deficit that had been increasingly characterized in the preceding decade.

Critique

The simplest observations are often the most prescient, and so it seems with the findings of Whitehouse et al. This study consolidated several lines of evidence to emphasize the importance of cholinergic networks in human memory, and their vulnerability in amnestic Alzheimer's disease. In establishing the 'cholinergic hypothesis of Alzheimer's disease' [29], a new direction for pharmacotherapeutics was enthusiastically embraced. Within a decade, a beneficial effect on cognition and functional capacity was demonstrated with the cholinesterase inhibitor, tacrine [30, 31], although adverse effects later led to withdrawal of the medication. Later, donepezil [32] and rivastigmine were also shown to be modestly effective. Even 30 years after the paper by Whitehouse et al., cholinesterase inhibitors remain the only pharmacological therapies proven to be beneficial in Alzheimer's disease, although their efficacy is, at best, modest.

10.4 **Neuropathological staging**

Main paper: Braak H, Braak E. Neuropathological staging of Alzheimer-related changes. *Acta Neuropathol* 1991; 82:239–59.

Background

As methods for detected brain amyloid became more advanced, and more sensitive, it became apparent that not all amyloid deposits were associated with dementia [33]. Indeed, a variety of different amyloid deposits were increasingly recognized—depending on the methods used in their detection—and the clinical relevance of such changes became difficult to decipher. Despite these challenges, the detection and quantification of so-called 'neuritic' or 'senile' plaques [34] formed the basis of the National Institute on Aging (NIA) criteria for the diagnosis of Alzheimer's disease, which were published in the mid-1980s [35]. An alternative set of diagnostic criteria, again based on the presence and frequency of plaques, was developed by the Consortium to Establish a Registry for Alzheimer's Disease (CERAD) which, for the first time, outlined a standardized schema for the diagnosis of 'possible', 'probable', and 'definite' Alzheimer's disease on pathological grounds [36].

Given the difficulties in classification of pathological neuritic plaques from other types of amyloid deposits, the German anatomist, Heiko Braak (b. 1937), together with his wife Eva (1939–2000), studied neurofibrillary tangles as an alternative marker of Alzheimer's disease stage. A detailed cross-sectional analysis of demented and non-demented individuals was performed using a neuroanatomical approach.

Methods

A total of 83 brains were obtained at autopsy and included in the study. Of these 83 cases, eight met clinical criteria for the diagnosis of Alzheimer's disease but did not meet the pathological criteria. A further 21 brains were from patients who met both clinical and pathological criteria for the diagnosis of Alzheimer's disease. The remaining 54 cases did not meet clinical or pathological criteria for the diagnosis of dementia. None of the cases included in the study had macroscopically detectable infarctions. The pathological examination included an assessment for the presence of amyloid deposits and neurofibrillary tangles in multiple brain regions, which were studied systematically.

Results

The two main features of Alzheimer's disease pathology, amyloid deposits and neurofibrillary tangles (Fig. 10.2), were mapped meticulously, and separate staging systems developed for both. With regard to the deposition of amyloid, three stages (A, B, and C) were described. In stage A, low densities of amyloid deposits were encountered in the basal portions of the frontal, temporal, and occipital lobes, but not the hippocampus. Stage B was characterized by medium densities of amyloid deposits in multiple cortical regions, but the primary sensory and primary motor cortices were spared. Finally, stage C was

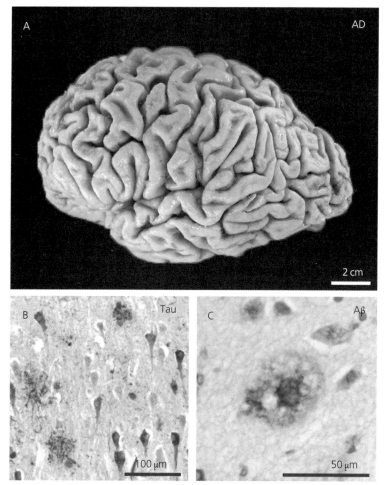

Fig. 10.2 The pathology of Alzheimer's disease. (**A**) On gross examination, generalized cerebral atrophy can be appreciated. (**B**) Neurofibrillary tangles, demonstrated using specific Tau staining. (**C**) Beta-amyloid staining demonstrates neuritic plaques.
Images provided courtesy of H. Cartwright and the Sydney Brain Bank, Sydney, Australia.

characterized by densely packed amyloid deposits in all cortical regions, as well as in some subcortical structures such as the thalamus and hypothalamus.

A six-level staging system for the distribution of neurofibrillary tangles was proposed. Stages I and II were defined by involvement of the entorhinal cortex and related structures, with little or no neocortical pathology. Stages III and IV were defined by increased involvement of limbic structures, with only mild neocortical pathology. By stage V, the neocortex was more definitely involved, whereas stage VI denoted extrapyramidal involvement.

Conclusions

This paper described, for the first time, a clear pattern of progression of Alzheimer's pathology based upon the distribution of neurofibrillary tangles. According to this staging system, the pathology begins in the transentorhinal region before spreading to the hippocampus, the neocortex, and then, finally, the extrapyramidal system. The use of neurofibrillary tangles, rather than neuritic plaques, was established as a useful marker of Alzheimer's disease stage.

Critique

The Braak and Braak system was adopted into revised diagnostic criteria in 1997, and remained an integral part of a further revision published in 2012 [18, 37]. The complexities in the classification of amyloid plaques is avoided altogether by using neurofibrillary tangles as a marker of pathology. Although the original system called for six stages, reducing the classification to four stages (no neurofibrillary tangles, stages I/II, stages III/IV, or stages V/VI) may improve inter-rater reliability [18].

The real genius of the Braak and Braak staging system is that the distribution and evolution of Alzheimer's pathology was carefully described. The model suggests an orderly, step-wise development of pathology from one brain region to the next [38]. Viewed in this context, clinical diseases stages such as 'pre-clinical', 'mild cognitive impairment', and 'dementia' can be more readily understood. Furthermore, subsequent studies confirmed a correlation between clinical features and Braak and Braak stage [39–41].

The study also focused attention on the medial temporal lobe complex, notably the hippocampus and entorhinal cortex, providing a link between neuropsychological investigations of cognitive impairment and neuropathological studies in Alzheimer's disease. It acted as a catalyst for the development of tests of episodic memory which depend upon this region, such as the paired associate learning test from the Cambridge Neuropsychological Test Automated Battery (CANTAB) battery which has proven sensitive for the early detection of the amnesia which characterizes typical Alzheimer's disease [42].

While the Braak and Braak staging system goes some way in explaining the progression of clinical features in so-called 'typical' Alzheimer's disease, 'atypical' phenotypes are now recognized [10, 43], including cases of posterior cortical atrophy, logopenic progressive aphasia [44], and corticobasal syndrome [45]. Clinicopathological correlation studies have suggested that the distribution of neurofibrillary tangles may differ in such atypical cases [11, 43, 46].

10.5 **A genetic link to beta-amyloid**

Main paper: Goate A, Chartier-Harlin MC, Mullan M, et al. Segregation of a missense mutation in the amyloid precursor protein gene with familial Alzheimer's disease. *Nature* 1991; 349:704–6.

Background

In the mid-1980s, amyloid was successfully purified from the brains of patients with extensive cerebral amyloidosis [47]. The same protein—later named beta-amyloid—was soon isolated from the brains of older individuals with Down's syndrome [48]. These two discoveries prompted the 'amyloid cascade' hypothesis of Alzheimer's disease (for review, see Tanzi [49]), which was most clearly outlined in 1992 [50]. In this context, several groups around the world searched frantically to find the gene encoding for beta-amyloid [51–54] and to link such a gene to the pathology of Alzheimer's disease and related conditions. Finally, mutations of the amyloid precursor protein gene (*APP*) were linked to intracerebral haemorrhage due to amyloid angiopathy in a Dutch cohort [55], setting the scene for discoveries in the field of Alzheimer's genetics.

Methods

The *APP* gene was studied in a single family of individuals who had pathologically proven early-onset Alzheimer's disease. A number of deoxyribonucleic acid (DNA) markers were used to narrow down the pathogenic mutation site on chromosome 21; this was made possible by comparing affected and unaffected family members. Once the pathogenic mutation site was shown to be in the vicinity of the *APP* gene, direct sequencing of exon 17 was performed. Exon 17 was selected as a possible mutation site first, since a mutation at this site had recently been detected in patients with hereditary intracerebral haemorrhage with amyloidosis [55].

Results

Sequence of exon 17 of the *APP* gene revealed a point mutation (from C to T) at base pair 2149, which caused a valine to isoleucine change at amino acid 717, in patients with early-onset Alzheimer's disease. This point mutation was not demonstrated in a cohort of 100 normal controls, nor in 14 cases of familial late-onset Alzheimer's disease.

Conclusions

This study demonstrated, for the first time, that early-onset Alzheimer's disease could be associated with a point mutation in the *APP* gene.

Critique

The identification of the first gene defect consolidated the association between Alzheimer's disease and abnormal amyloid protein processing and, critically, opened new avenues to diagnosis and therapeutics, notably via the creation of transgenic mice models of

Alzheimer's disease (for review see Tanzi [49]). While the finding is of critical importance to patients with early-onset familial Alzheimer's disease, mutations of *APP* are an infrequent cause of disease overall, and even in families with young-onset Alzheimer's disease, the second gene defect identified—*Presenilin 1*—turned out to be more common [56, 57]. The most common form of the disease—late-onset sporadic Alzheimer's disease—remains unexplained by these mutations. Furthermore, specific therapeutic strategies aimed at various aspects of amyloid processing have generally been disappointing and none have reached routine clinical practice, as yet.

10.6 **Semantic dementia**

Main paper: Hodges JR, Patterson K, Oxbury S, Funnell E. Semantic dementia: progressive fluent aphasia with temporal lobe atrophy. *Brain* 1992; 115:1783–806.

Background

In 1982, Mesulam published the cases of six patients with progressive speech and language disturbance which he called 'slowly progressive aphasia' [22]; this term was later altered to the general term 'primary progressive aphasia' [23]. Most of the cases presented in Mesulam's original description had *non-fluent* speech with difficulty naming objects (anomia) and word-finding difficulty, but relative preservation of other cognitive functions. The cases were associated with left peri-sylvian atrophy. Mesulam's study re-kindled interest in the focal dementia syndromes, which were first described by Arnold Pick more than a century ago [58, 59].

In this landmark paper, a progressive aphasic syndrome, with several distinct clinical and radiological features, was described. This phenotype was characterized by *fluent* aphasia, severe anomia, and progressive deterioration of semantic knowledge. This paper by Hodges et al. meticulously described the clinical, neuropsychological, and radiological features of the phenotype. The name 'semantic dementia', which was originally proposed by Snowden et al. [60], was reinforced for this fascinating and distinctive disorder.

Methods

The clinical, neuropsychological, and radiological profiles of five patients with semantic dementia were carefully described in detail. Case histories of each patient were described, as was the pattern of language disturbance encountered during the clinical assessment. The presence of severe anomia, semantic paraphrasias, and circumlocutions were reported, all in the context of fluent speech with preserved syntax and prosody.

A detailed discussion of neuropsychological performance was then presented. Specifically, performance on tests of memory (both verbal and visual), visuospatial function, problem solving, and reading was outlined. The semantic deficits were explored further using a number of carefully chosen tasks, which were combined into a 'semantic memory test battery'. These tasks included category fluency, object naming, picture sorting, picture pointing, and generation of verbal definitions.

Results

All five patients presented with complaints of difficulty naming people, places, or objects. On the whole, behavioural changes were mild, although one patient demonstrated marked disinhibition and another demonstrated rigid and obsessive behaviours. Their speech was fluent and retained normal prosody and syntax, although semantic paraphrasias, circumlocutions, and word-finding pauses were described to varying degrees. On clinic-based testing, moderate to severe anomia was universal, but—unlike other primary progressive aphasia syndromes—word knowledge was also found to be deficient; for example, patients had difficulty pointing to an object when given the name and were often unable to define a word or explain the use of an object. The patients with semantic dementia also demonstrated marked surface dyslexia—phonetic pronunciation of irregularly spelled words (e.g. 'pint' spoken as though it rhymed with 'mint').

On neuropsychological tests, patients were found to demonstrate impoverished category fluency, impaired object naming, impaired performance on picture pointing and sorting tasks, and an inability to provide verbal definitions. In contrast, non-verbal memory, working memory (as measured by forward and reverse digit span), and visuospatial function were preserved. Neuroimaging—which included structural (computed tomography—CT and magnetic resonance imaging—MRI) and functional (single-photon emission computed tomography—SPECT and positron emission tomography—PET) scans—revealed temporal atrophy and hypometabolism, more left-sided than right-sided (Fig. 10.3).

Conclusions

This paper clearly defines the clinical, neuropsychological, and radiological hallmarks of semantic dementia, a fascinating and quite distinctive phenotype of frontotemporal dementia. The defining features of the syndrome, including anomia with circumlocutions and semantic paraphrasias, in the context of impaired non-verbal semantic knowledge despite normal syntax and prosody, were described. The neuropsychological profile of semantic dementia was recognized as being distinct from that which one would expect in Alzheimer's disease, leading the authors to (correctly) suggest a non-Alzheimer's aetiology [61]. The marked anterior temporal involvement that is so characteristic of semantic dementia was identified. The authors drew attention to the similarity between their cases and those described by Arnold Pick and, many years later, by Elizabeth Warrington, who described 'selective loss of semantic memory' [62].

Critique

The study set the stage for the classification of the progressive aphasic syndromes within the broader rubric of frontotemporal dementia, by contrasting the features of semantic

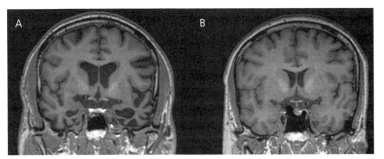

Fig. 10.3 The MRI appearance of semantic dementia. (**A**) Severe, asymmetrical, anterior temporal atrophy is present, worse on the left than the right. (**B**) An age-matched control subject demonstrating normal anterior temporal volume.

dementia to those found in progressive non-fluent aphasia, culminating in the formulation of the first international criteria for subtypes of frontotemporal dementia [63]. More recently, a third variant of progressive aphasia has been identified, so-called 'logopenic progressive aphasia', characterized by severe anomia but preserved semantic knowledge of word meaning, plus reduced sentence repetition and word span [20, 44].

The syndrome of semantic dementia has had an enormous impact for the study of semantic memory as it provides a unique model of progressive breakdown of this important aspect of human cognition in the context of otherwise well-preserved abilities. This has led to the formulation of influential models that posit a key role for the anterior temporal lobe in linking knowledge across cortical regions [64].

The classic syndrome of semantic dementia affects, predominantly, the left anterior temporal lobe, but right-sided cases are now recognized. Although the symptoms and neuropsychological deficits often overlap, prosopagnosia—an inability to recognize faces—and changes in behaviour typically dominate the clinical picture in such cases. Behavioural changes are now well characterized in semantic dementia.

10.7 **Identifying memory impairments**

Main paper: Petersen RC, Smith GE, Ivnik RJ, Kokmen E, Tangalos EG. Memory function in very early Alzheimer's disease. *Neurology* 1994; 44:867–72.

Background

By the early 1990s the main clinical characteristics of typical Alzheimer's disease were well described; clinical criteria for diagnosis had been developed [35, 36] and were in the process of being refined in the light of the Braak and Braak staging system [17]. Early and disproportionate memory disturbance was considered to be a critical feature of Alzheimer's disease and, as a consequence, memory impairment was a core feature of the diagnostic criteria. Nonetheless, there was some conjecture in the literature over the characteristic pattern of memory impairment in Alzheimer's disease. This issue gained critical importance when considering the diagnosis of early dementia. Could the type of memory impairment help define Alzheimer's disease on clinical grounds at an early stage?

This landmark paper explored aspects of memory impairment—especially, acquisition and delayed recall of new information—as potential markers of Alzheimer's disease, with a specific focus on cases with early dementia.

Methods

The paper used a novel memory task that involved multiple trials designed to maximize encoding of new information. Each subject was presented with 16 line drawings of everyday objects on individual cards. Each trial consisted of a verbal cue unique to each object. For example, 'an article of clothing', which would prompt the subject to identify and name the 'sweater'. Once all of the objects had been cued, identified, and named, the subject would be asked to recall, without prompting, as many of the objects as possible. Any missed objects would be cued once again (e.g. 'an article of clothing'). This procedure was repeated so that items not recalled initially were re-presented. Importantly, the study protocol included six trials, so that subjects had sufficient opportunity to learn the information. Delayed recall was assessed 30 minutes after the completion of the sixth trial.

Once the study protocol had been completed, a number of variables were calculated from the raw data. Several measures of information acquisition were defined and calculated for each individual patient. In addition, a measure of delayed recall was also recorded.

The study concentrated on two overlapping cohorts of patients and matched control subjects. Firstly, a large group of patients with Alzheimer's disease were compared to age- and education-matched controls. A second analysis was then performed, in which patients with early Alzheimer's disease, as defined by the Minimental Status Examination (MMSE) total score (24–26/30), were matched to controls with identical scores on the MMSE. These two groups—the early Alzheimer's disease group and the mildly impaired control group—were followed for 2 years; only patients who had been diagnosed with early Alzheimer's disease declined over that period of time.

Results

In total, 106 patients with Alzheimer's disease and an equivalent number of control subjects were included in the study. Both groups had a mean age of 80 years and mean duration of education of 12 years.

When compared to control subjects, patients with Alzheimer's disease consistently demonstrated reduced acquisition of new information—regardless of the method used to analyse the data. The mean number of items recalled across the six trials was significantly reduced (P < 0.0001) in the Alzheimer's disease group (23.8 +/– 14.0) compared to the control group (58.9 +/– 14.2). In addition, the sum of the freely recalled items and the cued items was also significantly reduced (P < 0.0001) in the Alzheimer's disease group (69.1 +/– 21.4) compared to the control group (94.5 +/– 3.41). Finally, the number of trials in which the subject recalled all 16 items—either by free or cued recall—was significantly reduced (P < 0.0001) in the Alzheimer's disease group (0.9 +/– 1.6) compared to the control group (5.1 +/– 1.3).

The study also considered performance on delayed recall (i.e. the number of items recalled after a delay of 30 minutes). Patients with Alzheimer's disease demonstrated impaired delayed recall compared to control subjects. Logistic analysis was used to determine the markers that were most useful in distinguishing Alzheimer's disease from control subjects. Measures of information acquisition were found to be the best predictors of Alzheimer's disease. This was demonstrated in the two study paradigms; when the total Alzheimer's disease group was compared to controls and when patients with early Alzheimer's disease were compared to slightly impaired control subjects.

Conclusions

Patients with Alzheimer's disease demonstrated impaired acquisition of new information, although the impairment became more obvious when multiple acquisition trials were used in the study protocol. Although patients with Alzheimer's disease also demonstrated impaired delayed recall, this was a less powerful predictor of Alzheimer's disease.

Critique

This landmark investigation used an elegant study protocol to explore the memory deficits encountered in typical Alzheimer's disease. One of the strengths of the study was the recognition that multiple memory trials may be necessary before early or subtle memory disturbance can be detected with confidence. The study reinforced the centrality of hippocampal dysfunction to the early presentation of typical or 'amnestic' Alzheimer's disease. The finding of significantly impaired episodic memory in very early Alzheimer's disease led the way to the conceptualization of mild cognitive impairment as a high-risk prodrome to more frank dementia, which characterizes the disease [65].

10.8 **A genetic link to tau**

Main paper: Hutton M, Lendon CL, Rizzu P, et al. Association of missense and 5'-splice-site mutations in tau with the inherited dementia FTDP-17. *Nature* 1998; 393:702–5.

Background

Following the purification of amyloid from the brains of patients with Alzheimer's disease in the mid-1980s [47], attention turned to the biochemical basis of neurofibrillary tangles. Several key studies in the subsequent few years demonstrated that the major constituent of neurofibrillary tangles was, in fact, hyper-phosphorylated tau [66–69]. Importantly, tau was soon confirmed to be the major constituent of inclusions identified in other neurode-generative diseases such as frontotemporal dementia (Fig. 10.4) and progressive supranuclear palsy [68], as well as corticobasal degeneration [70].

In this context, a new disease complex—initially termed, the Disinhibition-Dementia-Parkinsonism-Amyotrophy Complex—was described in a single family [71]. Members of this family presented with prominent behavioural disturbances suggestive of fronto-temporal dementia, but some later developed Parkinsonism or motor neuron disease. Pathological examination revealed a frontotemporal dementia with features distinct from those of Alzheimer's disease. In this important study, this clinical phenotype was linked to chromosome 17q21–22 [71]. This disorder was subsequently re-named frontotemporal dementia with Parkinsonism linked to chromosome 17 (FTDP-17).

Methods

In total, 40 individuals from families with FTDP-17 were combined for analysis. These individuals came from 22 English, 9 Scandinavian, 3 Dutch, 5 American, and 1 Australian family. Sequencing was performed of the entire *MAPT* gene, which encodes the tau protein, including flanking intronic regions.

Results

Three pathogenic single-point mutations were identified in the study. The first point mutation (P301L) was identified in both a Dutch and an American kindred of familial fronto-temporal dementia. The location of the P301L mutation, within exon 10, was expected to only affect 4-repeat tau isoforms, as exon 10 is spliced out of mRNA (messenger ribonucleic acid) that encodes 3-repeat tau. Consistent with this prediction, the brains of individuals who carried this mutation demonstrated accumulation of 4-repeat tau. The second point mutation (G272V), located within exon 9, was identified in a second Dutch kindred. Like the P301L mutation, the G272V mutation affects the microtubule-binding domain of the gene. A third missense point mutation (R406W) was identified in exon 13 in a single family from the USA.

In addition to the three missense mutations, a cluster of three mutations was identified in close proximity to the exon 10 5' splicing site. Subsequent analysis suggested that these

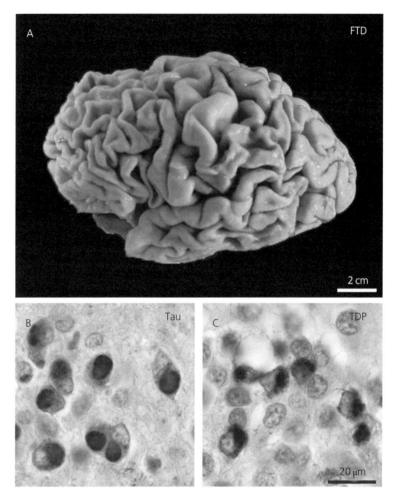

Fig. 10.4 The pathology of frontotemporal dementia. (**A**) Severe focal frontal atrophy is present—so-called 'knife edge' atrophy. (**B**) Tau positive intraneuronal inclusions. (**C**) TDP-43 positive intraneuronal inclusions.

Images provided courtesy of H. Cartwright and the Sydney Brain Bank, Sydney, Australia.

mutations resulted in alternative splicing of the gene, thus potentially increasing the proportion of 4-repeat tau production.

Conclusions

This study demonstrated that mutations of the *MAPT* gene were a cause of familial frontotemporal dementia. Several mutations, with different genomic consequences, were described in detail. Frontotemporal dementia could result from mutations affecting the proportion of 4-repeat tau production or by altering phosphorylation of tau isoforms, and abnormalities in microtubule-binding sites appeared to be important for the development of tauopathy.

Critique

This landmark of neurogenetics is important for a number of reasons. Although an association between several neurodegenerative diseases and accumulation of tau had been described in the decade prior to the publication of this study, some conjecture remained as to whether accumulation of tau was the *cause* or *consequence* of neuronal cell death. After the demonstration of single gene mutations in familial frontotemporal dementia, there was no doubt that alterations in tau biology were responsible for neurodegeneration, at least in those families that carried *MAPT* mutations. Furthermore, the study identified the two main mechanisms by which mutation of *MAPT* can result in tau pathology. Firstly, mutations affecting microtubule binding may lead to microtubule instability and subsequent neuronal cell death [72]. Secondly, mutations that alter the ratio of 3-repeat to 4-repeat tau isoforms, which are normally regulated through brain development, may also result in characteristic tau neuropathology. Specifically, an over-representation of 4-repeat tau appears to result in accumulation of tau in neurons and glia [73]. As with the discovery of the first mutation in Alzheimer's disease, this enabled the establishment of transgenic mice models [74, 75], which could then be used to explore therapeutic interventions, which are now progressing, to the stage of large-scale trials in humans.

In another fascinating parallel to Alzheimer's disease, the first mutation identified in familial frontotemporal dementia—although undoubtedly important—was ultimately overshadowed, in importance, by subsequent discoveries. Specifically, the *progranulin* gene, also on chromosome 17 [76, 77], and the *C9ORF72* hexamer repeat expansion on chromosome 9 [78, 79] may be more common causes of familial frontotemporal dementia than mutations of *MAPT* [80–82]. Unlike *MAPT* mutations, *progranulin* mutations and the *C9ORF72* hexamer repeat expansion are associated with TDP-43 positive intraneuronal inclusions.

10.9 **The concept of social cognition**

Main paper: Gregory C, Lough S, Stone V, et al. Theory of mind in patients with frontal variant frontotemporal dementia and Alzheimer's disease: theoretical and practical implications. *Brain* 2002; 125(Pt 4):752–64.

Background

In recent years, the full spectrum of behavioural disturbances encountered in frontotemporal dementia has been brought into focus. Attempts to document and characterize the patterns of behavioural change in frontotemporal dementia, and to determine the underlying neural substrates for these changes, have yielded fascinating insights into so-called 'social cognition'.

The behavioural disturbances encountered in behavioural variant frontotemporal dementia (bvFTD) typically include impaired executive function and altered social functioning, which may result in decreased empathy, loss of insight, and disinhibited behaviour [83]. Executive dysfunction has been linked to dorsolateral prefrontal cortex pathology, whereas deficits of social functioning have been associated with orbitomesial involvement [84]. Although patients with bvFTD may ultimately demonstrate both executive dysfunction and behavioural disturbances, the latter may predominate in the early stages. Unfortunately, while traditional neuropsychological tasks of executive dysfunction are sensitive to the disturbances encountered in neurodegenerative diseases, disturbances of social comportment may be difficult to measure. This apparent disconnect can present difficulties for diagnosis in the early stages of the disease.

One aspect of social cognition, first explored in developmental disorders associated with impaired social interaction such as autism and Asperger's syndrome [85], is so-called 'theory of mind'. Theory of mind is the ability of an individual to imagine the inner thoughts of another person, and this ability is normally acquired hierarchically throughout childhood and adolescence.

This landmark paper explored social cognition in patients with bvFTD and Alzheimer's disease, using neuropsychological tasks specifically designed to measure theory of mind. The neuroanatomical basis of disturbed theory of mind was investigated by correlation of performance on the tasks with the severity of orbitomesial atrophy on MRI.

Methods

Patients with bvFTD were compared to control subjects plus an Alzheimer's disease group. All study subjects completed a standardized neuropsychological battery that covered several cognitive domains including memory (verbal and visual), executive function, visuospatial function, object naming, word knowledge, and verbal fluency.

Patients with bvFTD underwent MRI scans of the brain, which included T1 sequences of the frontal and anterior temporal lobes, taken through the rectus gyrus, in the coronal plane. The degree of orbitofrontal atrophy was later assessed using a four-point visual rating scale (0 = no atrophy, 1 = mild, 2 = moderate, 3 = severe atrophy). Scans were rated on two separate occasions, with good agreement between the two assessments.

Four tasks designed to test theory of mind were administered. The first two tasks tested first- and second-order false belief. First-order false belief tasks require the subject to infer that another person may hold a different (and false) view to their own [86]. Second-order false belief tasks require the subject to infer what one person thinks another person is thinking. Developmentally normal children are generally able to correctly perform first-order false belief tasks by the age of 3–4 years, whereas the ability to perform second-order false belief tasks is only acquired after the age of 6 years. During the tasks, illustrated stories were presented and questions were used to probe the subjects understanding of them. The third task required the subject to detect a social '*faux pas*' from a collection of 20 short scenarios (10 included a social faux pas, and 10 did not). Ability to acquire a social *faux pas* is typically acquired between the ages of 9–11 years. The fourth and final task was the 'Reading the Mind in the Eyes' test, designed to assess whether subjects could infer complex emotions from the observation of facial expressions. During this task, subjects were shown 25 photographs of the eyes and asked to identify a corresponding meaning from two categories printed below each photograph.

Results

A total of 47 participants were included in the study; 19 with bvFTD, 12 with Alzheimer's disease, and 16 control subjects. Patients with bvFTD and Alzheimer's disease were matched for overall performance on the Addenbrooke's Cognitive Examination. As expected, patients with Alzheimer's disease had more significant memory impairment, whereas patients with bvFTD had more significant executive dysfunction. Patients with bvFTD performed significantly worse on all four theory of mind tasks compared to controls. In contrast, patients with Alzheimer's disease performed normally on three of the four tasks. In general, as the complexity of the theory of mind tasks increased, a greater proportion of patients with bvFTD demonstrated impairment. For example, 37% of bvFTD patients were impaired on the first-order false belief task, 47% were impaired on the second-order false belief task, and 74% were impaired on the social *faux pas* task. Interestingly, only 42% of bvFTD patients were impaired on the 'Reading the Mind in the Eyes' test. Patients with Alzheimer's disease performed at control level on all tasks, apart from the second-order false belief task—although, due to the design of the task, impairment in this group may have reflected impaired working memory rather than a true disturbance of theory of mind. MRI scans confirmed orbitomesial atrophy in the bvFTD group. The degree of atrophy, reflected in the visual rating scale scores, correlated with impaired performance on theory of mind tasks.

Conclusions

Patients with bvFTD showed impaired theory of mind, which appeared to mirror the behavioural changes they demonstrated. Patients with bvFTD can perform normally on standard executive tests traditionally used to assess frontal lobe function. Impaired theory of mind was shown to correlate with orbitomesial atrophy, reinforcing the critical role of this region which is affected early in bvFTD, in aspects of social cognition.

Critique

This was the first time that sophisticated measures of theory of mind had been applied to a group of patients with a neurodegenerative disorder. It paved the way for understanding the profound breakdown in social cognition demonstrated by such patients, which has been shown to produce extraordinary levels of burden and stress in their caregivers [87]. Subsequent studies have confirmed defects in theory of mind, as well as in moral decision making, empathy, and recognition of emotions, each of which appear to be associated with distinct neural networks [88–90]. This work has had a significant impact in terms of understanding the symptoms of patients with bvFTD but is yet to have a major impact in routine clinical practice, as the tests used in research studies are often complex in their administration and/or scoring, which hinders their applicability.

10.10 **Amyloid imaging**

Main paper: Klunk WE, Engler H, Nordberg A, et al. Imaging brain amyloid in Alzheimer's disease with Pittsburgh compound-B. *Ann Neurol* 2004; 55:306–19.

Background

One of the greatest difficulties in the diagnosis, management, and scientific study of patients with neurodegenerative diseases is making an early molecular diagnosis during life. Although clinical syndromes are well described, there is often marked variability and overlap in clinical presentations and patient prognosis, reflecting a myriad of underlying histopathologies. Accumulations of various intraneuronal inclusions such as TDP-43, tau, or amyloid have been identified pathologically, but making specific molecular diagnoses using only clinical and structural imaging tools is extremely difficult. Without a clear molecular target, the testing and implementation of specific drug therapies will be impossible.

Through a combination of detailed clinical phenotyping, neuropsychological evaluation, and structural imaging, an accurate diagnosis in neurodegenerative disease is often possible, at least in typical presentations [91]. Unfortunately, atypical cases, such as those presenting with progressive visual impairment (posterior cortical atrophy) or progressive aphasia, present diagnostic challenges. Clearly, specific biomarkers of underlying pathology are required. An ideal biomarker would be highly sensitive for pathology, allowing diagnosis at a very early stage of disease, but also specific for the pathology in question [92, 93]. Moreover, an ideal biomarker might also offer some information on patient prognosis—an issue of great significance to almost every patient diagnosed with neurodegenerative disease.

In this landmark paper, the PET ligand Pittsburgh compound B (PiB), which was derived from chemicals used to stain amyloid in histopathological specimens, was demonstrated to be a sensitive and specific marker of amyloid pathology in patients with mild to moderate Alzheimer's disease.

Methods

This study was composed of two parts. Firstly, the binding of PiB to brain amyloid was studied in an *in vitro* model. Secondly, the agent was given intravenously as a PET ligand, to detect cerebral amyloid *in vivo*. Patients and control subjects also underwent fluorodeoxyglucose PET imaging (FDG-PET) to determine areas of cortical hypometabolism.

In the first part of the study, fresh frozen pieces of frontal cortex from a patient with Alzheimer's disease and an age-matched control subject were incubated with PiB, and binding of the agent in grey and white matter was assessed. In the second part of the study, patients with mild to moderate Alzheimer's disease (MMSE total score 18–29)—diagnosed clinically—and a cohort of both young (21 years of age) and older (59–77 years of age) control subjects were recruited. All patients and controls underwent FDG-PET and PiB-PET scanning, and a large proportion of patients also had frequent blood sampling during PiB administration to assess uptake and clearance of the agent. The avidity of PiB binding was determined in reference to the cerebellum, defined as a standardized uptake value or SUV. The cerebellum was chosen as reference, as it is not normally subject to amyloid accumulation.

Results

Histopathological binding of PiB was assessed in two post-mortem specimens; one with documented Alzheimer's disease, and one age-matched control subject. Extensive PiB binding was documented within the cortex of the Alzheimer's disease specimen, but no significant cortical binding was identified in the age-matched control specimen. Minor binding of PiB was documented within the white matter of both specimens, but this was completely overshadowed by the degree of cortical binding in the Alzheimer's disease specimen.

In the imaging component of the study, 16 patients diagnosed with Alzheimer's disease and nine control subjects were recruited. Of the patients with Alzheimer's disease, 13 out of the 16 patients demonstrated marked cortical PiB binding (Fig. 10.5), compared to only

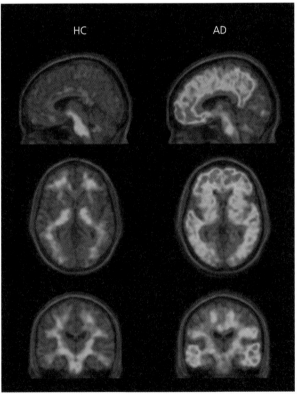

Fig. 10.5 Pittsburgh compound B (PiB) positron emission tomography. (**Left**) Healthy control subjects (HC) demonstrate little amyloid staining. (**Right**) Patients with Alzheimer's disease (AD) demonstrate avid PiB binding throughout the cerebral cortex.

Images provided courtesy of Profs Rowe and Villemagne, Austin Health, Melbourne, Australia.

one out of the nine control subjects. PiB binding was greatest in regions most affected by Alzheimer's disease pathology, such as the frontal and parietal cortices, but there was no significant PiB binding in the mesial temporal lobes. The degree of PiB binding did not correlate with symptom duration, anticholinesterase medication use, gender, or ApoE genotype.

Interestingly, the three PiB-negative patients who had been diagnosed with Alzheimer's disease had relatively preserved MMSE scores (28–29/30), despite follow-up of between 2 and 4 years. Furthermore, these three PiB-negative patients had normal FDG-PET scans. Remarkably, the single PiB-positive control subject was, in fact, the oldest subject studied, although this individual performed normally on screening neuropsychological testing. PiB metabolism was identical in patients with Alzheimer's disease and control subjects.

Conclusions

PiB-PET imaging was demonstrated to be a sensitive marker of amyloid pathology in a cohort of patients with Alzheimer's disease, as defined clinically. PiB was demonstrated to bind to cortical amyloid in pathologically proven Alzheimer's disease. As a PET ligand, the vast majority of patients with Alzheimer's disease were shown to be PiB-positive. The distribution of PiB binding corresponded to the pattern of amyloid pathology in Alzheimer's disease, but did not correlate with clinical factors such as disease duration or cognitive dysfunction, which have been shown to be more clearly related to the distribution and severity of neurofibrillary pathology. Unfortunately, the study also demonstrated that apparently normal elderly controls could also be PiB-positive.

Critique

For the first time, a sensitive and specific biomarker of molecular pathology was used successfully in a neurodegenerative disease. The study convincingly demonstrated avid cortical binding of PiB in pathological proven Alzheimer's disease, and PiB-PET positivity in a large percentage of patients diagnosed clinically with Alzheimer's disease.

The specificity of PiB-PET imaging reflects both an advantage and pitfall of the technology. For example, three patients in this study that met clinical criteria for the diagnosis of Alzheimer's disease had normal FDG-PET and PiB-PET scans, suggesting that a neurodegenerative disease in those cases was unlikely. On the other hand, the finding of PiB binding in an elderly control subject reinforces the old conundrum, which raises its head repeatedly throughout the clinical, pathological, and neuroimaging literature—how can Alzheimer's disease be distinguished from amyloid accumulation associated with normal ageing? One attractive hypothesis is that amyloid deposition precedes the development of cognitive decline, with an orderly progression from pre-clinical deposition, to mild cognitive impairment, and, finally, to established Alzheimer's disease [94–96]. Consistent with this model, PiB positivity does appear to increase the risk of conversion from mild cognitive impairment to established Alzheimer's disease [97]. On the other hand, the prevailing view of amyloidosis and Alzheimer's pathology may prove to be an oversimplification;

very recent studies have emphasized the fact that neuronal degeneration may, in fact, proceed in the absence of amyloid accumulation [98], suggesting that several inter-related factors may underlie the development of Alzheimer's pathology and clinical disease [99]. Further complicating the picture, recent studies have demonstrated that the relationship between amyloid load, hypometabolism on PET, and focal atrophy in atypical Alzheimer's phenotypes, such as logopenic progressive aphasia and posterior cortical atrophy, is very poor [100, 44].

Key unanswered questions

1 What initiates and propagates the accumulation of intraneuronal inclusions and neuronal loss in neurodegenerative disorders more widely?

2 How does clinical Alzheimer's disease fundamentally differ from the amyloid accumulation associated with ageing?

3 How can pathogenic processes be detected before significant neurodegeneration develops?

4 What strategies might then be used to delay or prevent neurodegeneration?

5 Can established neurodegeneration be reversed?

References

1 **Barbara J-G.** The physiological construction of the neurone concept (1891–1952). *C R Biol* 2006; **329**:437–49.

2 **Mazzarello P.** A unifying concept: the history of cell theory. *Nat Cell Biol* 1999; **1**:E13–E15.

3 **Pearce JMS.** Sir Charles Scott Sherrington (1857–1952) and the synapse. *J Neurol Neurosurg Psychiatry* 2004; **75**(4):544.

4 **Berrios, G. E.** (2010) A Conceptual History in the Nineteenth Century, *in Principles and Practice of Geriatric Psychiatry*, Third Edition (eds M. T. Abou-Saleh, C. Katona and A. Kumar), John Wiley & Sons, Ltd, Chichester, UK. doi: 10.1002/9780470669600.ch1

5 **Hodges JR.** Alzheimer's centennial legacy: origins, landmarks and the current status of knowledge concerning cognitive aspects. *Brain* 2006; **129**:2811–22.

6 **Kovacs GG.** Clinical stratification of subtypes of Alzheimer's disease. *Lancet Neurol* 2012; **11**:839–41.

7 **Rabinovici GD, Jagust WJ.** Amyloid imaging in aging and dementia: testing the amyloid hypothesis in vivo. *Behav Neurol* 2009; **21**:117–28.

8 **Alzheimer A.** Über eigenartige krankheitsfälle des späteren alters. *Z Gesamte Neurol Psychiatr* 1911; **4**:356–85.

9 **Kertesz A.** Frontotemporal dementia/Pick's disease. *Arch Neurol* 2004; **61**:969.

10 **Alladi S, Xuereb J, Bak T, et al.** Focal cortical presentations of Alzheimer's disease. *Brain* 2007; **130**:2636–45.

11 **Whitwell JL, Dickson DW, Murray ME, et al.** Neuroimaging correlates of pathologically defined subtypes of Alzheimer's disease: a case-control study. *Lancet Neurol* 2012; **11**:868–77.

12 **Blessed G, Tomlinson BE, Roth M.** Blessed-Roth Dementia Scale (DS). *Psychopharmacol Bull* 1988; **24**:705–8.

13 **Bak TH, Mioshi E.** A cognitive bedside assessment beyond the MMSE: the Addenbrooke's Cognitive Examination. *Pract Neurol* 2007; **7**:245–9.

14 **Mathuranath PS, Nestor PJ, Berrios GE, Rakowicz W, Hodges JR.** A brief cognitive test battery to differentiate Alzheimer's disease and frontotemporal dementia. *Neurology* 2000; **55**:1613–20.

15 **Mioshi E, Dawson K, Mitchell J, Arnold R, Hodges JR.** The Addenbrooke's Cognitive Examination Revised (ACE-R): a brief cognitive test battery for dementia screening. *Int J Geriatr Psychiatry* 2006; **21**:1078–85.

16 **Hyman BT, Van Hoesen GW, Damasio AR, Barnes CL.** Alzheimer's disease: cell-specific pathology isolates the hippocampal formation. *Science* 1984; **225**:1168–70.

17 **Braak H, Braak E.** Neuropathological staging of Alzheimer-related changes. *Acta Neuropathol* 1991; **82**:239–59.

18 **Hyman Bradley T, Phelps CH, Beach TG, et al.** National Institute on Aging—Alzheimer's Association guidelines for the neuropathologic assessment of Alzheimer's disease. *Alz Dement* 2012; **8**:1–13.

19 **Mrak RE, Griffin WST.** Dementia with Lewy bodies: definition, diagnosis, and pathogenic relationship to Alzheimer's disease. *Neuropsychiatr Dis Treat* 2007; **3**:619–25.

20 **Gorno-Tempini ML, Dronkers NF, Rankin KP, et al.** Cognition and anatomy in three variants of primary progressive aphasia. *Ann Neurol* 2004; **55**:335–46.

21 **Hodges JR, Patterson K, Oxbury S, Funnell E.** Semantic dementia. Progressive fluent aphasia with temporal lobe atrophy. *Brain* 1992; **115**:1783–806.

22 **Mesulam MM.** Slowly progressive aphasia without generalized dementia. *Ann Neurol* 1982; **11**:592–8.

23 **Mesulam MM.** Primary progressive aphasia. *Ann Neurol* 2001; **49**:425–32.

24 **Drachman DA LJ.** Human memory and the cholinergic system: a relationship to aging? *Arch Neurol* 1974; **30**:113–21.

25 **Bowen DM, Smith CB, White P, Davison AN.** Neurotransmitter-related enzymes and indices of hypoxia in senile dementia and other abiotrophies. *Brain* 1976; **99**:459–96.

26 **Davies P, Maloney AJ.** Selective loss of central cholinergic neurons in Alzheimer's disease. *Lancet* 1976; **2**:1403.

27 **Perry EK, Gibson PH, Blessed G, Perry RH, Tomlinson BE.** Neurotransmitter enzyme abnormalities in senile dementia. Choline acetyltransferase and glutamic acid decarboxylase activities in necropsy brain tissue. *J Neurol Sci* 1977; **34**:247–65.

28 **Whitehouse PJ, Price DL, Clark AW, Coyle JT, DeLong MR.** Alzheimer disease: evidence for selective loss of cholinergic neurons in the nucleus basalis. *Ann Neurol* 1981; **10**:122–6.

29 **Francis PT, Palmer AM, Snape M, Wilcock GK.** The cholinergic hypothesis of Alzheimer's disease: a review of progress. *J Neurol Neurosurg Psychiatry* 1999; **66**:137–47.

30 **Davis KL, Thal LJ, Gamzu ER, et al.** A double-blind, placebo-controlled multicenter study of tacrine for Alzheimer's disease. The Tacrine Collaborative Study Group. *N Engl J Med* 1992; **327**:1253–9.

31 **Farlow M, Gracon SI, Hershey LA, Lewis KW, Sadowsky CH, Dolan-Ureno J.** A controlled trial of tacrine in Alzheimer's disease. The Tacrine Study Group. *JAMA* 1992; **268**:2523–9.

32 **Rogers SL, Friedhoff LT.** The efficacy and safety of donepezil in patients with Alzheimer's disease: results of a US multicentre, randomized, double-blind, placebo-controlled trial. The Donepezil Study Group. *Dementia* 1996; **7**:293–303.

33 **Braak H, Braak E, Ohm T, Bohl J.** Alzheimer's disease: mismatch between amyloid plaques and neuritic plaques. *Neurosci Lett* 1989; **103**:24–8.

34 **McKeel DW, Burns JM, Meuser TM, Morris JC.** Chapter 3: Diagnosis of Alzheimer's disease: neuropathologic investigation methods. In: Oxford, United Kingdom: Clinical Publishing. *Dementia: An Atlas of Investigation and Diagnosis* 2007.

35 **Khachaturian ZS.** Diagnosis of Alzheimer's disease. *Arch Neurol* 1985; **42**:1097–105.

36 **Mirra SS, Heyman A, McKeel D, et al.** The Consortium to Establish a Registry for Alzheimer's Disease (CERAD). Part II. Standardization of the neuropathologic assessment of Alzheimer's disease. *Neurology* 1991; **41**:479–86.

37 **Montine TJ, Phelps CH, Beach TG, et al.** National Institute on Aging—Alzheimer's Association guidelines for the neuropathologic assessment of Alzheimer's disease: a practical approach. *Acta Neuropathol* 2012; **123**:1–11.

38 **Gold G, Bouras C, Kövari E, et al.** Clinical validity of Braak neuropathological staging in the oldest-old. *Acta Neuropathol* 2000; **99**:579–82; discussion 583–4.

39 **Bancher C, Braak H, Fischer P, Jellinger KA.** Neuropathological staging of Alzheimer lesions and intellectual status in Alzheimer's and Parkinson's disease patients. *Neurosci Lett* 1993; **162**:179–82.

40 **Bancher C, Jellinger K, Lassmann H, Fischer P, Leblhuber F.** Correlations between mental state and quantitative neuropathology in the Vienna Longitudinal Study on Dementia. *Eur Arch Psychiatry Clin Neurosci* 1996; **246**:137–46.

41 **Duyckaerts C, Hauw JJ.** Diagnosis and staging of Alzheimer disease. *Neurobiol Aging* 1997; **18**:S33–42.

42 **Swainson R, Hodges JR, Galton CJ, et al.** Early detection and differential diagnosis of Alzheimer's disease and depression with neuropsychological tasks. *Dement Geriatr Cogn Disord* 2001; **12**:265–80.

43 **Galton CJ, Patterson K, Xuereb JH, Hodges JR.** Atypical and typical presentations of Alzheimer's disease: a clinical, neuropsychological, neuroimaging and pathological study of 13 cases. *Brain* 2000; **123**(Pt 3):484–98.

44 Leyton CE, Villemagne VL, Savage S, et al. Subtypes of progressive aphasia: application of the International Consensus Criteria and validation using β-amyloid imaging. *Brain* 2011; **134**:3030–43.

45 Burrell, JR, Hornberger M, Villemagne VL, Rowe CC, Hodges JR. Clinical profile of PiB-positive corticobasal syndrome. *PloS One* 2013; **8**(4):e61025.

46 Kanne SM, Balota DA, Storandt M, McKeel DW Jr, Morris JC. Relating anatomy to function in Alzheimer's disease: neuropsychological profiles predict regional neuropathology 5 years later. *Neurology* 1998; **50**:979–85.

47 Glenner GG, Wong CW. Alzheimer's disease: initial report of the purification and characterization of a novel cerebrovascular amyloid protein. *Biochem Biophys Res Commun* 1984; **120**:885–90.

48 Masters CL, Simms G, Weinman NA, Multhaup G, McDonald BL, Beyreuther K. Amyloid plaque core protein in Alzheimer disease and Down syndrome. *Proc Natl Acad Sci USA* 1985; **82**:4245–9.

49 Tanzi RE. A brief history of Alzheimer's disease gene discovery. *J Alzheimers Dis* 2013; **33**(Suppl 1):S5–13.

50 Hardy JA, Higgins GA. Alzheimer's disease: the amyloid cascade hypothesis. *Science* 1992; **256**:184–5.

51 Goldgaber D, Lerman MI, McBride OW, Saffiotti U, Gajdusek DC. Characterization and chromosomal localization of a cDNA encoding brain amyloid of Alzheimer's disease. *Science* 1987; **235**:877–80.

52 Robakis NK, Ramakrishna N, Wolfe G, Wisniewski HM. Molecular cloning and characterization of a cDNA encoding the cerebrovascular and the neuritic plaque amyloid peptides. *Proc Natl Acad Sci USA* 1987; **84**:4190–4.

53 Robakis NK, Wisniewski HM, Jenkins EC, et al. Chromosome 21q21 sublocalisation of gene encoding beta-amyloid peptide in cerebral vessels and neuritic (senile) plaques of people with Alzheimer disease and Down syndrome. *Lancet* 1987; **1**:384–5.

54 Tanzi RE, Gusella JF, Watkins PC, et al. Amyloid beta protein gene: cDNA, mRNA distribution, and genetic linkage near the Alzheimer locus. *Science* 1987; **235**:880–4.

55 Levy E, Carman MD, Fernandez-Madrid IJ, et al. Mutation of the Alzheimer's disease amyloid gene in hereditary cerebral hemorrhage, Dutch type. *Science* 1990; **248**:1124–6.

56 Campion D, Dumanchin C, Hannequin D, et al. Early-onset autosomal dominant Alzheimer disease: prevalence, genetic heterogeneity, and mutation spectrum. *Am J Hum Genet* 1999; **65**:664–70.

57 Cruts M, Van Duijn CM, Backhovens H, et al. Estimation of the genetic contribution of presenilin-1 and -2 mutations in a population-based study of presenile Alzheimer disease. *Hum Mol Genet* 1998; **7**:43–51.

58 Pick A. Über die beziehungen der senilen hirnatrophie zur aphasie. *Prag Med Wochenschr* 1892; **17**:165–7.

59 Pick A. Über primäre progressive demenz bei erwachsenen. *Prag Med Wochenschr* 1904; **29**:417–20.

60 Snowden J, Goulding PJ, Neary D. Semantic dementia: a circumscribed form of cerebral atrophy. *Behav Neurol* 1989; **2**:167–82.

61 Davies RR, Hodges JR, Kril JJ, Patterson K, Halliday GM, Xuereb JH. The pathological basis of semantic dementia. *Brain* 2005; **128**:1984–95.

62 Warrington EK. The selective impairment of semantic memory. *Q J Exp Psychol* 1975; **27**:635–57.

63 Neary D, Snowden JS, Gustafson L, et al. Frontotemporal lobar degeneration: a consensus on clinical diagnostic criteria. *Neurology* 1998; **51**:1546–54.

64 Patterson K, Nestor PJ, Rogers TT. Where do you know what you know? The representation of semantic knowledge in the human brain. *Nat Rev Neurosci* 2007; **8**:976–87.

65 Flicker C, Ferris SH, Reisberg B. Mild cognitive impairment in the elderly: predictors of dementia. *Neurology* 1991; **41**:1006–9.

66 Crowther T, Goedert M, Wischik CM. The repeat region of microtubule-associated protein tau forms part of the core of the paired helical filament of Alzheimer's disease. *Ann Med* 1989; **21**:127–32.

67 Delacourte A, Defossez A. Alzheimer's disease: tau proteins, the promoting factors of microtubule assembly, are major components of paired helical filaments. *J Neurol Sci* 1986; **76**:173–86.

68 Pollock NJ, Mirra SS, Binder LI, Hansen LA, Wood JG. Filamentous aggregates in Pick's disease, progressive supranuclear palsy, and Alzheimer's disease share antigenic determinants with microtubule-associated protein, tau. *Lancet* 1986; **2**:1211.

69 Wischik CM, Novak M, Thøgersen HC, et al. Isolation of a fragment of tau derived from the core of the paired helical filament of Alzheimer disease. *Proc Natl Acad Sci USA* 1988; **85**:4506–10.

70 Uchihara T, Mitani K, Mori H, Kondo H, Yamada M, Ikeda K. Abnormal cytoskeletal pathology peculiar to corticobasal degeneration is different from that of Alzheimer's disease or progressive supranuclear palsy. *Acta Neuropathol* 1994; **88**:379–83.

71 Wilhelmsen KC, Lynch T, Pavlou E, Higgins M, Nygaard TG. Localization of disinhibition-dementia-parkinsonism-amyotrophy complex to 17q21–22. *Am J Hum Genet* 1994; **55**:1159–65.

72 Hasegawa M, Smith MJ, Goedert M. Tau proteins with FTDP-17 mutations have a reduced ability to promote microtubule assembly. *FEBS Lett* 1998; **437**:207–10.

73 Goedert M, Spillantini MG, Crowther RA, et al. Tau gene mutation in familial progressive subcortical gliosis. *Nat Med* 1999; **5**:454–7.

74 Spittaels K, Van den Haute C, Van Dorpe J, et al. Prominent axonopathy in the brain and spinal cord of transgenic mice overexpressing four-repeat human tau protein. *Am J Pathol* 1999; **155**:2153–65.

75 Tesseur I, Van Dorpe J, Spittaels K, Van den Haute C, Moechars D, Van Leuven F. Expression of human apolipoprotein E4 in neurons causes hyperphosphorylation of protein tau in the brains of transgenic mice. *Am J Pathol* 2000; **156**:951–64.

76 Baker M, Mackenzie IR, Pickering-Brown SM, et al. Mutations in progranulin cause tau-negative frontotemporal dementia linked to chromosome 17. *Nature* 2006; **442**:916–9.

77 Cruts M, Gijselinck I, Van der Zee J, et al. Null mutations in progranulin cause ubiquitin-positive frontotemporal dementia linked to chromosome 17q21. *Nature* 2006; **442**:920–4.

78 DeJesus-Hernandez M, Mackenzie IR, Boeve BF, et al. Expanded GGGGCC hexanucleotide repeat in noncoding region of C9ORF72 causes chromosome 9p-linked FTD and ALS. *Neuron* 2011; **72**:245–56.

79 Renton AE, Majounie E, Waite A, et al. A hexanucleotide repeat expansion in C9ORF72 is the cause of chromosome 9p21-linked ALS-FTD. *Neuron* 2011; **72**:257–68.

80 Dobson-Stone C, Hallupp M, Bartley L, et al. C9ORF72 repeat expansion in clinical and neuropathologic frontotemporal dementia cohorts. *Neurology* 2012; **79**:995–1001.

81 Simón-Sánchez J, Dopper EGP, Cohn-Hokke PE, et al. The clinical and pathological phenotype of C9ORF72 hexanucleotide repeat expansions. *Brain* 2012; **135**:723–35.

82 Van der Zee J, Gijselinck I, Dillen L, et al. A pan-European study of the C9orf72 repeat associated with FTLD: geographic prevalence, genomic instability, and intermediate repeats. *Hum Mutat* 2013; **34**:363–73.

83 Burrell JR, Hodges JR. From FUS to Fibs: what's new in frontotemporal dementia? *J Alzheimers Dis* 2010; **21**:349–60.

84 **Hornberger M, Savage S, Hsieh S, Mioshi E, Piguet O, Hodges JR.** Orbitofrontal dysfunction discriminates behavioral variant frontotemporal dementia from Alzheimer's disease. *Dement Geriatr Cogn Disord* 2010; **30**:547–52.

85 **Baron-Cohen S, O'Riordan M, Stone V, Jones R, Plaisted K.** Recognition of faux pas by normally developing children and children with Asperger syndrome or high-functioning autism. *J Autism Dev Disord* 1999; **29**:407–18.

86 **Baron-Cohen S.** Perceptual role taking and protodeclarative pointing in autism. *Brit J Devel Psychol* 1989; **7**:113–27.

87 **Mioshi E, Bristow M, Cook R, Hodges JR.** Factors underlying caregiver stress in frontotemporal dementia and Alzheimer's disease. *Dement Geriatr Cogn Disord* 2009; **27**:76–81.

88 **Kipps CM, Nestor PJ, Acosta-Cabronero J, Arnold R, Hodges JR.** Understanding social dysfunction in the behavioural variant of frontotemporal dementia: the role of emotion and sarcasm processing. *Brain* 2009; **132**:592–603.

89 **Manes FF, Torralva T, Roca M, Gleichgerrcht E, Bekinschtein TA, Hodges JR.** Frontotemporal dementia presenting as pathological gambling. *Nat Rev Neurol* 2010; **6**:347–52.

90 **Shany-Ur T, Poorzand P, Grossman SN, et al.** Comprehension of insincere communication in neurodegenerative disease: lies, sarcasm, and theory of mind. *Cortex* 2012; **48**:1329–41.

91 **Snowden Julie S, Thompson JC, Stopford CL, et al.** The clinical diagnosis of early-onset dementias: diagnostic accuracy and clinicopathological relationships. *Brain* 2011; **134**:2478–92.

92 **Sonnen JA, Montine KS, Quinn JF, Kaye JA, Breitner JC, Montine TJ.** Biomarkers for cognitive impairment and dementia in elderly people. *Lancet Neurol* 2008; **7**:704–14.

93 **Turner MR, Kiernan MC, Leigh PN, Talbot K.** Biomarkers in amyotrophic lateral sclerosis. *Lancet Neurol* 2009; **8**:94–109.

94 **Fripp J, Bourgeat P, Acosta O, et al.** Appearance modeling of 11C PiB PET images: characterizing amyloid deposition in Alzheimer's disease, mild cognitive impairment and healthy aging. *Neuroimage* 2008; **43**:430–9.

95 **Pike KE, Savage G, Villemagne VL, et al.** Beta-amyloid imaging and memory in non-demented individuals: evidence for preclinical Alzheimer's disease. *Brain* 2007; **130**:2837–44.

96 **Villemagne VL, Pike KE, Darby D, et al.** Abeta deposits in older non-demented individuals with cognitive decline are indicative of preclinical Alzheimer's disease. *Neuropsychologia* 2008; **46**:1688–97.

97 **Villemagne VL, Pike KE, Chételat G, et al.** Longitudinal assessment of Aβ and cognition in aging and Alzheimer disease. *Ann Neurol* 2011; **69**:181–92.

98 **Knopman DS, Jack CR Jr, Wiste HJ, et al.** Brain injury biomarkers are not dependent on β-amyloid in normal elderly. *Ann Neurol* 2013; **73**:472–80.

99 **Chételat G.** Alzheimer disease: Aβ-independent processes—rethinking preclinical AD. *Nat Rev Neurol* 2013; **9**:123–4.

100 **Lehmann M, Ghosh PM, Madison C, et al.** Diverging patterns of amyloid deposition and hypometabolism in clinical variants of probable Alzheimer's disease. *Brain* 2013; **136**:844–58.

Chapter 11

Mitochondrial diseases

Gráinne S. Gorman and Patrick F. Chinnery

11.0 **Introduction**

Mitochondrial diseases are a diverse group of neurometabolic disorders manifesting important genotypic phenotypic heterogeneity. Since the initial discovery of 'sarcosomes' within muscle cells, more than 150 years ago, mitochondria have held scientific intrigue for microbiologists, biochemists, pathologists, and geneticists alike.

This chapter chronicles the discovery of the structural and functional complexity of mitochondria, and the increasing recognition of human diseases caused by both mutations in mitochondrial and nuclear DNA. We review the first clinical description of mitochondrial disease, so-called 'Luft's disease' [1] that marks the development of mitochondrial medicine. Over the ensuing decades and coinciding with the complete sequencing of human mitochondrial DNA, the rapid expansion of human chemical pathology as a clinical academic discipline prompted the reporting of more than one hundred multi-system patient syndromes assigned to mitochondrial dysfunction. By 1986, this culminated in the publication of the first large-scale study, led by John Morgan Hughes and colleagues in London, that meticulously phenotyped an extensive case series of patients with mitochondrial disease. This seminal paper, defining the pre-molecular era of mitochondrial medicine, supports the concept of a varied, overlapping spectrum of mitochondrial diseases as opposed to distinct clinical entities only, which 35 years later, has been affirmed by the molecular characterization of these disorders.

We follow the rapid developments of mitochondrial medicine and evolution of the molecular era and review, firstly, the pivotal steps in our understanding of the genetic basis of mitochondrial diseases including the discovery of the first pathogenic mutation in mitochondrial (mt)DNA and of the first pathogenic mtDNA point mutation; the identification of the genetic basis of the most common form of mitochondrial disease (a point mutation of the tRNA $^{Leu(UUR)}$ gene in mitochondrial myopathy, encephalopathy, lactic acidosis, and stroke-like episodes (MELAS)) and of the most common nuclear-mitochondrial disease gene (encoding mitochondrial polymerase γ (*POLG*); and confirmation of Mendelian inheritance and characterization of a new group of disorders of mtDNA maintenance described by muscle-restricted mtDNA deletions.

We critique cardinal papers documenting the minimum prevalence of adult mitochondrial disease, crucial to the evaluation of interventions and planning of future services, and appraise the first large randomized controlled therapeutic trial in a mitochondrial disorder—in a group of diseases with few effective treatments and no known cures. Finally, we recount the current key developments in mitochondrial medicine today, with the advent of next-generation sequencing that is in the process of revolutionizing our approach to the diagnosis of mitochondrial disease. However, 25 years after the discovery of the first genetic causes of mitochondrial disease, the fastidious clinical and biochemical characterization of patients remains cogent to diagnostic yield—reminiscent of the pre-molecular era.

11.1 **The first description of mitochondrial disease**

Main paper: Luft R, Ikkos D, Palmieri G, Ernster L, Afzelius B. A case of severe hypermetabolism of non-thyroid origin with a defect in the maintenance of mitochondrial respiratory control: a correlated clinical, biochemical and morphological study. *J Clin Invest* 1962; 41:1776–804.

Background

In 1962, a Swedish endocrinologist, Rolf Luft (1914–2007), meticulously described a 35-year-old woman with severe hypermetabolism from the age of 7 years, associated with profuse perspiration, polydipsia without polyuria, progressive asthenia, and a svelte body habitus. The patient had a high basal metabolic rate with normal thyroid function.

Results

The main laboratory finding was consistent with an oxygen uptake of between 140 and 210% that was unchanged following 6 days of administration of 100 μg triiodothyronine (see Fig. 11.1). Skeletal muscle biochemistry showed a high cytochrome oxidase activity, a high RNA content, and a relatively low level of coenzyme Q. Electron microscopy revealed the perinuclear accumulation of variable-sized mitochondria and paracrystalline inclusions. Respiration, phosphorylative efficiency, and ATPase activity were measured in the patient and in a control subject. The findings indicated that the mitochondria were not able to adjust their respiration in response to the available phosphate and/or phosphate acceptor. On the other hand, the mitochondria had a normal capacity for coupled phosphorylation when both substrates were present. Based on these findings, the authors used the term 'loose coupling' (between respiration and phosphorylation), to describe the first pathogenic mitochondrial defect.

Conclusions

This is now considered to be the first clinical description of a possible mitochondrial disorder, so-called 'Luft's disease', and marked the development of mitochondrial medicine.

Critique

In 1857, Swiss anatomist, Rudolph Albert Von Kölliker (1817–1905), first described 'sarcosomes' as granular cytoplasmic compartments, with their own membrane, present in skeletal muscle. [2] The term 'mitochondrion' was first proposed by the German microbiologist, Carl Benda (1857–1932), in 1898, derived from the Greek words 'mitos' meaning 'thread' and 'chondron' meaning 'grain' [3], and became widely accepted, from the 1930s onwards, to describe these granular organelles [2].

During the 'golden age' of biological electron microscopy, numerous important discoveries were made. The Romanian biologist, George Emil Palade (1912–2008), who with Albert Claude and Christian de Duve pioneered biological electron microscopy, determined mitochondria were 'isolated' organelles. These images showed the structure of mitochondria

A   B

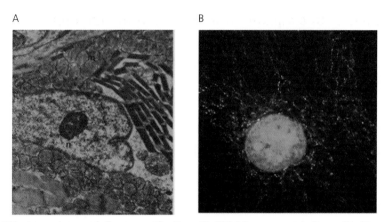

Fig. 11.1 Electron micrograph (low magnification: 10,000x) from a muscle fibre of Luft's hypermetabolic patient showing a nucleus (n) surrounded by numerous mitochondria (m).
(B): Contemporary live cell imaging showing human fibroblast cells labelled for mitochondria (red, TMRM) and DNA material (nucleus and nucleiods; green, picogreen) to identify the mitochondrial network.

Reproduced from *Journal of Clinical Investigation*, 41, Luft R, Ikkos D, Palmieri G, Ernster L, Afzelius B, A case of severe hypermetabolism of non-thyroid origin with a defect in the maintenance of mitochondrial respiratory control: a correlated clinical, biochemical and morphological study, p. 1776–1804, Copyright (1962), with permission from the American Society for Clinical Investigation.

and were even able to visualize what were later identified as the ATPase molecules [4]. At the same time, mitochondria were determined as functionally independent with the demonstration of β-oxidation, the Krebs cycle, and oxidative phosphorylation occurring within these structures [5]. Other significant breakthroughs in human chemical pathology around the time of Luft's publication [1] were the discovery of DNA within mitochondria, by electron microscopy [6], and its subsequent biochemical verification [7], paving the way for the biochemical and molecular studies of human mitochondrial diseases.

Although Luft's disease was first described in 1962, it was a further 14 years before the second case was described [8]. Five decades on, the genetic cause for this hypermetabolic disorder still has not been elucidated. However, this detailed case report—characterized by euthyroid hypermetabolism, histological features of mitochondrial dysfunction, and high oxygen consumption (200 times normal)—provided the first clear evidence of the link between disordered function of a cell organelle in man and human disease. Curiously, there have been very few descriptions of similar patients over the last half-century.

In a symposium given by Luft years later, entitled the 'Development of mitochondrial medicine', he explained how he linked the patient's clinical presentation to that of mitochondrial dysfunction. He noted:

> The idea of involvement of the mitochondria came to me when I looked into textbooks of biochemistry where, almost exclusively, studies on rat liver mitochondria were the basis for views of energy metabolism. I suggested that some error of the coupling of oxidation to phosphorylation might explain the patient's enormous oxygen consumption. [9]

11.2 The first large study describing the clinical features of mitochondrial diseases

Main paper: Petty RK, Harding AE, Morgan-Hughes JA. The clinical features of mitochondrial myopathy. *Brain* 1986; 109:915–38.

Background

The description of Luft's disease, in 1962, coincided with the rapid expansion of human chemical pathology as a clinical academic discipline [1], and precipitated several clinical reports describing human diseases associated with mitochondrial dysfunction. This was fuelled by the complete sequencing of human mtDNA and, by 1988, over 120 patient syndromes had been described in the literature, purported to be due to mitochondrial dysfunction [10]. With an expanding and complicated phenotypic spectrum, British neurologist, Anthony Schapira, and colleagues [11] first coined the phrase 'mitochondrial encephalomyopathy' to reflect the recognition of the multi-system nature of mitochondrial disorders associated with structurally and/or functionally abnormal mitochondria. However, in this landmark paper [12], a team led by British neurologist, John Morgan-Hughes (1932–2012), described the first large case series of patients with mitochondrial disease, based on their observations at the National Hospital for Nervous Diseases at Queen Square, London.

Methods

This was a single-centre, clinical characterization of 66 patients (35 women) between 1969 and 1984, with histologically defined mitochondrial myopathy as classified by the presence of 4% or more of muscle fibres showing peripheral mitochondrial accumulations (according to published criteria) [13]. Forty-seven cases (nine previously reported) were reviewed by the authors and a further 19 patients, from review of clinical records only (four deceased).

Results

Data published included the history and clinical examination, serum creatine kinase and metabolic profiles, neurophysiological assessments (electromyography—EMG), electroretinopathy (ERG), electroencephalography (EEG), brain imaging, cerebrospinal fluid (CSF) analysis, cycle ergometry, and cardiac investigations (see Fig. 11.2). Thirty-three patients underwent *in vitro* biochemical studies of mitochondrial metabolism, to include assessment of defects in complexes I to V, as described in Methods in the literature [14].

Clinical phenotype

Three distinct clinical phenotypes were described:

1 ophthalmoplegia and limb weakness (36 patients);

2 proximal weakness with fatigability (12 patients); and

3 predominantly or exclusively a central nervous system (CNS) disease (18 patients).

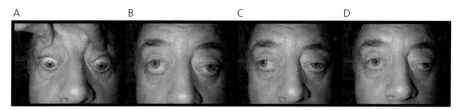

Fig. 11.2 Canonical clinical features of a patient with mitochondrial chronic progressive external ophthalmoplegia (PEO). Bilateral ptosis is evident and extra ocular motility in cardinal directions of gaze is severely reduced, with relative preservation of down gaze as the patient is asked to look down (a), up (b), right (c) and left (d).

Thirty-seven patients presented with ptosis (three with isolated ptosis), with or without progressive external ophthalmoplegia (PEO), two patients had facial muscle weakness, 12 patients reported dysarthria, and 13 patients complained of dysphagia.

Thirteen patients presented with a pure limb myopathy causing proximal muscle weakness and exercise intolerance. Twenty-four patients had CNS features that were severe in three, but mild in 21. Cerebellar ataxia was observed in 27 patients with mitochondrial myopathy (10 cases were reported as severe, and seven were associated with concomitant dysarthria). Seven patients manifested general seizures; three, myoclonic jerks; and five had a movement disorder (four, chorea; one, dystonia). Dementia was reported in 13 patients with seven reported as having severe cognitive impairment. Other eye features included pigmented retinopathy (24 patients) with concomitant CNS disease (15 patients) and optic atrophy (five patients). Other systemic features included peripheral neuropathy (eight patients), short stature (13 patients), growth hormone deficiency (one patient), mild scoliosis (two patients), and pes cavus (one patient).

Investigations

Physiological parameters: Serum creatine kinase was normal in 48 patients (65 patients tested). Blood lactate was normal (<1.5 mmol/l) in 35 patients (50 patients tested). Cycle ergometry (29 patients tested) showed abnormal lactate handling in 20 patients. Renal function was normal, except for an individual with hypertension and known renal disease who had previously undergone renal transplantation. Two patients were diabetic, two had hypothyroidism, and two had been investigated for infertility.

Neurophysiological assessments: EMG (61 patients tested) was normal in 16 individuals and consistent with myopathy in 38 patients and neuropathy in seven patients. ERG (14 patients tested) was abnormal in all manifesting pigmented retinopathy (11 patients) and in one patient without retinopathy. EEG (32 patients tested) was normal in 16 patients and revealed paroxysmal changes associated with known epilepsy in seven patients. Nine patients had evidence of non-specific diffuse slow wave activity, seven of whom also had clinical evidence of CNS disease.

Brain imaging: Computed tomography (CT) brain imaging (35 patients tested) was normal in 17 patients; 18 patients had evidence of cerebral atrophy, 12 patients had documented cerebellar atrophy, and only four patients had evidence of basal ganglia calcification.

CSF analysis: CSF analysis (28 patients tested) revealed an elevated protein in eight patients and one individual in whom CSF protein fluctuated during episodes of inter-current illness. No patient had raised CSF oligoclonal IgG.

Cardiac screening: Eleven patients had evidence of cardiac involvement—nine exhibiting cardiac conduction defects on ECG, and two requiring insertion of a permanent pacemaker.

Biochemical analysis: Thirty-three patients were studied. This disclosed evidence of complex I deficiency (18 patients), complex III deficiency (nine patients), combined complex III and IV deficiency (one patient), complex V deficiency (one patient), and four further cases within whom an identifiable defect could not be pinpointed.

Conclusions

This was the first large study describing the clinical features of mitochondrial diseases in the pre-molecular era. Cohorts like this were a ripe test-bed for new genetic techniques that were in their infancy.

Critique

This paper was the first to crystallize the phenotypic heterogeneity of a large cohort of patients with mitochondrial disorders. The authors defined three distinct clinical phenotypes of mitochondrial disease but favoured the concept of overlap syndromes with 'variations on a common theme' [15], as opposed to the theory of distinct clinical syndromes. The emergence of mitochondrial DNA diseases over the subsequent decade seemed to contradict this view, with apparently specific genetic defects in patients with known clinical syndromes (including myoclonic epilepsy, lactic acidosis, stroke-like episodes (MELAS) [16]; myoclonic epilepsy, ragged red fibres (MERRF); [17] Kearns-Sayer syndrome (KSS [18]; and Leber's hereditary optic neuropathy (LHON) [19]. However, 35 years later, the ongoing molecular dissection of mitochondrial diseases has reaffirmed their conclusions. Mitochondrial disorders include a wide, overlapping spectrum of diseases, with some groups having distinguishing features.

11.3 **Discovery of the first pathogenic mutation in mitochondrial DNA**

Main paper: Holt IJ, Harding AE, Morgan-Hughes JA. Deletions of muscle mitochondrial DNA in patients with mitochondrial myopathy. *Nature* 1988; 331(6158):717–9.

Background

Chronic progressive external ophthalmoplegia (CPEO), pigmentary retinopathy, and cardiac conduction abnormalities were first described in a case report of two patients in 1958 by American neuro-ophthalmologists, Thomas P. Kearns and George Pomeroy Sayre [20]. Two years later, Jager and colleagues published another case of a 13-year old boy with the same clinical features [21]. However, it was not until 1965, when Kearns published a further nine unrelated cases with this classical triad, that the condition was definitively defined [18].

In 1980, British biochemist, Fred Sanger, and colleagues, published the first sequence of human mitochondrial DNA [22], paving the way for the molecular investigation of suspected mitochondrial diseases. The sequence was derived from a human placenta, and some regions were so difficult to sequence that bovine DNA was used to fill in the gaps [23]. Harnessing emerging DNA recombinant techniques, Ian Holt—a graduate student working with British neurologist, Anita Harding (1952–1995)—John Morgan-Hughes, and John Clarke began looking for mtDNA mutations. By studying muscle DNA from their large series of patients, the group made a landmark breakthrough in mitochondrial pathophysiology by demonstrating single large-scale mtDNA deletions in sporadic human encephalomyopathies, including KSS. This heralded the advent of the molecular era in mitochondrial medicine.

Methods

Leukocyte DNA from 38 patients with mitochondrial myopathy, 44 unaffected relatives, and 35 control subjects was digested using 28 restriction endonucleases and hybridized to fragments to radio-labelled HeLa-cell mtDNA by Southern blotting. Muscle DNA from 25 patients with mitochondrial myopathy and 18 control subjects was analysed by enzymes cleaving at either one or two sites. The deletions were mapped by further restriction enzyme analysis and hybridization with 14 small fragments of HeLa-cell mtDNA.

Results

When muscle mtDNA from nine patients with mitochondrial myopathy was studied, two large fragments hybridized to labelled HeLa-cell whole mtDNA, revealing the first partial deletion (see Fig. 11.3). Further mapping showed different deletions in two patients: a male with complex 1 deficiency who harboured an abnormal mtDNA which was 11.6 kilobases (kb) in length compared to 16.5 kb (normal band); and a patient with

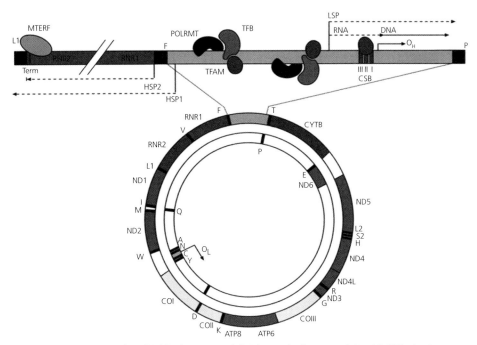

Fig. 11.3 Human mitochondrial (mt) genome. (A) Schematic diagram of the 16.6 kb circular, double-stranded human mitochondrial genome with an enhanced, linear view of the D-loop and transcription termination regions. The outer circle represents the heavy (H) strand of the genome and the inner circle, the light (L) strand. Human mtDNA encodes the two mt-rRNA genes—RNR1 (12S rRNA) and RNR2 (16S rRNA), 22 mt-tRNAs identified by their single letter abbreviation, and 13 essential respiratory chain polypeptides: seven subunits (ND1–ND6 and ND4L) of complex I, CYTB of complex III, three catalytic subunits (COI–COIII) of complex IV, and ATP6 and ATP8 of complex V. Major non-coding regions of the genome include the origin of L-strand replication (O_L) and the 1.1 kb D-loop in which the origin of H-strand replication (O_H) and regulatory elements and binding sequences for key factors involved in mtDNA transcription initiation and termination are located.

complex 3 defect and a deletion of muscle mtDNA of approximately 5.9 kb. The area of deletion included the sequences coding for three subunits of complex I, cytochrome oxidase subunits II and III (complex IV), two subunits of mitochondrial ATPase, and eight tRNAs. The other seven patients with mitochondrial myopathy had similar but not duplicate deletions of this region: four patients exhibited complex I deficiency; one patient, complex II deficiency; and two patients, normal biochemistry. Densitometry showed that the proportion of deleted mtDNA ranged from 18% to 79% in these nine patients (see Fig. 11.4).

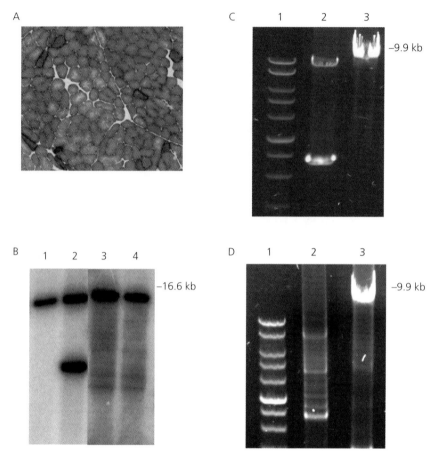

Fig. 11.4 Histological and histochemical assessments of skeletal muscle. The analysis of skeletal muscle still remains the 'gold standard' test in determining mtDNA involvement in disease pathology. (A) Sequential COX-SDH histochemistry from a patient's quadriceps muscle biopsy is often the first line of investigation and may show the presence of scattered COX-deficient fibres (dark) amongst normal fibres (light). (B) Southern blotting of muscle DNA is often used to detect single and multiple mtDNA deletions. Figure shows analysis observed in a control (lane 1), a patient with a heteroplasmic, single large-scale mtDNA deletion (lane 2), and patients with multiple mtDNA deletions (lanes 3 and 4). (C) Long-range PCR amplification of muscle DNA is also routinely used to detect single and multiple mtDNA deletions and this clearly shows a smaller amplification product in addition to the wild type product; this smaller product represents a single mitochondrial DNA deletion (lane 2). Also shown is a control (lane 3) and DNA size markers (lane 1). (D) Long-range PCR amplification of muscle DNA shows significant evidence of multiple mitochondrial DNA deletions (lane 4) when compared to a wild type control (lane 3). Also shown are DNA size markers (lane 1).

Conclusions

This work identified the first pathogenic mutation of mtDNA causing human disease, and showed that the mutation was heteroplasmic, with varying proportions of mutant and wild-type mtDNA in different individuals.

Critique

This work provided a pivotal step in understanding mitochondrial disease. The investigation of suspected mtDNA deletions is now routine, and numerous different deletions in mtDNA have been linked to KSS. Subsequent work has shown that different levels of mtDNA heteroplasmy are present in different tissues, and that mtDNA deletions are rarely detectable in leukocyte DNA. Had the investigators limited their observations to blood samples, their conclusions would have been very different. This paper illustrates the importance of building a well-phenotyped clinical cohort linked to a biobank of pathologically affected tissue. Subsequent work on another large clinical cohort at Columbia University Medical Center, New York, showed that large-scale mtDNA rearrangements were associated with various forms of PEO, and not only Kearns-Sayre syndrome [24, 25].

11.4 **Discovery of the first pathogenic mitochondrial DNA point mutation**

Main paper: Wallace DC, Singh G, Lott MT, et al. Mitochondrial DNA mutation associated with Leber's hereditary optic neuropathy. *Science* 1988; 242:1427–30.

Background

Leber's hereditary optic neuropathy (LHON; also, Leber's optic atrophy) is a maternally inherited degeneration of retinal ganglion cells and their axons, first reported by the German ophthalmologist, Theodor Karl Gustav von Leber (1840–1917) in 1871 [19]. His seminal paper described abrupt central visual loss in young men from four families, initially thought to be X-linked, but subsequently shown to be strictly maternally inherited [26]. Using the recently published human mtDNA reference sequence [22], American geneticist, Doug Wallace, and co-workers, identified the first pathogenic point mutation in the gene encoding subunit four of complex I (ND4) in a family with LHON.

Methods

Wallace and colleagues sequenced 85% of the LHON mtDNA-coding region from a proband from a large pedigree of blind individuals, compared with normal controls. Pathogenicity was inferred if the mutation:

1 changed a highly conserved amino acid;

2 was frequently found in patients with LHON; and

3 was not found in disease-free controls from the general population.

Results

A guanine to adenine transition mutation at nucleotide pair 11,778 of the mtDNA was found in patients with LHON. Unlike mtDNA deletions, the first point mutation was homoplasmic (i.e. all of the mtDNA carried the mutation) (see Fig. 11.5).

Conclusions

m.11778A>G is now recognized to be the most common mtDNA mutation causing LHON, and probably the most common pathogenic mtDNA mutation worldwide [27]. These findings catalysed the large-scale sequencing of mtDNA in other patients with mitochondrial disease that did not harbour a deletion in skeletal muscle.

Critique

Proving pathogenicity was not straightforward because both affected and unaffected individuals were in the same family. A key step was the observation of the same mutation in different LHON pedigrees on different genetic backgrounds. This indicated that the mutation had occurred on multiple different occasions, and each time it was associated with LHON. Wallace recognized that the mtDNA mutation was essential for the development

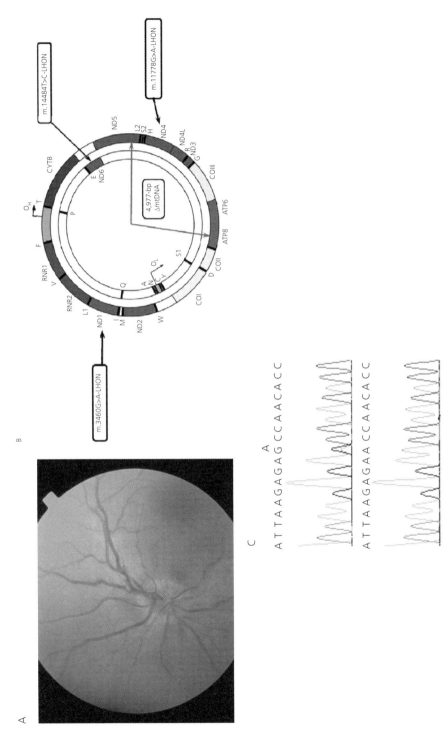

Fig. 11.5 Ocular and molecular abnormalities associated with Leber hereditary optic neuropathy (LHON). (A) The acute, cardinal, fundal appearance in LHON showing tortuosity of the retinal vessels, disc hyperaemia, and parapapillary nerve fibre layer swelling. (B) Depiction of the circular, double-stranded human mitochondrial genome delineating the sites of the *three* primary mtDNA mutations associated with LHON (mutations in the *MTND1*, *MTND4*, and *MTND6* genes). (C) A DNA sequencing chromatogram, which is a visual representation of a patient's DNA sample showing a heteroplasmic m.11778G>A (p. Arg340His) *MTND4* mutation.

of LHON, but that additional factors must be involved in modulating the phenotypic expression of the disorder. The three primary pathogenic mtDNA mutations reported in >90% of individuals with LHON within one large study [28] were: m.11778G>A (MT-ND4) [29], m.14484T>C (MT-ND6) [30], and m.3460G>A (MT-ND1) [31]. In the North East of England, these three primary LHON mtDNA mutations account for almost 50% of all mitochondrial disease in adults, with 1 in 9000 people carrying this mutation and causing blindness in approximately 1 in 14,000 adult males [27], with a founder effect seen in French Canadians with m.14484T>C [32].

Perhaps more crucially, it is also recognized that other genetic and environmental factors are critical in modulating disease expression including X chromosomal changes [33], haplogroup [34], heteroplasmy [35], and environmental toxins [36], particularly cigarette smoking [37].

11.5 **Mendelian inheritance of mitochondrial disorders**

Main paper: Zeviani M, Servidei S, Gellera C, Bertini E, DiMauro S, DiDonato S. An autosomal dominant disorder with multiple deletions of mitochondrial DNA starting at the D-loop region. *Nature* 1989; 339:309–11.

Background

Shortly after the detection of the first single large-scale deletions of mtDNA in CPEO, it became clear that some patients had multiple different deletions of mtDNA in skeletal muscle. Some of these affected individuals had a family history consistent with both maternal and paternal transmission of the inherited trait, questioning the dogma that human mtDNA was exclusively inherited down the maternal line [38].

Methods

Four patients (two sisters, cousin, and aunt) from one pedigree with PEO, myopathy, cataracts, and early death, presented with a late-onset form of mitochondrial myopathy, associated with autosomal dominant pattern of inheritance in familial cases with deletions of mtDNA in skeletal muscle. Deletions were detected by restriction mapping analysis [39] and by sequencing of the breakpoint regions by polymerase chain reaction (PCR) amplification [40].

Results

Zeviani and colleagues confirmed the presence of multiple mtDNA deletions affecting the same mtDNA region, starting at the 5' end of the mtDNA D-loop template, in all four patients with mitochondrial myopathy (see Fig. 11.4).

Conclusions

These findings suggested that, although central to the diagnosis and the pathogenesis, the deletions themselves were not inherited. This implicated an unknown nuclear gene defect that was transmitted as an autosomal dominant trait and predisposed an individual to the secondary deletion formation.

Critique

This paper was the first to confirm the autosomal dominant inheritance of a mitochondrial disease, and opened up a new category called 'disorders of mtDNA maintenance'. The authors fortuitously proposed that the deleterious effects were cumulative over time, as exemplified by the late-onset and progressive nature of the disorder. Two years later, a second form of mitochondrial disease with Mendelian transmission was described with the first quantitative defect of mtDNA (mtDNA depletion) in patients with autosomal recessive disorders affecting muscle or liver [41]. Subsequent linkage and candidate gene analysis have now identified several nuclear genes responsible for this group of disorders characterized by PEO and these include *POLG1* [42], *POLG2* [43], *SLC25A4* [44], *C10orf2* [45], *RRM2B* [46], *TK2* [47], *MFN2* [48], *OPA1* [49], and, more recently, *DNA2* [50].

11.6 **Identification of a point mutation of the tRNA Leu(UUR) gene in MELAS**

Main paper: Goto Y, Nonaka I, Horai SA. Mutation in the tRNA Leu(UUR) gene associated with the MELAS subgroup of mitochondrial encephalomyopathies. *Nature* 1990; 348(6302):651–3.

Background

In the late 1980s and early 1990s, mitochondrial encephalomyopathies were recognized as distinct clinical syndromes, and soon linked to specific defects of the mitochondrial subunits of the respiratory chain complexes. Pavlakis and colleagues [16] described two patients with mitochondrial myopathy, encephalopathy, lactic acidosis, and stroke-like episodes, with similar blood and muscle findings, and coined the acronym MELAS for this condition. The cause of this syndrome was not clear for some time, and although Pavlakis presumed that there was an underlying biochemical defect in the mitochondria, it would be eight years later before a genetic diagnosis would be made. By 1990, it had already been established that dysfunction of the tRNA Lys gene caused MERRF [51]—a severe mitochondrial disorder characterized by myoclonic epilepsy and cardinal histological features of mitochondrial dysfunction. Goto and colleagues, in Tokyo, postulated tRNA abnormalities in MELAS were also the likely genetic basis of this syndrome, given histological similarities and frequent biochemical defects congruent to that observed in MERRF.

Methods

Restriction endonuclease, *Apa*I, was applied to identify the postulated pathogenic mutation and Southern blot analysis was performed to confirm mtDNA heteroplasmy.

Results

An adenine to guanine transition mutation at nucleotide pair 3243 in the dihydrouridine loop of mitochondrial tRNA Leu(UUR) was identified in 26 out of 31 independent MELAS patients and one out of 29 patients with CPEO in whom a family history was consistent with mitochondrial myopathy. The mutation was not detected in 50 control subjects and five patients with MERRF (see Fig. 11.6).

Conclusions

For the first time, Goto and colleagues identified the genetic basis of MELAS, one of the most common forms of mitochondrial myopathy, and at the same time devised a simple molecular diagnostic test.

Critique

This paper was the first to recognize the association of MELAS with a heteroplasmic point mutation in the tRNA Leu(UUR) gene. At the time, the authors were unsure how abnormalities of the tRNA caused the functional and morphological changes of mitochondria

A

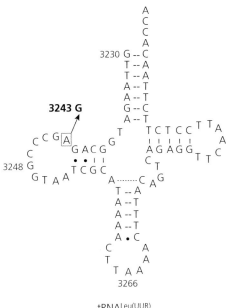

tRNALeu(UUR)

B

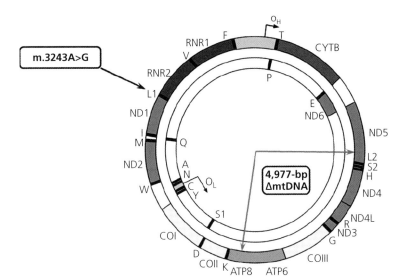

Fig. 11.6 Illustrations of the tRNA Leu(UUR) gene in MELAS. (A) The cloverleaf structure of human mttRNA Leu(UUR) is illustrated with the m. 3243A > G mutation, first recognized by Goto et al. [69] to be associated with MELAS; highlighted. It is now recognized that up to three-quarters of all MELAS cases harbour this adenine to guanine transition at position 3243. (B) This illustration of the circular, double-stranded human mitochondrial genome depicts the m.3243A>G mutation in the mtDNA MT-TL1 gene coding for mttRNA Leu(UUR). (C) This DNA sequencing chromatogram shows a heteroplasmic m.3243A>G *MTTL1* mutation and the location of the mutation within the mt-tRNA Leu(UUR) molecule.

Acknowledgements for images: RW Taylor, Eve Simcox, Emma Blakeley, Patrick Yu-Wai-Man, and Charlotte Alston.

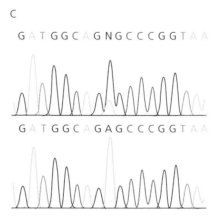

Fig. 11.6 (continued)

which they observed. It is now recognized that approximately 80% of all cases of MELAS harbour this adenine to guanine transition at position 3243 mutation [52]. This paved the way for the subsequent identification of more than 23 other pathogenic tRNA mutations in patients with MELAS in the same tRNA Leu(UUR) gene [53], and heralded the hunt for novel pathogenic tRNA gene mutations. The m.3243A>G mutation was shown to reduce tRNA Leu(UUR) aminoacylation and the modification of its anti-codon wobble position. This resulted in defective mitochondrial protein synthesis and reduced activities of respiratory chain complexes, providing a possible target site for therapeutic intervention. Human *trans*mitochondrial cybrid cell studies have recently demonstrated that mitochondrial targeting of recombinant tRNAs can rescue the phenotype caused by the MELAS mutation, suggesting tRNA specificity manipulation holds great potential as an innovative therapeutic strategy in patients with mitochondrial tRNA disorders [54].

11.7 **The prevalence of mtDNA disease and pathogenic mtDNA mutations in the North East of England**

Main paper: Chinnery PF, Johnson MA, Wardell TM. The epidemiology of pathogenic mitochondrial DNA mutations. *Ann Neurol* 2000; 48(2):188–93.

Background

By the late 1990s, mitochondrial myopathies were recognized as a heterogeneous group of genetic disorders, resulting in significant morbidity and disability. Although new mtDNA mutations and novel phenotypes were being catalogued in the literature, as a group they were considered to be very rare—perhaps only affecting one or two per million of the population. Studying patients referred to the regional neurology centre in Newcastle-upon-Tyne, British neurologist, Patrick Chinnery, and colleagues, comprehensively defined the extent and spectrum of mitochondrial disease in the adult population for the first time [55].

Methods

Clinical, biochemical, and genetic studies were carried out on adult patients with suspected mitochondrial disease, referred to a single centre in the North East of England between 1990 and 1999. Family members and affected relatives living within the study region were also traced and included in the study. The minimum point prevalence of mitochondrial disease in adults of working age, and the minimum prevalence of adults and children at risk of developing mitochondrial disease was calculated for a population of 2,122,290 individuals in mid-August 1997. Further family tracing in unaffected individuals enabled an estimation of the unaffected carrier rate for the same mid-year period.

Results

6.57 per 100,000 (95% CI = 5.30–7.83/100,000) adult individuals of working age had mitochondrial disease, and 7.59 per 100,000 (95% CI = 6.23–8.94/100,000) adults and children were at risk of developing mitochondrial disease. These findings, overall, reflected that 12.48 per 100,000 adults and children in the general population either had or were at risk of developing a mitochondrial disorder.

Conclusions

This study showed that at least ~1 in 10,000 adults would be affected by a mitochondrial disorder, placing the disease among the most common inherited disorders.

Critique

The first *population-based* study of a single pathogenic mtDNA mutation was carried out in northern Ostrobothnia in Finland, in 1998 [56]. Majamaa and colleagues, using molecular genetic testing of the probands followed by careful family tracing, estimated the frequency of the m.3243A>G mutation in the general population of 245,201 individuals as an adult point disease prevalence of 16.3/100,000 (95% CI = 11.3–21.4/100,000) or 1 in 6135. Higher incidences of the m.3243A>G mutation were noted in those with specific clinical phenotypes including deafness, hypertrophic cardiomyopathy, ophthalmoplegia, deafness, and occipital stroke.

There were clear discrepancies between the results of these two population-based studies. In Finland, the prevalence of the 3243A>G appeared to be 10-fold greater than that in northern England. This may in part have been due to the make-up of the population assessed. It is now recognized, with the development of new molecular diagnostic techniques, that the original prevalence figures were an under-estimation. A follow-up prevalence study by the Newcastle group revised their minimum prevalence figures for mtDNA disease and identified that 9.2 in 100,000 people had clinically manifested mtDNA disease, and a further 16.5 in 100,000 children and adults were at risk for the development of mtDNA disease—findings commensurate to mtDNA disease being one of the most common inherited neuromuscular disorders [57]. Moreover, the original study was based on adults presenting to a neurology clinic. Individuals with a predominantly non-neurological phenotype (e.g. diabetes and deafness) could have been missed in this study. In addition, childhood presentations with a fatal clinical course would not have been captured in this study [58]. Finally, the clinical and genetic spectrum of mitochondrial disease has continued to expand, revealing new phenotypes and new genotypes not recognized at the time of the original study. Of particular importance, mutations in the mtDNA polymerase *POLG* have emerged as a major cause of adult mitochondrial disease, so a revised estimate of the disease prevalence is probably closer to 1 in 5000.

11.8 **Identification of the most common nuclear mitochondrial disease gene**

Main paper: Van Goethem G, Dermaut B, Löfgren A, Martin JJ, Van Broeckhoven C. Mutation of *POLG* is associated with progressive external ophthalmoplegia characterized by mtDNA deletions. *Nat Genet* 2001; 28(3):211–2.

Background

Around the year 2000, genetic linkage and positional cloning had identified autosomal dominant missense mutations in the adenine nucleotide translocator (*ANT1*) [44] and mutations in *C10ORF2* [45] as a cause of autosomal dominant progressive external ophthalmoplegia (*ad*PEO), but it was clear that the major genetic cause had yet to be defined. Mutations in these genes had been excluded in three Belgian PEO pedigrees: one family who showed an inheritance pattern consistent with *ad*PEO, one family with recessive PEO (*ar*PEO), and another in whom the inheritance pattern could not be determined as both parents of the patient were deceased prior to review.

Methods and results

A 10-cM genome-wide scan and genotyping of additional microsatellite markers identified a candidate region at 15q22-q26, which included the gene encoding mitochondrial polymerase γ (*POLG*), in the adPEO pedigree. Subsequent Basic Local Alignment Search Tool (BLAST) alignment of *POLG* mRNA alignment and sequencing of its 22 codons identified a heterozygous mutation (Y955C) that was later confirmed to definitively co-segregate with adPEO in this family. In the other two families, *POLG* was sequenced revealing two compound heterozygous missense mutations: A467T and L304R in family B, and the A467T and R3P in family C. Although three of the 229 control subjects were heterozygous for A467T, neither the R3P or L304R mutations were observed.

Conclusions

This study identified probably the most important nuclear gene responsible for mitochondrial disease, and showed that different mutations could cause either a recessive or dominant disorder.

Critique

POLG-related disorders are now recognized as a group of nuclear genetic disorders characterized by phenotypic and genotypic heterogeneity, as well as highly variable age of onset. These disorders are characterized by secondary mtDNA defects in clinically affected tissues including multiple mtDNA deletions or the loss of mtDNA (mtDNA depletion). Alpers-Huttenlocher syndrome presents early in childhood with a severe clinical course characterized by progressive encephalopathy, intractable seizures, and liver failure, culminating in early mortality [59]. Ataxia neuropathy phenotypes include additional features such as ophthalmoplegia and seizures, but morbidity relates predominantly to the core features of ataxia and neuropathy [60]. Other recognized clinical phenotypes include late-onset ataxia [61]. Over a decade on, and although genotype–phenotype patterns are now rapidly emerging in *POLG*-related disorders, the mechanisms of pathogenesis still remain to be fully elucidated.

11.9 The first large randomized controlled therapeutic trial in a mitochondrial disorder

Main paper: Klopstock T, Yu-Wai-Man P, Dimitriadis K, et al. A randomized placebo-controlled trial of idebenone in Leber's hereditary optic neuropathy. *Brain* 2011; 134:2677–86.

Background

Despite the increase in understanding of the molecular basis of mitochondrial disease, and hundreds of case reports describing benefits from a wide variety of different vitamin supplements and co-factors, Cochrane systematic reviews in 1996 and 2011 found no objective evidence that any treatment was beneficial in mitochondrial disease (see Fig. 11.5). The vast majority of the published reports of treatment were based on small open-labelled case series and used biomarkers of dubious clinical relevance. Although there had been 12 randomized controlled trials in mitochondrial diseases, these had been small or inconclusive. A key step was to establish international consortia to build the clinical cohorts required for an adequately powered randomized, placebo-controlled trial.

Methods

The authors conducted a 24-week, multi-centre, double-blind, randomized, placebo-controlled trial of 900 mg per day of idebenone in a 2:1 ratio, in 85 patients with LHON harbouring one of the three primary mitochondrial DNA mutations (m.3460A>G, m.11778G>A, or m.14484T>C). The pre-defined end points were:

Primary end point: best recovery in visual acuity between baseline and week 24;

Secondary end point: change in best visual acuity; changes in visual acuity of the best eye at baseline; and changes in visual acuity for both eyes in each patient.

Colour contrast sensitivity and retinal nerve fibre layer thickness were also measured in subgroups.

Results

Idebenone was shown to be safe and well tolerated in patients with LHON. In the *intention to treat* group, the *primary* end point was not achieved. However, in patients with discordant visual acuities at baseline, post hoc interaction analysis showed a difference in response to idebenone with all *secondary* end points achieving statistically significant differences between the drug and placebo groups, with the largest treatment effect among patients harbouring the m.11778G>A and m.3460G>A mutations.

Conclusions

This study demonstrated the importance of multi-centre collaboration to develop new treatments for mitochondrial diseases. Idebenone holds therapeutic promise for patients with these disorders, with the greatest response perhaps in genotype-dependent mitochondrial diseases.

Critique

The speculative benefits of idebenone in patients with LHON was first proposed in 1992 [62], but it would be almost a decade later until this first complete randomized, placebo-controlled trial evaluating this therapeutic intervention in patients with mitochondrial disease [63]. Historically, endeavours to develop therapeutic strategies in such rare genetic disorders are often hampered by recruitment of patients to such drug studies and the annotation of meaningful outcome measures for both the patient and investigator [64]. To date, no pharmacological agent has proven to meet anticipated primary end points in patients with mitochondrial disorders. This may, in part, reflect the therapeutic attributes of the drug under investigation, but may also relate to the validity and appropriateness of the outcome points conscripted.

Supportive evidence of the therapeutic benefits of idebenone in patients with LHON continues to mount. Carelli et al. [65], in a response to Klopstock's publication, retrospectively reviewed patients' responses to 'off-label' idebenone administration at a specialist centre in Italy. Visual recovery was greater in the idebenone-treated group, with the duration and timing of therapy affecting the degree of recovery. These beneficial effects of idebenone appear to persist following discontinuation of treatment, for a median of 30 months [66], but further large-scale trials are needed.

11.10 Targeted next-generation sequencing in mitochondrial medicine

Main paper: Calvo SE, Compton AG, Hershman SG, et al. Molecular diagnosis of infantile mitochondrial disease with targeted next-generation sequencing. *Sci Transl Med* 2012; 25:118.

Background

Bioinformatic and experimental work implicates over 1000 nuclear genes in mitochondrial biogenesis and maintenance [67]. All of these genes are a potential cause of mitochondrial disease. This presents a major challenge diagnostically, because the time and effort needed to sequence all potential disease genes using traditional 'Sanger' based techniques would be prohibitive in each family or patient. Next-generation sequencing has the potential to revolutionize the diagnostic approach, with a single genetic test possible, in the clinic, for many patients with a suspected mitochondrial disorder. Vamsi Mootha and colleagues at Harvard Medical School, Boston, USA have been the vanguard of these technological developments. Based on *in silico* predictions of mitochondrial localization (MitoCarta), they developed an array to capture the sequence of more than 1000 genes thought to be important for mitochondrial function.

Methods

Forty-two genetically undetermined and unrelated infants with mitochondrial diseases were studied. All fulfilled the clinical and biochemical criteria for oxidative phosphorylation (OXPHOS) disease before 2 years of age. mtDNA and all coding exons of 1034 nuclear genes encoding mitochondrial proteins were sequenced in each child with targeted next-generation sequencing. DNA differences detected in the patients and that were rare in the general population, predicted to disrupt protein function and suggestive of recessive mendelian inheritance, were evaluated and compared to 371 healthy controls.

Results

Ten patients were determined to harbour recessive mutations in eight genes previously linked to mitochondrial disorders (*ACAD9, POLG, BCS1L, COX6B1, GFM1, TSFM, GFM1, TYMP*) and *AARS2*. Pathogenicity was established in nine of these ten patients by demonstrating:

1 allele segregation with disease in a family;

2 that the identified mutations were rare in controls; and/or

3 that the genes identified caused reduced cellular abundance of full-length mRNA transcripts, protein products, or OXPHOS subunits and assembly factors.

Fifteen candidate genes (*ACAD8, ACADSB, AGK (2), AKR1B15, C1orf31, C6orf125, C7orf10, EARS2, LYRM4, MTCH1, MTERF, MTHFD1L, NDUFB3, UCP1, and UQCR10*) were identified in 13 patients. Twelve patients had recessive mutations in nuclear genes not previously ascribed to disease, and one patient harboured a large 7.2 kb mtDNA deletion. Pathogenicity was determined in two of the twelve cases, in which the infants harboured either the *NDUFB3* or *AGK* mutations.

Conclusions

Next-generation sequencing can provide a molecular diagnosis in up to a quarter of genetically undetermined cases of mitochondrial myopathies, and potentially determine a further 25% in the coming decade as more genes causing mitochondrial myopathies are elucidated.

Critique

Next-generation sequencing is in the process of revolutionizing the approach to diagnosis of mitochondrial disease, moving the goal posts from sequence detection to the functional validation of new mutations. The targeted gene approach used by Calvo and colleagues delivered a step-change in mutation discovery, but, inevitably, the targeted capture of suspected disease genes limits the potential to find totally unexpected disease genes which could only affect mitochondria through an indirect mechanism. These technical issues have been partially addressed using whole exome capture, leading to new disease gene discovery [68], and, ultimately, through whole genome sequencing. However, 25 years after the discovery of the first genetic causes of mitochondrial disease, the diagnostic yield is still critically dependent on the meticulous clinical and biochemical characterization of patients.

Key unanswered questions

1 What is the way forward to providing a comprehensive diagnosis?

Despite major advances in understanding the molecular basis of mitochondrial diseases, identifying and confirming the diagnosis still remains a challenge. Part of the difficulty is identifying patients with milder phenotypes within the context of a busy general neurology clinical practice. With the expanding spectrum of phenotypes, this is becoming more and more difficult. Once the diagnosis is considered, then, at present, the investigations are often highly specialized and complex. Initial clinical evaluation detailing the personal and family history, using clinical investigations to document the extent of the phenotype, is the key to building the evidence base in support of the diagnosis. This may lead to a particular phenotype or syndrome which implicates a specific gene defect. Often though, this is not the case, and the clinician must take a systematic approach involving a biopsy of the affected tissue, if appropriate. This leads on to the histochemical and biochemical evaluation in mitochondrial function, which can help target the genetic investigations.

Currently, diagnosis is only possible in approximately two-thirds of patients thought to have mitochondrial disease. The implementation of next-generation whole exome and whole genome sequencing, over the next 5 years, is likely to drastically modify the diagnostic approach, leading to a diagnosis based on a blood DNA analysis in the outpatient clinic. However, interpreting the huge genetic diversity present in the exome and the genome will be challenging, and a biopsy may still be needed to prove that the underlying punitive pathogenic variants are actually causing the mitochondrial disorder. Also, it is important to remember that, for mitochondrial DNA disorders, the molecular defect may not be detectable in a blood sample. Urinary epithelium and buccal mouth swabs may provide an alternative to an invasive muscle or liver biopsy for mtDNA analysis.

2 What is the relationship between genotype and phenotype?

Ultimately, all mitochondrial disorders are thought to arise from a defect of adenosine triphosphate (ATP) synthesis linked to the process of oxidative phosphorylation. It is, therefore, utterly remarkable that this final common pathway can cause such a huge variation of clinical phenotypes. On the one hand, the same genetic defect can cause different phenotypes in different members of the same family. On the other hand, a similar phenotypic spectrum can be seen with different genetic lesions in the nuclear or the mitochondrial DNA. For mtDNA diseases, the concept of heteroplasmy further complicates the situation, with different percentage levels of mutation in different cells within the same organ, and different levels between different organs in the same individual. A further complication arises when we consider the segregation pattern of some common mtDNA diseases, such as LHON. The pattern of affected and unaffected individuals in the same family implicates nuclear genetic modifiers that interact with the mtDNA defect to cause the disease. It may well be that some of the phenotypic variability arises from a complex interaction between the nuclear genome and the mitochondrial genome in all mitochondrial disorders. This is important because understanding this mechanism may provide the key to finding an effective treatment. In the short term, understanding this interaction will help provide guidance to the patient and the clinician about the future prognosis and disease prevention.

3 How can we prevent mtDNA disease transmission?

A comprehensive molecular diagnosis encompassing all known nuclear mitochondrial genes will be the key to providing accurate recurrence risks and pre-implantation genetic diagnosis for mendelian mitochondrial disorders. A greater understanding of the disease penetrance and of potential genetic modifiers will refine this, over time. For many mtDNA diseases, mtDNA heteroplasmy makes the situation more complex. MtDNA is exclusively inherited down the maternal line, but there can be major differences in the inherited level of heteroplasmy between different siblings. This creates uncertainty in the clinic because it is very difficult to predict the outcome of pregnancy. Mothers can have either severely affected children, unaffected children, or a whole range in between. Attempts to understand this mechanism at the basic science level have made substantial progress in recent years, but the precise cellular mechanisms of the 'mitochondrial genetic bottleneck' have yet to be ascertained. Understanding this basic biology will, hopefully, lead to mechanisms that can be manipulated in order to prevent transmission of the pathogenic mtDNA defect.

In the short term, there has been great recent interest in the possibility of preventing the transmission of mtDNA disease through nuclear or chromosomal spindle transfer. These approaches involve the manipulation of early embryos *in vitro* and have the potential to change the germ line indefinitely. This has been a source of great controversy, and the treatment is, as at 2013, illegal. However, researchers on both sides of the Atlantic have been studying the early stages of human development *in vitro*, and the approach appears to have great potential to prevent the transmission of mtDNA diseases. Current work is focused on preclinical studies aimed at demonstrating that the technical aspects of the procedure are safe. Following a public consultation in early 2013, in the United Kingdom, the Human Embryology and Fertilization Authority reached the conclusion that such procedures are an acceptable way of trying to prevent mtDNA disease transmission.

4 What is the next step in developing effective treatment?

There is no treatment proven to be effective for mitochondrial diseases. Some disorders do have a potential treatment, such as co-enzyme Q10 replacement in defects of Q10 biosynthesis, or allergenic stem cell transplantation in mitochondrial neurogastrointestinal encephalopathy (MNGIE). However, these treatments are likely to have a very specific indication, and, in any case, they have not been formally evaluated in a clinical trial. With the establishment of both North American and European consortia, major clinical and research groups are coming together to pool their patients. This is a key step in developing natural history studies to underpin interventional trials which will hopefully deliver new therapies in the near future.

References

1 **Luft R, Ikkos D, Palmieri G, Ernster L, Afzelius B.** A case of severe hypermetabolism of nonthyroid origin with a defect in the maintenance of mitochondrial respiratory control: a correlated clinical, biochemical, and morphological study. *J Clin Invest* 1962; **41**:1776–804.

2 **Liesa M, Palacin M, Zorzano A.** Mitochondrial dynamics in mammalian health and disease. *Physiol Rev* 2009; **89**(3):799–845.

3 **Benda C.** Ueber dier spermatogenese de verbebraten und höherer evertebraten, II. Theil: die histiogenese der spermien. *Arch Anat Physiol* 1898; **73**:393–8.

4 **Palade GE.** The fine structure of mitochondria. *Anat Rec* 1952; **114**(3):427–51.

5 **Lehninger AL.** Fatty acid oxidation and the Krebs trocarboxylic acid cycle. *J Biol Chem* 1945; **161**:413.

6 **Nass MM, Nass S.** Intramitochondrial fibers with DNA characteristics. I. Fixation and electron staining reactions. *J Cell Biol* 1963; **19**:593–611.

7 **Schatz G.** The isolation of possible mitochondrial precursor structures from aerobically grown baker's yeast. *Biochem Biophys Res Commun* 1963; **12**:448–51.

8 **DiMauro S, Bonilla E, Lee CP, et al.** Luft's disease. Further biochemical and ultrastructural studies of skeletal muscle in the second case. *J Neurol Sci* 1976; **27**(2):217–32.

9 **Luft R.** The development of mitochondrial medicine. *Proc Natl Acad Sci USA* 1994; **91**(19):8731–8.

10 **Scholte HR.** The biochemical basis of mitochondrial diseases. *J Bioenerg Biomembr* 1988; **20**(2):161–91.

11 **Shapira Y, Harel S, Russell A.** Mitochondrial encephalomyopathies: a group of neuromuscular disorders with defects in oxidative metabolism. *Isr J Med Sci* 1977; **13**(2):161–4.

12 **Petty RK, Harding AE, Morgan-Hughes JA.** The clinical features of mitochondrial myopathy. *Brain* 1986; **109**(Pt 5):915–38.

13 **Morgan-Hughes JA, Mair WG, Lascelles PT.** A disorder of skeletal muscle associated with tubular aggregates. *Brain* 1970; **93**(4):873–80.

14 **Morgan-Hughes JA, Darveniza P, Kahn SN, et al.** A mitochondrial myopathy characterized by a deficiency in reducible cytochrome b. Brain 1977; **100**(4):617–40.

15 **Dimauro S.** A history of mitochondrial diseases. *J Inherit Metab Dis* 2011; **34**(2):261–76.

16 **Pavlakis SG, Phillips PC, DiMauro S, De Vivo DC, Rowland LP.** Mitochondrial myopathy, encephalopathy, lactic acidosis, and strokelike episodes: a distinctive clinical syndrome. *Ann Neurol* 1984; **16**(4):481–8.

17 **Fukuhara N, Tokiguchi S, Shirakawa K, Tsubaki T.** Myoclonus epilepsy associated with ragged-red fibres (mitochondrial abnormalities): disease entity or a syndrome? Light- and electron-microscopic studies of two cases and review of literature. *J Neurol Sci* 1980; **47**(1):117–33.

18 **Kearns TP.** External ophthalmoplegia, pigmentary degeneration of the retina, and cardiomyopathy: a newly recognized syndrome. *Trans Am Ophthalmol Soc* 1965; **63**:559–625.

19 **Leber T.** Uber hereditare und congenital-angelegte sehnervenleiden. *Graefe's Arch Ophthalmol* 1871; 17:249–91.

20 **Kearns TP, Sayre GP.** Retinitis pigmentosa, external ophthalmophegia, and complete heart block: unusual syndrome with histologic study in one of two cases. *AMA Arch Ophthalmol* 1958; **60**(2):280–9.

21 **Jager BV, Fred HL, Butler RB, Carnes WH.** Occurrence of retinal pigmentation, ophthalmoplegia, ataxia, deafness and heart block. Report of a case, with findings at autopsy. *Am J Med* 1960; **29**:888–93.

22 Anderson S, Bankier AT, Barrell BG, et al. Sequence and organization of the human mitochondrial genome. *Nature* 1981; **290**(5806):457–65.

23 Andrews RM, Kubacka I, Chinnery PF, Lightowlers RN, Turnbull DM, Howell N. Reanalysis and revision of the Cambridge reference sequence for human mitochondrial DNA. *Nat Genet* 1999; **23**(2):147.

24 Zeviani M, Moraes CT, DiMauro S, et al. Deletions of mitochondrial DNA in Kearns-Sayre syndrome. *Neurology* 1988; **38**(9):1339–46.

25 Moraes CT, DiMauro S, Zeviani M, et al. Mitochondrial DNA deletions in progressive external ophthalmoplegia and Kearns-Sayre syndrome. *N Engl J Med* 1989; **320**(20):1293–9.

26 Erickson RP. Leber's optic atrophy, a possible example of maternal inheritance. *Am J Hum Genet* 1972; **24**(3):348–9.

27 Man PY, Griffiths PG, Brown DT, Howell N, Turnbull DM, Chinnery PF. The epidemiology of Leber hereditary optic neuropathy in the North East of England. *Am J Hum Genet* 2003; **72**(2):333–9.

28 Mackey DA, Oostra RJ, Rosenberg T, et al. Primary pathogenic mtDNA mutations in multigeneration pedigrees with Leber hereditary optic neuropathy. *Am J Hum Genet* 1996; **59**(2):481–5.

29 Wallace DC, Singh G, Lott MT, et al. Mitochondrial DNA mutation associated with Leber's hereditary optic neuropathy. *Science* 1988; **242**(4884):1427–30.

30 Johns DR, Neufeld MJ, Park RD. An ND-6 mitochondrial DNA mutation associated with Leber hereditary optic neuropathy. *Biochem Biophys Res Commun* 1992; **187**(3):1551–7.

31 Howell N, McCullough D, Bodis-Wollner I. Molecular genetic analysis of a sporadic case of Leber hereditary optic neuropathy. *Am J Hum Genet* 1992; **50**(2):443–6.

32 Macmillan C, Kirkham T, Fu K, et al. Pedigree analysis of French Canadian families with T14484C Leber's hereditary optic neuropathy. *Neurology* 1998; **50**(2):417–22.

33 Hudson G, Carelli V, Horvath R, Zeviani M, Smeets HJ, Chinnery PF. X-inactivation patterns in females harboring mtDNA mutations that cause Leber hereditary optic neuropathy. *Mol Vis* 2007; **13**:2339–43.

34 Hudson G, Carelli V, Spruijt L, et al. Clinical expression of Leber hereditary optic neuropathy is affected by the mitochondrial DNA-haplogroup background. *Am J Hum Genet* 2007; **81**(2):228–33.

35 Chinnery PF, Andrews RM, Turnbull DM, Howell NN. Leber hereditary optic neuropathy: does heteroplasmy influence the inheritance and expression of the G11778A mitochondrial DNA mutation? *Am J Med Genet* 2001; **98**(3):235–43.

36 Cyrus-Hajmassy M. Bilateral visual deterioration in excessive tobacco and alcohol consumption. *Ophthalmologe* 2012; **109**(9):901–6.

37 Kirkman MA, Yu-Wai-Man P, Korsten A, et al. Gene-environment interactions in Leber hereditary optic neuropathy. *Brain* 2009; **132**(Pt 9):2317–26.

38 Giles RE, Blanc H, Cann HM, Wallace DC. Maternal inheritance of human mitochondrial DNA. *Proc Natl Acad Sci USA* 1980; **77**(11):6715–9.

39 Sherrington R, Brynjolfsson J, Petursson H, et al. Localization of a susceptibility locus for schizophrenia on chromosome 5. *Nature* 1988; **336**(6195):164–7.

40 Endicott J, Forman JB, Spitzer RL. Research approaches to diagnostic classification in schizophrenia. *Birth Defects Orig Artic Ser* 1978; **14**(5):41–57.

41 Moraes CT, Shanske S, Tritschler HJ, et al. mtDNA depletion with variable tissue expression: a novel genetic abnormality in mitochondrial diseases. *Am J Hum Genet* 1991; **48**(3):492–501.

42 Van Goethem G, Dermaut B, Lofgren A, Martin JJ, Van Broeckhoven C. Mutation of POLG is associated with progressive external ophthalmoplegia characterized by mtDNA deletions. *Nat Genet* 2001; **28**(3):211–2.

43 **Longley MJ, Clark S, Yu Wai Man C, et al.** Mutant POLG2 disrupts DNA polymerase gamma subunits and causes progressive external ophthalmoplegia. *Am J Hum Genet* 2006; **78**(6):1026–34.

44 **Kaukonen J, Juselius JK, Tiranti V, et al.** Role of adenine nucleotide translocator 1 in mtDNA maintenance. *Science* 2000; **289**(5480):782–5.

45 **Spelbrink JN, Li FY, Tiranti V, et al.** Human mitochondrial DNA deletions associated with mutations in the gene encoding Twinkle, a phage T7 gene 4-like protein localized in mitochondria. *Nat Genet* 2001; **28**(3):223–31.

46 **Tyynismaa H, Ylikallio E, Patel M, Molnar MJ, Haller RG, Suomalainen A.** A heterozygous truncating mutation in RRM2B causes autosomal-dominant progressive external ophthalmoplegia with multiple mtDNA deletions. *Am J Hum Genet* 2009; **85**(2):290–5.

47 **Tyynismaa H, Sun R, Ahola-Erkkila S, et al.** Thymidine kinase 2 mutations in autosomal recessive progressive external ophthalmoplegia with multiple mitochondrial DNA deletions. *Hum Mol Genet* 2012; **21**(1):66–75.

48 **Rouzier C, Bannwarth S, Chaussenot A, et al.** The MFN2 gene is responsible for mitochondrial DNA instability and optic atrophy "plus" phenotype. *Brain* 2012; **135**(Pt 1):23–34.

49 **Hudson G, Amati-Bonneau P, Blakely EL, et al.** Mutation of OPA1 causes dominant optic atrophy with external ophthalmoplegia, ataxia, deafness and multiple mitochondrial DNA deletions: a novel disorder of mtDNA maintenance. *Brain* 2008; **131**(Pt 2):329–37.

50 **Ronchi D, Di Fonzo A, Lin W, et al.** Mutations in DNA2 link progressive myopathy to mitochondrial DNA instability. *Am J Hum Genet* 2013; **92**(2):293–300.

51 **Shoffner JM, Lott MT, Lezza AM, Seibel P, Ballinger SW, Wallace DC.** Myoclonic epilepsy and ragged-red fiber disease (MERRF) is associated with a mitochondrial DNA tRNA(Lys) mutation. *Cell* 1990; **61**(6):931–7.

52 **Sproule DM, Kaufmann P.** Mitochondrial encephalopathy, lactic acidosis, and strokelike episodes: basic concepts, clinical phenotype, and therapeutic management of MELAS syndrome. *Ann NY Acad Sci* 2008; **1142**:133–58.

53 **Schon EA, DiMauro S, Hirano M.** Human mitochondrial DNA: roles of inherited and somatic mutations. *Nat Rev Genet* 2012; **13**(12):878–90.

54 **Karicheva OZ, Kolesnikova OA, Schirtz T, et al.** Correction of the consequences of mitochondrial 3243A>G mutation in the MT-TL1 gene causing the MELAS syndrome by tRNA import into mitochondria. *Nucleic Acids Res* 2011; **39**(18):8173–86.

55 **Chinnery PF, Johnson MA, Wardell TM, et al.** The epidemiology of pathogenic mitochondrial DNA mutations. *Ann Neurol* 2000; **48**(2):188–93.

56 **Majamaa K, Moilanen JS, Uimonen S, et al.** Epidemiology of A3243G, the mutation for mitochondrial encephalomyopathy, lactic acidosis, and strokelike episodes: prevalence of the mutation in an adult population. *Am J Hum Genet* 1998; **63**(2):447–54.

57 **Schaefer AM, McFarland R, Blakely EL, et al.** Prevalence of mitochondrial DNA disease in adults. *Ann Neurol* 2008; **63**(1):35–9.

58 **Skladal D, Halliday J, Thorburn DR.** Minimum birth prevalence of mitochondrial respiratory chain disorders in children. *Brain* 2003; **126**(Pt 8):1905–12.

59 **Naviaux RK, Nguyen KV.** POLG mutations associated with Alpers' syndrome and mitochondrial DNA depletion. *Ann Neurol* 2004; **55**(5):706–12.

60 **Hakonen AH, Heiskanen S, Juvonen V, et al.** Mitochondrial DNA polymerase W748S mutation: a common cause of autosomal recessive ataxia with ancient European origin. *Am J Hum Genet* 2005; **77**(3):430–41.

61 **Craig K, Ferrari G, Tiangyou W, et al.** The A467T and W748S POLG substitutions are a rare cause of adult-onset ataxia in Europe. *Brain* 2007; **130**(Pt 4): E69; author reply E70.

62 **Mashima Y, Hiida Y, Oguchi Y.** Remission of Leber's hereditary optic neuropathy with idebenone. *Lancet* 1992; **340**(8815):368–9.

63 **Klopstock T, Yu-Wai-Man P, Dimitriadis K, et al.** A randomized placebo-controlled trial of idebenone in Leber's hereditary optic neuropathy. *Brain* 2011; **134**(Pt 9):2677–86.

64 **Pfeffer G, Majamaa K, Turnbull DM, Thorburn D, Chinnery PF.** Treatment for mitochondrial disorders. *Cochrane Database Syst Rev* 2012; **4**:CD004426.

65 **Carelli V, La Morgia C, Valentino ML, et al.** Idebenone treatment in Leber's hereditary optic neuropathy. *Brain* 2011; **134**(Pt 9):e188.

66 **Klopstock T, Metz G, Yu-Wai-Man P, et al.** Persistence of the treatment effect of idebenone in Leber's hereditary optic neuropathy. *Brain* 2013; **136**(Pt 2):e230.

67 **Pagliarini DJ, Calvo SE, Chang B, et al.** A mitochondrial protein compendium elucidates complex I disease biology. *Cell* 2008; **134**(1):112–23.

68 **Haack TB, Haberberger B, Frisch EM, et al.** Molecular diagnosis in mitochondrial complex I deficiency using exome sequencing. *J Med Genet* 2012; **49**(4):277–83.

69 **Goto Y, Nonaka I, Horai SA.** Mutation in the tRNA $^{Leu(UUR)}$ gene associated with the MELAS subgroup of mitochondrial encephalomyopathies. *Nature* 1990; **348**(6302):651–3.

Chapter 12

Myology

Michael Swash

12.0 **Introduction**

As in other areas of medicine, advances in myology have in large measure followed technical innovations and consequent new concepts in scientific understanding of muscle anatomy, physiology, and pathology. Myopathology, in particular, has changed out of all recognition in this period with the advent, firstly, of the technique of frozen sections enabling the application of enzyme histochemistry to individual sections of muscle tissue, followed by the use of monoclonal antibodies to delineate the distribution and expression of individual proteins in muscle cells, and also in characterizing the inflammatory response. More recently, the advent of molecular genetics has transformed our understanding of the classification of muscle disorders.

The traditional approach to investigation of a patient with a neuromuscular disease used the classical clinical methods of the neurological history and examination, later supplemented by electrophysiological studies, especially electromyography (EMG) and muscle biopsy [1]. This methodology therefore involved clinical, physiological, and pathological assessments that were evaluated as separate, but complementary techniques, each providing related information. All these techniques remain in use but, currently, molecular evaluation of the biopsy and genetic studies are proving most revealing. Detailed studies of molecular genetics and muscle proteins have fundamentally altered the boundaries of clinical diagnosis. Some syndromes formerly regarded as definite entities, with clearly defined criteria for their diagnosis, are now regarded as complex groups of related disorders, defined by their molecular basis. This has led to confusion in relation to determination of diagnosis and prognosis and, especially, in explaining to patients and their families exactly the nature of the diagnosis. One cannot tell a patient and family with a limb-girdle muscular dystrophy that they suffer from a 'mutation on chromosome so and so'; to do so simply invites the question 'But, doctor, what disease is it?' Of course, this is not unique to muscle disorders, but it is starkly evident in this specialty.

In considering how these fundamental changes in clinical practice came about, one must acknowledge many important contributions. Contemporary neuroscience so often involves contributions from a number of investigators, working in collaboration in different institutions and different countries. Frequently, several groups of investigators work in the same general area and their contributions overlap, but all are important.

Early publications described clinical syndromes of muscle disease as a distinct group of disorders that required clinical separation from spinal root, motor nerve, or anterior horn cell disorders [2]. The fundamental concept of disease of muscle as a primary disorder, as so often with new concepts in medicine, was enshrined in several major textbooks in the nineteenth and early twentieth centuries [3–5] following their eponymous descriptions. This group of muscle diseases was termed the muscular dystrophies, a phrase often used synonymously with the word myopathy, but the phrase 'muscular dystrophy' became associated with inherited causation. This group of disorders included conditions such as Duchenne and Becker muscular dystrophies, facio-scapulo-humeral (Landouzy-Dejerine), myotonic (Steinert), and distal muscular dystrophy (Gowers) [3]. Limb-girdle muscular dystrophy was a term introduced in 1954 in the seminal clinical study from Newcastle by Walton and Nattrass [6].

In their monograph on the history of Duchenne muscular dystrophy, Emery and Emery [7] noted that a wasting disease of muscle was recognized in an 18-year-old man by the Scottish anatomist, Sir Charles Bell (1774–1842), as recorded in his monograph *The Nervous System of the Human Body* in 1830 [8]. The prototypical muscle disease, Duchenne muscular dystrophy, was described independently in Italy, Britain, Germany, and France, before achieving recognition as a diagnostic entity. The contribution of French neurologist, Guillaume Duchenne (1806–1875), was especially important because he introduced his 'muscle harpoon' method of achieving muscle biopsy, thus allowing correlation of clinical features with myopathology [9]. Nonetheless, the myopathic nature of Duchenne's disease was first clearly set out by Wilhelm Erb (1840–1921), who emphasized the distinction between spinal grey matter disease and muscle disease in patients presenting with muscular weakness and wasting in 1884 [10].

Following these early concepts, the chapter on muscle disease in the second edition of the book by British neurologist, Samuel Kinnier Wilson (1878–1937) [2], published in 1954, was based on this nineteenth-century clinical classification. The subsequent major advances in myopathic disorders that have transformed clinical practice commenced with the Walton and Nattrass paper [6], also published in 1954, but first, there was a major and startling advance in what have become known as 'the metabolic myopathies'.

12.1 **Metabolic myopathies**

Main paper: McArdle B. Myopathy due to a defect in muscle glycogen breakdown. *Clin Sci Mol Med* 1951; 10:13–33.

Background

This report, by the British neurologist, Brian McArdle (1911–2002), working at Guy's Hospital, London, was the first description of a myopathy due to a recognized enzyme defect [11]. It set the scene for all subsequent studies of the group of disorders known as 'metabolic myopathies' and was a landmark for metabolic studies of disease in other bodily systems. It was especially important since the disorder of function identified was limited to one tissue—a defect of myophosphorylase in skeletal muscle; thus illustrating the importance of subspecialization of metabolic pathways within individual tissues of the human body.

Methods and results

McArdle's report represented a new approach to the study of muscle disorders associated with fatigue, exercise-induced power failure, and muscle cramp. It illustrated the application of biochemical knowledge to a focused investigation at a time when muscle histochemistry was not established, and microscopy was more or less limited to formalin-fixed, paraffin-embedded sections. Electron microscopy was then in its infancy. The biochemistry of the Krebs cycle and of energy metabolism and its relation to adenosine triphosphate (ATP) in the initiation of muscular contraction was then relatively new knowledge.

It was these concepts that were applied by McArdle to the study of a rare, recessively inherited disorder characterized by muscle aches and exercise-induced cramp and weakness. He demonstrated that the disorder was accompanied by a failure to produce lactate on muscular exertion, and devised the standardized ischaemic lactate test to demonstrate the metabolic disorder—failure of the venous blood lactate levels to rise during ischaemic exercise—in venous blood derived from the biceps brachii muscle exercising with its arterial supply occluded by a blood pressure cuff. He correctly surmised, from the clinical and histological features, that the underlying defect was absence of muscle myophosphorylase, leading to reduction in ATP production through the Krebs cycle and dependence on fat breakdown for energy production. Excess muscle fibre glycogen was recognized in muscle biopsies in the disorder.

Conclusions and critique

Subsequently, single enzyme defects have been defined at most points in the Krebs cycle, each with a recognizable phenotype, and most with recognizable clinical presentations in childhood (early onset) but with different presentations in adult life (late-onset) [12]. In addition, metabolic muscle weakness is well described in association with mitochondrial enzyme mutations in muscle (see Chapter 11), causing disorders in the electron transport system and leading to lipid deposition in muscle fibres—the lipid storage myopathies. In these disorders, often associated with progressive ophthalmoplegia, mitochondria show highly characteristic 'parking lot' inclusions in ultrastructural studies [13].

Myopathies with intermittent hyperpyrexia, often exercise-induced [14] or induced by general anaesthesia, due to dissociation of energy production from contraction resulting in heat emission from muscle, occur especially in the context of myopathies with cores (see earlier). At first, these myopathies were usually diagnosed by metabolic studies on muscle biopsies, or by searching for raised venous blood lactate levels in mitochondrial myopathies. Now, these disorders, as well as McArdle's myophosphorylase deficiency, are more usually diagnosed by DNA (deoxyribonucleic acid) studies aimed at detecting specific mutations in the relevant gene [15]. Three mutations account for nearly 90% of cases.

The exercise-induced myoglobinurias [16] are a somewhat less well-understood group of disorders characterized by relatively rapid onset of potentially fatal myoglobinuria, often in the context of heavy exercise under adverse conditions, especially in very hot environments, with associated dehydration. Myoglobinuria is not a specific syndrome; mitochondrial disorders with lipid storage may also present with myoglobinuria. Most cases occur in young men, and a specific biochemical causation is often difficult to establish.

Regrettably, despite the high level of understanding regarding the metabolic disorder in most of these syndromes, little of practical utility is available in respect of therapy. Furthermore, the initial hope, even expectation that elucidation of the biochemical anomalies in these myopathies associated with specific defects in muscle enzyme function would lead to understanding of weakness in the muscular dystrophies themselves, has not been fulfilled. The latter are specific cell proteinopathies, not involving muscle enzymes important for contraction and relaxation of muscle.

12.2 **Clarification of classification**

Main paper: Walton JN, Nattrass FJ. On the classification, natural history and treatment of the myopathies. *Brain* 1954; 77:169–231.

Background

Although, in the mid-twentieth century, the five major clinical syndromes (see section 12.0) were reasonably well delineated as clinical entities, nothing was known as to their pathogenesis. More importantly, when this paper was published in 1954, there were many other patients with muscular weakness, evidently due to primary myopathic disease, that could not be characterized within this simple clinical classification. John Walton (born 1922) and Frederick Nattrass (1891–1979) (Fig. 12.1) commented that:

> The great majority of cases are genetic in origin, though the exact pathogenesis of the muscle wasting remains a mystery . . . the mode of inheritance of the various forms is not fully understood . . . (as a result of) the lack of any general agreement concerning classification.

In this paper, Walton and Nattrass conducted a detailed review of the historical background and then used data from 105 personally studied cases to derive a new classification of muscle disease.

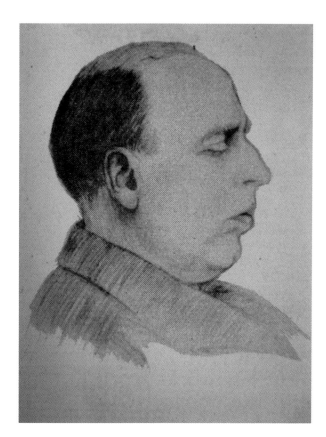

Fig. 12.1 (A) Frederick J. Nattrass (1891–1979), neurologist and Professor of Medicine, University of Newcastle.

Silhouette from the Medical Pilgrims, reproduced under the Creative Commons Act 4.0.

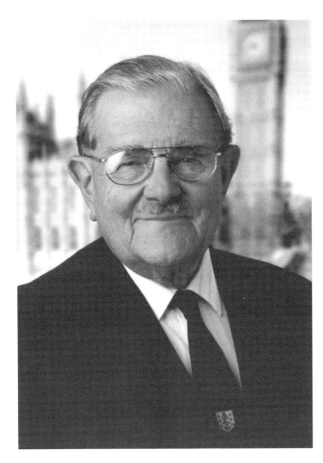

Fig. (B) John N. Walton (born 1922), Emeritus Professor of Neurology, University of Newcastle; now Lord Walton of Detchant.
Reprinted with permission from Lord Walton.

Methods and results

The 105 patients were all independently examined by the two authors, all had EMG studies, and all had muscle biopsy to establish the pathological changes; the clinical diagnosis of primary muscle disease was therefore verified. In addition, as many family members as possible were interviewed and when necessary, they were examined by one of the authors. An attempt was made to ascertain all patients with primary muscle disease in the population served by the Newcastle hospital services—the counties of Northumberland and Durham. Among this group of patients, there were 84 cases of pseudohypertrophic muscular dystrophy. Having recognized these patients as suffering from the disorder described by Duchenne [9], Walton and Nattrass suggested that this disorder should be termed 'Duchenne muscular dystrophy', terminology that rapidly became universally used. Most of these cases were young boys, but in three families, the disease seemed to take a slower course, and in one, the disease commenced at age 26 years, and he was still alive aged 44 years. Presumably, these were examples of Becker X-linked muscular dystrophy, although this was not then recognized. In three girls, there were similar clinical features, but these defied explanation at that time. Eighteen patients in the families studied had facioscapulohumeral muscular dystrophy, including three asymptomatic family members—a finding that was later acknowledged as important in genetic counselling.

Two patients had progressive distal myopathy and one had ocular myopathy. A further 18 cases had 'limb-girdle muscular dystrophy' (LGMD). This was defined as a disorder with predominant involvement of proximal limb-girdle musculature, usually beginning in the third decade, with relatively slow progression. Muscle hypertrophy was infrequent in this group. The syndrome of LGMD could occur in men or women. There was considerable variation in the natural history, usually with slow but sometimes more rapid progression. Walton and Nattrass thought most cases of limb-girdle myopathy were inherited as an autosomal recessive trait. In addition, Walton and Nattrass recognized Sir Jonathan Hutchinson's description of progressive ocular myopathy [17], sometimes with progression to proximal upper limb muscles.

Conclusions and critique

Walton and Nattrass commented that this classification, shown in Table 12.1, 'was much too unwieldy for routine use' since it included many conditions of 'extreme rarity' and others of possibly artificial definition. They considered that 'menopausal muscular dystrophy', which was usually steroid-responsive, was probably a form of indolent late-onset polymyositis. At this time, there was uncertainty as to whether myotonia congenita was an early stage of dystrophia myotonica, or a separate entity, and the various clinical forms of the myotonic syndromes and their modes of inheritance were not then recognized.

It was thought that the pathological changes in muscle in all these disorders was constant and universal, but this was the era in which histopathological studies were limited to formalin-fixed, paraffin-embedded tissue, so that it was not possible to study cell metabolism or cell microstructure by microscopy. These revelations awaited enzyme histochemistry and the electron microscope. Walton and Nattrass suggested that:

> The great majority of the commonly occurring cases of myopathy can be classified, using traditional criteria, into one of the remaining groups (pseudohypertrophic—Duchenne; atrophic pelvifemoral—Leyden-Moebius; juvenile scapulohumeral—Erb; facioscapulohumeral—Landouzy-Dejerine; late juvenile—Nevin; distal—Gowers).

Walton and Nattrass noted a controversy in the contemporary literature concerning classification, especially between Bell [35], whose work was based on a careful study of 1228 published cases and 113 patients gleaned from the records at Queen Square, and Tyler and Wintrobe [36] who, with Stevenson [37], considered that all cases of muscular dystrophy could be defined as of childhood onset or facioscapulohumeral types. They regarded pseudohypertrophy as an unreliable criterion upon which to base a classification of a disease entity. However, Bell [35] had gone further, and noted that there were families with sex-linked recessive, autosomal dominant and autosomal recessive patterns of inheritance of muscle disease and that these patterns of inheritance were found in pseudohypertrophic

Table 12.1 Classification of muscle disorders according to Walton and Nattrass [6]

1. Pseudohypertrophic muscular dystrophy [9, 18]
2. The pelvic girdle atrophy type [19, 20]
3. The juvenile (scapulohumeral) type [10]
4. The facioscapulohumeral type [21]
5. The distal type [22]
6. The late juvenile type [23]
7. The Barnes type [24]
8. Myotonia congenital [25] and paramyotonia congenital [26]
9. Dystrophia myotonia [27, 28]
10. The simple atrophic type of amyotonia congenita [29, 30]
11. The local myopathies [31, 32]
12. Benign childhood myopathy (probably polymyositis) [6]
13. Unusual myopathies of metabolic origin [11, 34]
14. Thyrotoxic myopathy
15. 'Myasthenic myopathy'
16. Atypical myopathy

Reproduced from *Brain*, 77, Walton JN, Nattrass FJ, On the classification, natural history and treatment of the myopathies, p. 169–231, Copyright (1954), with permission from Oxford University Press.

cases, atrophic cases, and myopathies with facial involvement, indicating a likely much more complex pathogenesis for this group of diseases. Indeed, Stevenson [37] recognized that the pseudohypertrophic form was a discrete entity and defined its clinical characteristics as a disease of young boys. Walton and Nattrass [6] described a group of patients with, what they termed, limb-girdle dystrophy, a disorder that had been subsumed by Stevenson within a group of 'autosomal limb-girdle dystrophies' that included facioscapulohumeral dystrophy. Walton and Nattrass recognized that the latter disorder was inherited in an autosomal dominant fashion, and that most cases of limb-girdle dystrophy were of autosomal recessive inheritance, when any pattern of inheritance could be determined. On the other hand, they stated that they considered myotonia and dystrophia myotonica to be variants of the same disease process.

In the second half of their paper, Walton and Nattrass described their clinical, electrocardiographic (ECG), and radiological studies in considerable detail, together with the negative results of various therapies, including alpha-tocopherol (vitamin E) in 105 patients from the Newcastle region. ECG abnormalities were reported in 12 of 48 cases of Duchenne dystrophy and in 4 of 15 cases of dystrophia myotonica. EMG and pathological data were given in separate reports.

This paper was fundamentally important in reconciling the earlier descriptions with careful clinico-pathological observations in a group of patients taken from a defined area of the UK. It proved possible to redefine the limits of several of these genetic disorders, to cast doubt on the issue of classification and nosology of a late-onset muscle disease mainly affecting women and responsive to steroid therapy, and to set out, with clarity, problems requiring future research. For John Walton (later appointed a life peer as Baron Walton of Detchant) himself, this paper proved the catalyst to a lifetime concerned with studies of muscle disease, in many different aspects. He has played a vital role in encouraging clinical and basic science studies in this group of disorders, and in the organization of care pathways in the UK and, by example, abroad. His organizational skills have proved invaluable in other national aspects of medical policy, beyond the muscular dystrophies.

12.3 **The myosin ATPase method—key to technique**

Main paper: Padykula HA and Herman E. The specificity of the histochemical method for adenosine triphosphatase. *J Histochem Cytochem* 1955; 3170–89.

Background

This report by Helen Padykula and Edith Herman, from the Department of Anatomy at Harvard, provided the scientific basis for the application of their method to study the distribution of ATPase in skeletal muscle and, indeed, in other tissues [38]. They noted the previous uncertainty concerning the specificity of the reaction in previous studies dating from the 1930s and later. They noted further uncertainties regarding the use of the Gomori medium for the reaction and the requirement for a sulfhydryl (SH) group in the enzyme reaction, pointing out that the SH group had been found to inhibit the action of alkaline phosphomonoesterases.

Methods and results

They used fresh, frozen cryostat sections of tissue from adult albino rats. Their method required a short pre-incubation of 15–20 minutes in a medium containing ATP adjusted to pH 9.4. They commented that in skeletal muscle, the enzyme reaction occurred on myofibrils, not in the sarcoplasm. They noted earlier literature strongly supporting co-localization of ATPase with myofibrils and with mitochondria, but concluded that 'true ATPase of striated muscle occurs in the myofibrils and probably not in the mitochondria or sarcoplasm', whereas in other tissues, ATPase is localized in mitochondria.

Conclusions and critique

This histochemical method and the observations themselves provided the basis for all subsequent enzyme histochemical studies in skeletal muscle biopsies, thus leading to recognition of different fibre types and to understanding of fast and slow contracting and fatiguing muscle fibres in human muscle. The implications for the organization of the motor system at spinal level rapidly became apparent when it was discovered that in reinnervation (chronic partial denervation) there was 'grouped atrophy', indicating that muscle fibres denervated by degeneration of their nerve supply could attract innervation from neighbouring healthy axons by axonal sprouting, causing grouping of muscle fibres of the same histochemical type in the muscle. A new era of histological studies of muscle was born.

12.4 **Childhood-onset myopathies**

Main paper: Gonatas NK, Shy GM, Godfrey EH. Nemaline myopathy; the origin of nemaline structures. *New Engl J Med* 1966; 274:535–9.

Background

In the late 1960s, there was a sudden efflorescence of understanding regarding non-dystrophic myopathies in childhood. As so often in science, this new research was driven by new technology.

Methods and results

At that time, the laboratory of George Milton Shy (1919–1967) in Bethesda, Maryland, USA, where the young W. King Engel was also working, was in the forefront of the application of enzyme histochemistry in the study of muscle biopsies. In 1963, they reported a new congenital myopathy in a child, and described it as 'nemaline myopathy', alluding to the characteristic rod-like bodies found in the cytoplasm of skeletal muscle fibres in the disease [39]. The child was floppy and weak, but the disorder was not rapidly progressive. Sadly, Milton Shy, remembered by those who knew him as a brilliant lecturer and master of the multiple slide projector technique, passed away suddenly, shortly after this seminal contribution.

A second case of nemaline myopathy was described by Engel et al. in the following year [40]. Familial occurrence of the disease was reported in 1965 [41]. The report of 1966 by Gonatas et al. [42] set the scene for many subsequent studies of non-dystrophic childhood myopathies associated with intra-fibre inclusions and vacuoles by identifying the likely nature of the protein constituent of the rod bodies as tropomyosin B. This was a reference to the ultrastructural work of Huxley [43], describing the orientation of the contractile proteins of skeletal muscle in terms of the sliding hypothesis of the actin–myosin interaction, and its organization around the Z-band interface.

Conclusions and critique

Thus there was the possibility that some myopathies might be due to abnormalities in muscle contractile proteins and muscle structural proteins, although this realization was perhaps not immediately apparent to all those involved in trying to understand muscle disease. In modern terminology, this was a disease with 'proteinaceous inclusions' in muscle fibres [44] (Table 12.2).

Childhood-onset myopathies [45, 46] are characterized by onset early in life, with generalized proximally predominant weakness (which may be very mild or rather severe), hypotonia (associated with head lag), and dysmorphic features. The latter largely reflect weakness of muscles during development, for example, of the face and palate. Some childhood-onset myopathies are associated with flexion contractures. They are usually relatively non-progressive and some may improve with maturity, perhaps because of

Table 12.2 Classification of childhood-onset (congenital) myopathies

Myopathies with proteinaceous inclusions
Nemaline myopathy
Myosin storage myopathy
Cap disease
Reducing body myopathy
Myopathies with cores
Central core disease (sometimes with rods)
Multicore disease (ryanodine mutations)
Myopathies with central nuclei
Myotubular myopathy
Centronuclear myopathy
Myopathies with increased fibre size variation
Congenital fibre type disproportion

the normal increase in muscle bulk and strength in adolescence. These myopathies are inherited.

Subtle differences in phenotype are used by experienced clinicians to suggest the underlying causation [46]. The childhood-onset or congenital myopathies have been classified in various ways, but the most obvious method relies on the pathology in the muscle biopsy (Table 12.2). This, however, has been largely superseded by a genetic classification based on mutational analysis, which recognizes that the variable clinical and pathological features in any one of these clinical syndromes are determined by specific mutations, together with, as yet unknown, modifier genes. Some, for example *ryr* mutations with multicore formation, may be associated with cardiomyopathy.

12.5 **The motor unit**

Main paper: Edström L, Kugelberg E. Histochemical composition, distribution of muscle fibres and fatiguability of single motor units. *J Neurol Neurosurg Psychiatry* 1968; 31424–33.

Background

In the 1960s, there was an anatomical problem that delayed understanding of muscle pathology in denervating disorders that stemmed from the motor unit construct of German-born neurophysiologist, and later Danish citizen, Fritz Buchthal (1907–2003). Buchthal [47] initially considered motor units as discrete, closely related groups of muscle fibres, that he termed subunits, a concept that was derived from analysis of EMG recordings using conventional concentric needle electrodes, and also from special multi-electrode recordings. This suggestion was countered by Lars Edström and Erik Kugelberg (1913–1983) [48], working in Uppsala, Sweden, who demonstrated that the distribution of muscle fibres belonging to an individual unit in a muscle was quasi-random.

Necrosis and regeneration of single muscle fibres or of small clusters of muscle fibres in muscular dystrophies and inflammatory myopathies was already well-known from classical pathological studies [49, 50], but the process of remodelling of the motor unit in denervation/reinnervation was not understood at this time.

Methods and results

Edström and Kugelberg [48] stimulated single motor nerve fibres in the anterior roots of adult albino rats innervating the tibialis anterior muscle, using a tetanus of 10 Hz for 10 minutes. The relevant muscle was then removed for histological examination and sections were stained using the succinic dehydrogenase, esterase, phosphorylase, and glycogen methods. Cross-sectional analysis of the muscle showed that there were two principal fibre types, which at this time—before the current histochemical nomenclature was devised, as discussed by Engel [51], using the method of Padykula and Herman [38]—were termed A fibres (equivalent to white muscle) and B fibres (equivalent to red muscle). They recognized that some motor units, as determined by their study, consisted wholly of A fibres, and others wholly of B fibres. The distribution of fibres within an individual motor unit was shown best in the Periodic acid-Schiff diastase (PAS) glycogen preparations (Fig. 12.2).

These fibres were scattered, usually isolated, but sometimes two to four together and occasionally up to six in a straight or curved row (Fig. 12.1). The fibres were irregularly spaced with no signs of grouping. The density of fibres was somewhat greater in the centre of the unit than in the periphery. It was also noted that there was considerable overlap in the distribution of different motor units in any muscle, and that single motor units did not necessarily extend along the whole length of the muscle. The researchers also studied the

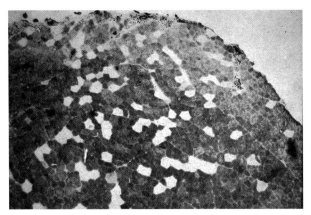

Fig. 12.2 Distribution of the muscle fibres belonging to a single motor unit in rat tibialis anterior muscle, as shown by Edstrom and Kugelberg, using the glycogen depletion technique [48].

Reproduced from *Journal of Neurology, Neurosurgery & Psychiatry*, 31, Edstrom L, Kugelberg E, Histochemical composition, distribution of muscle fibres and fatiguability of single motor units, p. 424–433, Copyright (1968), with permission from the BMJ Publishing Group Ltd.

twitch and fatigue characteristics of individual motor units, and showed that they corresponded to the expected type A or type B fibre properties.

Conclusions and critique

This work showed conclusively that the muscle fibres making up individual motor units in a healthy muscle were diffusely distributed in different areas of the muscle, and that individual motor units consisted of muscle fibres of identical histochemical and physiological type. They drew attention to observations in the earlier literature in neurogenic disorders, especially in motor neurone disease (amyotrophic lateral sclerosis). Slauck [52] had suggested, in 1921, that groups of atrophic fibres of different sizes in this disease represented individual denervated motor units, but Wohlfart [53] later pointed out that the number of fibres in an atrophic group was much smaller than the calculated number of fibres belonging to a motor unit, so that one motor unit probably corresponded to several atrophic groups. Wohlfart and Wohlfart showed that physiological overlapping of different motor units would explain this phenomenon [54]. Edstrom and Kugelberg refer to electrophysiological data concordant with this view in their paper.

This precise anatomical demonstration of the territory of the motor unit proved of fundamental importance in the interpretation of muscle pathology in neurogenic disorders, since it led to the concepts of grouped atrophy and of fibre type grouping as features of denervation and of reinnervation, respectively. Further, these concepts led to the development of quantitative aspects of motor unit physiology in clinical electromyography essential to diagnostic evaluation of EMG recordings [55]. These ideas were consonant with the supravital methylene blue studies of Coers and Woolf [56], showing axonal sprouting at the terminal axon branches and at the motor end plates themselves in denervating disorders. Ultrastructural studies further defined these changes, and were accompanied by studies of the distribution of acetylcholine receptors at the motor endplates and in the extrajunctional regions after muscle fibre denervation, leading to understanding of the trophic response to denervation in determining the arrival of regenerating sprouts of motor axons into the endplate region. After this work, muscle pathology was assessable in terms of a known normal motor unit anatomy.

12.6 **Fibre type definition and nomenclature**

Main paper: Engel WK. Fibre-type nomenclature of human skeletal muscle for histochemical purposes. *Neurology* 1974; 24:344–8.

Background

In the late 1960s, enzyme histochemical methods in histology were beginning to be developed to visualize enzymatic activity in biological tissues. These methods proved especially interesting in studies of striated muscle. It was already known that there were two types of muscle fibres, particularly well recognized in the white and red muscle tissues of birds and certain invertebrates, and that there were both fast contracting and slow contracting muscle fibres in human skeletal muscle tissue [57]. Indeed, the slower contraction properties of red muscle had earlier been observed by the French anatomist, Louis-Antoine Ranvier (1835–1922), and it was understood that slowly contracting muscle fibres contained more lipid droplets than fast contracting fibres [58].

King Engel's report [51] represented a coherent, well-argued statement concerning the classification of muscle fibres in histological preparations, using the frozen section technique that had, by then, replaced the time-honoured, formalin-fixed and paraffin-embedded methodology for processing muscle biopsy specimens (Fig. 12.3). These methods had been developed during the preceding decade in King Engel's Bethesda laboratory, at first in conjunction with G. Milton Shy, and then with a series of enthusiastic collaborators. Others also contributed, especially Victor Dubowitz in Sheffield (then London), Michel Fardeau in Paris, and Lars Edström and colleagues in Uppsala, Sweden. Key to this endeavour was the method of Padykula and Herman for demonstrating adenosine triphosphatase in skeletal muscle [38].

Conclusions and critique

The report received the imprimatur of the World Federation of Neurology's Research Group on Neuromuscular Disorders and, therefore, established a sequence of data that set

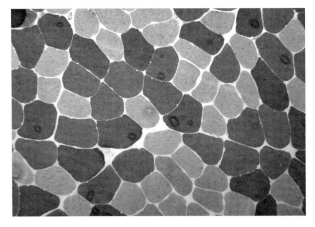

Fig. 12.3 The normal fibre type mosaic seen in an ATPase preparation preincubated at pH9.4; type 1 and type 2 fibres.

the scene for subsequent studies in muscle pathology laboratories across the world. King Engel has been known throughout his career for his intuitive insights and this review of 1974 illustrates his wide-ranging pattern of thought. He states that

> ... for several years we have been using a two-fiber-type nomenclature for human skeletal muscle, 'type I' and 'type II' fibers, based on fiber identification with the myofibrillar adenosine triphosphatase reaction at pH9.4

thus indicating the fundamental importance of Padykula and Herman's contribution from 1955 [38].

He recognized, however, that this two-fibre type system had been criticized on the grounds that fibre type might be mutable under certain conditions (for example, change in innervation or with physical training) or that it might, in fact, oversimplify the variety of fibre types found in muscle. He quoted Burke as suggesting two subtypes of fast contracting type II fibres [59]. He also drew attention to the value of this system of fibre typing in recognizing pathological change in muscle biopsies in various disorders. Brooke and Engel had described these changes in a seminal series of papers published in 1969, in which they considered myopathology of upper and lower motor neuron disorders, in children and adults, and in myotonias and myasthenia gravis [59–62]. This series of papers was especially important since it introduced measurement of fibre size, with statistical analysis of the frequency distribution of the various fibre types, into muscle biopsy pathology.

Although the two-fibre type classification was then thought to be probably unduly simple, it has stood the test of time with the modification that three subsets of type II fibres—type 2A, type 2B, and type 2C—were recognized, following the description by Brooke and Kaiser [63], a year after this review of Engel's. Reversal of the staining characteristics in the ATPase reaction when preincubation was carried out at acid pH (pH4.35) was described by Engel in his review [64]. Engel discussed the utility of classification of fibre types on the basis of ATPase reactivity versus other enzymatic reactions, such as the NADH reductase reaction (then termed the DPN reaction) or the phosphorylase reaction, and noted the stability of the ATPase reaction. The issue of the influence of innervation on muscle fibre typing was addressed, subsequently, by several investigators, using cross-innervation studies, which demonstrated its dependence on the innervation rather than on an intrinsic property of the muscle fibres themselves [65, 66]. The muscle fibre type histological properties with various enzyme reactions were tabulated in the review, a table that has been utilized by every investigator and pathologist in the field (Table 12.3).

The enzymatic characteristics of these fibre types were subsequently correlated with their physiological characteristics. In this correlation, Type 1 fibres are described as 'slow-twitch; oxidative' and slow contracting; Type 2A fibres as 'fast-twitch; oxidative-glycolytic' and fast contracting, fatigue resistant; and Type 2B fibres as 'fast-twitch; glycolytic' and fast contracting, fast fatiguing [59].

Table 12.3 Histochemical classification of muscle fibre types, modified to reflect usual practice at the time of their description in 1969 [58–63]

Reaction	Type I	Type II
DPN dehydrogenase	high	low
TPN dehydrogenase	high	low
Succinate dehydrogenase	high	low
Cytochrome oxidase	high	low
Phosphorylase	low	high
Glycogen	low	high
ATPase pH9.4	low	high
ATPase pH 4.35	high	low
Oil red O	high	low

Reproduced from *Science*, 174(4010), Burke RE, Levine DN, Zajac FE, et al., Mammalian motor units: pathological-histochemical correlation in three type of cat gastrocnemius muscle, p. 709–712, Copyright (1971), with permission from the American Society for Clinical Investigation.

The distribution of fibre types in different human muscles was studied in detail by investigators in Newcastle, England, providing the basis for statistical analysis of pathological change in biopsies from different sites [67], although there are variations in different portions of a single muscle.

12.7 **Inflammatory muscle disease**

Main paper: Pearson CM, Bohan A. The spectrum of polymyositis and dermatomyositis. *Med Clin North Am* 1977; 61:439–57.

Background

The early history of the origin of the concept of polymyositis and its overlap with dermatomyositis [68] illustrates the difficulty in deciding whether there were major differences between the two syndromes that continued for 100 years following the original description of polymyositis by Ernst Wagner (1829–1888) in Germany [69].

Methods and results

Walton and Adams had recognized four clinical groups of patients with inflammatory muscle disease. In the first group, disease was limited to muscles, without evidence of involvement of other tissues, although cases of childhood or adult onset were recognized in this group. In the second group, there were minor associated features of skin involvement or of 'collagen disease'. In the third group, muscle involvement was relatively slight, occurring in the context of severe collagen-vascular disease, and, in the fourth group, there was an association of dermatomyositis with cancer [70]. Pearson and Bohan [71], working in Boston, Massachussetts, developed five major criteria for diagnosis of polymyositis/dermatomyositis (PM/DM):

1 Symmetrical proximal weakness progressing over weeks or months

2 Muscle biopsy showing necrosis and regeneration of muscle fibres with inflammatory cell exudates

3 Raised serum skeletal muscle enzyme levels

4 Characteristic EMG findings

5 Typical cutaneous rash of dermatomyositis.

Conclusions and critique

These simple criteria acknowledged the overlapping relationship of the syndromic variability presented by inflammatory myopathy. They provided a framework for later studies of the immunological and pathological features of this group of disorders. An important distinction was drawn by Banker and Victor at this time, working at Case-Western Reserve University in Cleveland, Ohio, who reported that DM of childhood, a disorder with a high mortality even with steroid therapy, was associated with a capillary angiopathy at the edges of muscle fascicles [72]. This feature differed from the myopathology associated with PM in adults, but was later found to be similar to the muscle biopsy features of acute DM in adults. However, muscle biopsy is a selective procedure, and there was evidence of overlap of the DM and PM syndromes in adults.

There was also controversy concerning the reported association of inflammatory muscle disease with cancer, except perhaps for DM in adults [73]. A classification of this group of disorders, now generally termed simply 'inflammatory myopathies', has subsequently arisen that largely reconciles these views:

1 Idiopathic inflammatory myopathy

2 Secondary inflammatory myopathy occurring in association with other systemic or connective tissue disorders, or with bacterial, viral, or parasitic infections

3 Infantile, childhood, or congenital forms

4 Miscellaneous forms.

Idiopathic inflammatory myopathy is considered to include the distinct subsets of PM, DM, and inclusion body myositis (IBM). PM has an autoimmune pathogenesis, as shown by its association with other autoimmune disorders and evidence for T-cell mediated damage to muscle fibres. In DM, the disorder is due to complement-mediated microangiopathy [72, 73]. The more recently described entity of IBM, also generally considered a form of inflammatory muscle disease, but of late onset and with a distal upper limb predilection, differs in that there are 'degenerative features' in affected muscle fibres and the inflammatory response is relatively sparse [74].

In DM, a cascade of immunopathic processes is unleashed following complement activation on vascular endothelial cells with release of cytokines and chemokines that are active against muscle cell membranes, specifically against molecules that serve as ligands for integrins; cell adhesion molecules such as VCAM and ICAM. In PM, CD8+ cells invade major histocompatibility complex (MHC) class-1 expressing muscle fibre, and a similar process appears to occur in IBM, although the latter disorder fails to respond, even to intensive immunosuppressive therapy. Clearly, there is much yet to be learned about these clinical syndromes [75].

12.8 **Duchenne muscular dystrophy—a mystery understood at last**

Main paper: Hoffman EP, Brown RH, Kunkel LM. Dystrophin: the protein product of the Duchenne muscular dystrophy locus. *Cell* 1987; 51:919–28.

Background

Duchenne muscular dystrophy (DMD) is the exemplar of the muscular dystrophies—genetically determined degenerations of skeletal muscle usually associated with muscle fibre necrosis and secondary interstitial fibrosis. The history of ideas regarding the fundamental defects in this group of disorders, which includes those disorders reclassified by Walton and Nattrass [6] in 1954, is complex and involves almost every possible mechanism, including myopathic, neurogenic, and vascular causations. These have been reviewed in detail by Emery and Emery [7].

The description of focal plasma membrane (sarcolemmal) defects in both non-necrotic and necrotic muscle fibres in DMD, accompanied by delta-shaped areas of myofibrillar rarefaction underlying these deficits, shown in electron microscopic preparations by Mokri and Andrew Engel, in 1975, at the Mayo Clinic [76], initially failed to convince the scientific community of the fundamental importance of the observation, even though the authors showed that peroxidase penetrated into the interior of the muscle fibre in these delta lesions. Up to that time, research had been dominated by earlier concepts, including a neurogenic hypothesis, but this new suggestion of a primary cell membrane defect opened an avenue that eventually led to the discovery of the membrane structural protein dystrophin and related cell structural proteins.

A controversy ensued as to the significance of hypercontracted fibres and hyaline fibres in DMD muscle biopsies, settled by Andrew Engel and collaborators as a feature of the membrane leakiness they had described [77]. Allen Roses and colleagues, at Duke University, went further and showed abnormalities in other cell membranes, for example erythrocytes, in DMD [78].

The Duchenne gene was localized to the Xp15 region (on the short arm of the X chromosome) by linkage to various associated disorders, including the allelic disorder, Becker muscle dystrophy, although the latter disorder had erroneously been linked to colour blindness and, therefore, to a putative locus on the long arm of the X chromosome. Linkage to chronic granulomatous disease and to the Kell blood group proved relevant [79], and genetic marker studies gradually localized, more precisely, the relevant DNA sequences using restriction fragment length polymorphisms (RFLPs) and complementary DNAs (cDNAs), leading to detection of deletions in the gene itself in patients with DMD [80–82]. This achievement represented the culmination of the work of many investigators across the world and was dependent on the rapidly evolving technology of DNA analysis.

Methods and results

Kunkel's group used polyclonal antibodies against fusion proteins derived from cDNAs using bacteria as a substrate to identify the protein product of the Duchenne locus. Following established naming terminology, they called this protein dystrophin—which was, of course, the protein product of this gene in normal boys, whereas in DMD patients, the protein product was itself absent or grossly abnormal. The dystrophin molecule was shown to be a large rod-shaped protein consisting of 3685 amino acids [83]. It constitutes only 0.002% of muscle protein, yet is fundamentally important for muscle fibre function because of its biological role in the maintenance of cell membrane structure. This triumph of molecular biology represented the first successful discovery of a functional biological protein disorder in a disease, without prior knowledge as to the basic cause of the disease. Dystrophin was shown to be an essential component of the muscle fibre plasmalemma, consisting of a costameric protein that formed a lattice in the membrane.

In the muscular dystrophy eponymously attributed to German physician, Peter Emil Becker (1908–2000), dystrophin was present in reduced quantity and abnormal morphology associated with a deletion, especially in the rod domain. In DMD itself, dystrophin was present at levels generally less than 10% of normal, and often less than 5%. Frequently, the C-terminal domain was affected by deletions [84]. Mutations that disrupted the reading frame of the normal DNA nucleotide triplets were more likely to result in DMD, and in-frame deletions were more likely to cause Becker dystrophy [85]. The relation of dystrophin to the muscle fibre membrane was elucidated by Campbell and Kahl [86] who reported that dystrophin was closely associated with a glycoprotein in the membrane, forming a dystrophin-associated glycoprotein complex, an observation that subsequently proved important in understanding the LGMDs. Dystrophin was, therefore, not directly attached to the sarcolemma, but formed an attachment with glycoproteins in the membrane, which were themselves related to the extracellular matrix. This concept led to the elucidation of the molecular defects underlying a number of additional myopathic disorders associated with specific defects in one or other of these glycoproteins, thus revealing a generic membrane defect causation for many of these disorders [87].

Conclusions and critique

It is interesting to note, however, that the question as to the progressive nature of the muscular disorder in DMD is not necessarily revealed by these studies. However, recurrent focal muscle cell damage associated with the membrane defect, leading to segmental muscle cell necrosis associated with calcium influx, results in progressive loss of contractile function, progressive increase in interstitial fibrosis with stiffening and increased viscosity of the muscle tissue, and, therefore clinical progression. The rate of progression of muscle damage in DMD can be slowed by low-dose steroid therapy, presumably as a result of a non-specific stabilization of the muscle fibre membrane or perhaps a reduction in the associated necrosis-induced inflammatory response [88].

These studies of the molecular genetic basis of DMD and its associated disorders have made it possible to offer definite testing for genetic risk in women in families affected by DMD, with accuracy both in predicting the risk of carrier status and, equally importantly, for excluding such risk, thus obviating the uncertainty associated with the older methods that were dependent on CK determinations and muscle biopsy. There remains a need to search for point deletions, but even this initially difficult task can now be automated. The discovery of the link between the dystrophin gene in the muscle fibre membrane and membrane-associated glycoproteins, in particular, provided an explanation and a research tool for elucidating the causative defects underlying a number of hitherto poorly defined clinical myopathies of limb-girdle type (LGMD) as recognized by Walton and Nattrass more than 50 years ago.

12.9 **Myotonic and ion channel syndromes**

Main paper: Brook JD, McCurrah ME, Harley HG, et al. Molecular basis of myotonic dystrophy: expansion of a trinucleotide (CTG) repeat at the 3^l end of a transcript encoding a protein kinase family member. *Cell* 1992; 68:799–808.

Related paper: Fu YH, Pizzuti A, Fewick RG, et al. An unstable triplet repeat in a gene related to myotonic muscular dystrophy. *Science* 1992; **255**:1256–8.

Background

Myotonic dystrophy is a unique clinical syndrome [89] that varies in severity from case to case. In many cases, the diagnosis is not suspected until a complicating cardiac conduction abnormality, or respiratory disorder linked to infection, draws attention to frontal baldness and distal weakness, with very mild facial weakness, cataract, and a history of gastrointestinal (GI) disturbance, associated with myotonia exacerbated by cold. Infants of only mildly and perhaps undiagnosed myotonic mothers are often severely affected by a floppy infant syndrome, with mental retardation [90]. The diagnosis is, therefore, at first often missed. Characteristic abnormalities in intrafusal muscle fibres in muscle spindles have been described, but remain poorly understood [91].

Methods and results

These two papers [92, 93] appeared simultaneously from two different laboratories. Both identified a trinucleotide (CTG) repeat sequence associated with the condition. Myotonic dystrophy type 1 (DM1) disease tends to occur earlier in successive generations in affected families—the phenomenon of genetic anticipation. This genetic instability is characteristic of DNA repeat syndromes. As in other trinucleotide repeat syndromes, the repeats occur in so-called simple sequence repeats in the genome; in DM1, this DNA repeat is on chromosome 19. Curiously, much of the expansion in this region of the gene seems to occur in postnatal life. In DM1, the myotonia itself probably principally results from alternative splicing of the muscle-specific chloride channel, leading to reduced chloride conductance across the muscle fibre membrane—a channelopathy. The phenotype of DM1 is likely to be due mainly to alternative splicing of RNA (ribonucleic acid), itself secondary to the underlying CTG DNA repeat [94]. A similar molecular abnormality leads to insulin resistance in the disease.

Conclusions and critique

The discovery of the genetic basis of DM1 led to major advances in comprehending the relation between genetic disorder and clinical manifestations of the disease that have proven applicable to other genetic disorders. Indeed, the similarity of the clinical features of classical DM1 to proximal myotonic myopathy (PROMM)—termed DM2—associated with an untranslated CCTG expansion on chromosome 3, has suggested a similar biochemical mechanism involving a disturbance in RNA metabolism. In DM2, there is a similar instability in the number of DNA repeats, accounting for different phenotypes in different individuals.

Although treatment with acetazolamide may improve myotonia in the disease, this is not the source of the major deficits, which are due to muscle weakness (causing ventilatory disorder), limb and trunk weakness, and central nervous system (CNS) abnormalities (leading to sleep apnoea). These cannot, thus far, be modified by medical intervention.

Ion channel disorders have been found to cause other forms of myotonia—the non-dystrophic myotonias. In these disorders, myotonia results from mutations in sodium or chloride channels in the muscle fibre membrane that disrupt the orderly opening and closing sequence of these channels during their excitation, initiated in response to propagation of the action potential along the muscle fibre membrane and through the T-tubular system, following neural excitation by acetyl choline. Several different patterns of clinical abnormality have been recognized by their clinical features, by EMG analysis [95], and by molecular studies—in particular, cold-induced myotonia, myotonia induced by exercise (paramyotonia) or relieved by exercise (myotonia congenital), familial hypokalaemic or hyperkalaemic periodic paralysis, and thyrotoxic periodic paralysis. Specific genetic tests are available for these disorders, reflecting developing knowledge of the proteins involved, at channel level, in causing the functional disorders characteristic of these syndromes [96, 97].

The discovery of expansion of a CTG trinucelotide repeat sequence in the non-coding region of the DMPK gene in DM1 opened a door to the concept that other genetic disorders, involving the CNS, might result from a similar abnormality. Thus, the molecular basis of Huntington's disease, the spinocerebellar atrophies, and other disorders began to be understood. Most of these disorders show proteinaceous inclusions in the nuclei or cytoplasm of affected cells.

12.10 **Limb-girdle muscular dystrophies—dystroglycanopathies**

Main paper: Muntoni F, Brockington M, Blake DJ, Torelli S, Brown SC. Defective glycosylation in muscular dystrophy. *Lancet* 2002; 360:1419–21.

Background

The limb-girdle muscular dystrophies (LGMD), as tentatively classified by Walton and Nattrass [6], remained ill-defined until relatively recently. Although clearly not a single nosological entity but, rather, a group of related but discrete disorders characterized by progressive proximal lower and upper limb weakness, with subtly different phenotypes, different rates of progression, cardiomyopathy in some cases, and either autosomal recessive or autosomal dominant patterns of inheritance, these disorders remained a challenge. In a few families, the disorder seemed to follow a pattern of sporadic occurrence and, in others, a pattern of X-linked recessive inheritance. Some were of late onset, but most seemed to develop in childhood or adolescence.

Methods and results

Muntoni et al. [98] noted an evolving discovery of genes encoding sarcolemmal, extracellular matrix, sarcomeric, and nuclear envelope proteins. They emphasized the importance of defective assembly of these related proteins associated with mutations encoding for putative glycosyltransferases, leading to aberrant glycosylation of α-dystroglycan, an external membrane protein expressed in muscle, brain, and other tissues. This defective glycosylation results in loss of interactions with extracellular matrix partner proteins causing myopathy—LGMD syndromes (Fig. 12.4). This new understanding of the link between dystrophin and other membrane-associated glycoproteins injected fresh impetus into research in this group of disorders, and the new information concerning them led to consolidation of a classification of these LGMDs that had been set out in a consensus conference held in 1995 [99]. This conference determined classification of this group of disorders based not on clinical appearances but on their underlying genetic disorders. From this classification, it became possible to study phenotypic variation and to assess prognostic variables.

   The conference delegates (from Europe, Brazil, Tunisia, and the USA) reviewed published work reporting LGMD syndromes, noting certain clinical pointers to diagnosis within the classification that could be used to direct molecular studies, leading to precise diagnosis. At the time, the conferees were concerned by the heterogeneity of the LGMD syndromes. They noted the range of mutations that could occur in a single gene in different families, and the likelihood that a separate, unlinked 'modifier gene' might determine the phenotype by modifying the expression of the disordered gene. A classification, based on the data reported, described one form of autosomal dominant LGMD and five autosomal recessive syndromes, using the nomenclature 'LGMD1' to describe the autosomal dominant disorder and 'LGMD2A' etc. to describe the autosomal recessive syndromes. DMD was recognized as an X-linked disorder. At the time of this conference, no definite diagnosis

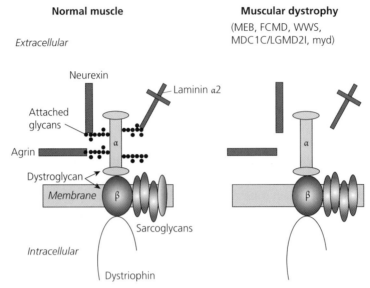

Fig. 12.4 Dystrophin-glycoprotein complex in muscular dystrophies [98].

In normal muscle, glycans attached to α-dystroglycan link the dystrophin-glycoprotein complex to extracellular proteins, including agrin and laminin, across the cell membrane and basal lamina. Loss of glycosylation of α-dystroglycan in muscular dystrophies disrupts the link to these extracellular proteins.

(MEB: muscle-eye-brain disease; FCMD: Fukuyama congenital muscular dystrophy; WWS: Walker-Warburg syndrome; MDC1C/LGMD2I: variants of Fukutin-related LGMD; Myd: myodystrophy mouse)

Reproduced from *Lancet*, 360, Muntoni F, Brockington M, Blake DJ, et al., Defective glycosylation in muscular dystrophy, p. 1419–1421, Copyright (2002), with permission from Elsevier.

could be offered in counselling a family with a sporadic case of LGMD. However, the majority of cases are inherited as autosomal recessive disorders.

As genetic studies matured and became more generally available, further syndromes were identified, and by 2007 [100], three autosomal dominant syndromes (LMGD1A–1C) and eight autosomal recessive syndromes (LGMD2A–2K) were recognized, in all of which the molecular basis was described. The genes involved were genes for myotilin, lamina/C (a nuclear envelope protein), caveolin 3 (a plasma membrane gene), calpain 3, dysferlin (a plasma membrane repair protein), four separate sarcoglycans (localized as part of the dystrophin glycoprotein complex), telethonin (localized in the sarcomeres), TRIM 32 (a ubiquitin ligase), FKRP (fukutin: a substrate of alpha dystroglycan), titin (a component of the sarcomere), and POMT (a glycosyl transferase). Clinical manifestations ranged from distal presentation (LGMD1A), focal muscle involvement LGMD2B), cardiomyopathy (LGMD1A, 1B, 2C–F, and 2I), respiratory failure, muscle hypertrophy resembling Becker dystrophy or DMD (LGMD2I), and mental retardation with microcephaly (LGMD2K).

Many of these disorders were first reported in restricted, inbred populations, for example in Tunisia [101] or on the island of Réunion [102]. Myopathies with mutations in the fukutin gene are particularly interesting in that the disorder, causing a severe and progressive congenital myopathic syndrome, appears relatively common in Japan, and has been reported in European populations as a milder allelic variant to LGMD2I [103].

Conclusions and critique

A suggested plan for assessment clinically, and then by muscle biopsy, was set out in the later consensus document [100]. Most of these disorders present in childhood, but milder forms may present later in life. Various diagrammatic depictions of the relationships of the various proteins involved in these syndromes have been prepared (see Fig. 12.2), which illustrate their integral relationship to the sarcolemma and to structural proteins within the cell (the so-called cytoskeletal proteins). These proteins, and proteins of the contractile apparatus making up myofilaments, are themselves involved in a number of other inherited myopathies. Although many of the publications concerning this group of LGMD syndromes hint at the possibility that knowledge of their molecular pathogenesis might lead to treatment by, for example, stem cell transfer, there are no suggestions so far of therapeutic success.

The development of ideas about this group of diseases, still difficult to manage, illustrates the slow progress from initially incomplete clinical descriptions that often led to controversy, especially regarding the specificity and limits of the disorder described. Progress depended on the application of new ideas derived from novel techniques of investigation. In most disorders, the first such methodology was pathology (Fig. 12.5), a discipline that has itself evolved beyond recognition over the last 150 years. Paraffin-embedding methods have given way to celloidin embedding and, latterly, to the use of thin frozen sections. The

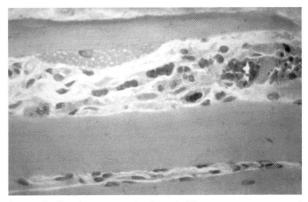

Fig. 12.5 A necrotic muscle fibre in a myopathy. Muscle fibre remnants are seen in the centre of the fibre space, associated with a macrophage response, and an active satellite cell, with foamy cytoplasm, at the periphery initiating the regenerative response. This process is often focal and segmental, not involving the muscle fibre throughout its length.

latter technique opened up the new field of enzyme histochemistry, and of immunological methods, allowing demonstration of cell metabolites and specific proteins. Electron microscopy, initially an important technique in the period 1950–1970, has assumed less relevance since the advent of innovative methods in light microscopy.

Electrophysiological techniques continue to have a role in clinical investigation and also in research into specific problems in muscle and CNS disorders (such as ALS and SMA). Muscle imaging, by magnetic resonance imaging (MRI) and, increasingly, by real-time ultrasound, has only recently found a routine role in the clinical investigation of muscle disorders. It provides a measure that can be used for comparison in follow-up studies. Clearly, there are areas where knowledge is incomplete, especially in applying information from genetic studies in inherited disorders to therapy, and also in understanding how to modify and even prevent immunologically mediated disease. Muscle disorders are ideal in many respects for such research, given the ready availability of muscle tissue for biopsy studies.

Key unanswered questions

1 Why do muscle disorders usually predominantly affect proximal muscles, or show discrete patterns of muscle involvement?

2 What determines genotype–phenotype interactions in the hereditary myopathies?

3 Is there a practical technological solution to the problem of gene replacement therapy in Duchenne muscular dystrophy and related disorders?

4 Are there preferred points of progression in the different muscle diseases at which specific therapies ideally should be applied?

5 What triggers the onset of autoimmune inflammatory myopathy?

References

1 Swash M, Schwartz MS. *Neuromuscular Diseases—A Practical Approach to Diagnosis and Management*, 3rd ed. London: Springer-Verlag; 1997; 1–541.

2 Kinnier Wilson SA. *Neurology*, 2nd ed. London: Butterworth; 1954; 1105–34 and 1168–83.

3 Gowers WR. *Manual of Diseases of the Nervous System*. 2nd ed. London: J&A Churchill; 1899 Vol 1. 1–616; Vol 2. 1–1068.

4 Erb WH. *Handbuch der Krankheiten des Nervensystems (2 volumes)*. Leipzig: FCW Vogel; 1876–8.

5 Oppenheim H. *Lehrbuch der Nervenkrankheiten*. Berlin: S Karger; 1894.

6 Walton JN, Nattrass FJ. On the classification, natural history and treatment of the myopathies. *Brain* 1954; **77**:169–231.

7 Emery AEH, Emery MLH. *The History of a Genetic Disease: Duchenne Muscular Dystrophy or Meryon's Disease*. London: Royal Society of Medicine Press; 1995; 9–24.

8 Bell C. *The Nervous System of the Human Body*. London: Longman; 1830.

9 Duchenne GBA. Recherches sur la paralysie musculaire pseudo-hypertrophique ou paralysie myo-sclérosique. *Arch Gen de Méd* 1868; 11:5–25, 179–209, 305–21, 421–43, 552–88.

10 Erb WH. Über die 'juvenile form' der progressiven muskelatrophie und ihre beziehungen zur sogenannten pseudohypertrophie der muskeln. *Dtsch Arch Klin Med Leipzig* 1884; **34**:467–519.

11 McArdle B. Myopathy due to a defect in muscle glycogen breakdown. *Clin Sci Mol Med* 1951; **10**:13–33.

12 Di Mauro S, Tonin P, Servidei S. Metabolic myopathies. In: Rowland LP, Di Mauro S (eds). *Handbook of Clinical Neurology*. Amsterdam: Elsevier; 1992; **62**:479–526.

13 Olson W, Engel WK, Walsh GO, et al. Oculocraniosomatic neuromuscular disease with 'ragged red fibres'. Histochemical and ultrastructural changes in limb muscles of a group of patients with idiopathic progressive ophthalmoplegia. Arch *Neurol* 1972; **26**:193–211.

14 Denborough MA, Lovell RRH. Anaesthetic deaths in a family. *Lancet* 1960; **2**:45.

15 Tsujino S, Shanske S, Di Mauro S. Molecular genetic heterogeneity of myophosphorylase deficiency (McArdle's disease). *N Engl J Med* 1993; **329**:241–5.

16 Tonin P, Lewis P, Servidei S, et al. Metabolic causes of myoglobinuria. *Ann Neurol* 1990; **27**:181–5.

17 Hutchinson J. On ophthalmoplegia externa or asymmetrical immobility (partial) of the eyes (with ptosis). *Med Chir Trans* 1899; **62**:307–29.

18 Gowers WR. Clinical lectures on pseudo-hypertrophic muscular paralysis. *Lancet* 1879; **2**:1–2, 37–9, 73–5, 113–6.

19 von Leyden E. *Hereditare Formen der Progressiven Muskelatrophie; die Lipomatose Muskelatrophie. Klinik der Ruckenmarkskrankheiten. Vol 2*. Berlin: A Hirschwald; 1876; 525–40.

20 Moebius PJ. Ueber die hereditaren Nervenkrankheiten ll. Die hereditare oder degenerative Muskelatrophie. Sammlung Lin VOrtrage in verbindung mit Deutschen Kinikern, herausgegeben von Richard Volkmann (Leipzig). *Innere Medicin* 1879; No 57:1510–31.

21 Landouzy L, Dejerine J. De la myopathie atrophique progressive Myopathie sans neuropathie debutant ordinaire dans l'enfance, par la face. *Rev Med* 1885; **5**:81–117.

22 Gowers WR. A lecture on myopathy and a distal form. *BMJ* 1902; **2**:89–92.

23 Nevin S. Two cases of muscular degeneration occurring in late adult life with a review of the recorded cases of late progressive muscular dystrophy (late progressive myopathy). *Quart J Med* 1936; **5**:51–68.

24 Barnes S. Myopathic family, with hypertrophic, pseudohypertrophic, atrophic and terminal (distal in upper extremities) stages. *Brain* 1932; **5**:1–46.

25 **Thomsen J.** Tonische krampfe in willkurlich beweglichen muskeln in folge von ererbter psychischer disposition. *Arch Psychiatr Nervenkr* 1876; **6**:702.

26 **Eulenberg A.** Ueber eine familiar durch 6 generationen verfolgbare form congenitaler paramyotonie. *Neurol Centralbl* 1886; **55**:265–72.

27 **Steinert H.** Über das klinische und anatomische bild des muskelschwunds der myotoniker. *Dtsch Z Nervenheilkd* 1909; **37**:58–104.

28 **Batten FE, Gibb HP.** Myotonia atrophica. *Brain* 1909; **32**:187–205.

29 **Aldren Turner JW.** The relationship between amyotonia congenita and congenital myopathy. *Brain* 1940; **63**:163–77.

30 **Walton JN.** Amyotonia congenita: a follow-up study. *Lancet* 1956; **267**:1023–8.

31 **Bramwell E.** Observations on myopathy. *Proc Roy Soc Med* 1922; **16**:1–12.

32 **Denny-Brown D.** Myopathic weakness of quadriceps. *Proc Roy Soc Med* 1939; **32**:867–9.

33 **Swash M, Heathfield KWG.** Quadriceps myopathy; a variant of limb-girdle dystrophy syndrome. *J Neurol Neurosurg Psychiatry* 1983; **46**:355–7.

34 **Acheson D, McAlpine D.** Muscular dystrophy associated with paroxysmal myoglobinuria and excessive excretion of ketosteroids. *Lancet* 1953; **262**:372–5.

35 **Bell J.** Dystrophia myotonica and allied diseases. In Penrose LS (Ed) The Treasury of Human Inheritance. *Nervous diseases and muscular dystrophies*. London. Cambridge University Press. 1947; **4**:343–410.

36 **Tyler FH, Wintrobe MM.** Studies in disorders of muscle: 1. The problem of progressive muscular dystrophy. *Ann Intern Med* 1950; **32**:72–9.

37 **Stevenson AC.** Muscular dystrophy in Northern Ireland: 1. An account of the condition in 51 families. *Ann Eugenics* 1953; **18**:50–91.

38 **Padykula HA, Herman E.** The specificity of the histochemical method for adenosine triphosphatase. *J Histochem Cytochem* 1955; **3**:170–95.

39 **Shy GM, Engel WK, Somers JF, Wanko T.** Nemaline myopathy: a new congenital myopathy. *Brain* 1963; **86**:793–810.

40 **Engel WK, Wanko T, Fenichel GM.** Nemaline myopathy: second case. *Arch Neurol* 1964; **11**:22–39.

41 **Spiro AJ, Kennedy C.** Hereditary occurrence of nemaline myopathy. *Arch Neurol* 1965; **13**:155–9.

42 **Gonatas NK, Shy GM, Godfrey EH.** Nemaline myopathy; the origin of nemaline structures. *New Engl J Med* 1966; **274**:535–9.

43 **Huxley HF.** Electron microscope studies on structure of natural and synthetic protein filaments from striated muscle. *J Molec Biol* 1963; **7**:281–308.

44 **Goebel HH, Blaschek A.** Protein aggregation in congenital myopathies. *Semin Pediatr Neurol* 2011; **18**:272–6.

45 **Dubowitz V.** *Muscle Disorders in Childhood*, 2nd ed. London: WB Saunders; 1995; 1–540.

46 **Brooke MH.** *A Clinician's View of Neuromuscular Diseases*. Baltimore: Williams and Wilkins; 1977.

47 **Buchthal F, Guld C, Rosenfalck F.** Multi-electrode study of the territory of a motor unit. *Acta Physiol Scandinavica* 1957; **39**:83–104.

48 **Edstrom L, Kugelberg E.** Histochemical composition, distribution of muscle fibres and fatiguability of single motor units. *J Neurol Neurosurg Psychiatry* 1968; **31**:424–33.

49 **Greenfield JG, Shy GM, Alvord EC, Berg L.** *An Atlas of Muscle Pathology in Neuromuscular Disease*. Edinburgh: E & S Livingstone; 1957; 1–104.

50 **Walton JN.** *Polymyositis*. Edinburgh: E & S Livingstone; 1958; 1–270.

51 **Engel WK.** Fibre-type nomenclature of human skeletal muscle for histochemical purposes. *Neurology* 1974; **24**:344–8.

52 Slauck A. *Beitrage fur kenntniss der muskelpathologie. Ztschr ges Neurol Psychat* 1921; **71**:352–6.

53 Wohlfart G. Muscular atrophy in diseases of the lower motor neuron. Contribution to the anatomy of the motor units. *Arch Neurol Psychiat* 1949; **61**:599–620.

54 Wohlfart S, Wohlfart G. Mikroskopische untersuchungen und progressive muskelatrophien. *Acta Med Scand* 1935; 1–137.

55 Stalberg E, Schwartz MS, Thiele B, Schiller HH. The normal motor unit in man—single fibre multielectrode investigation. *J Neurol Sci* 1976; **27**:291–301.

56 Coers C, Woolf AL. *The Innervation of Muscle: A Biopsy Study*. Charles C Thomas; 1959; 1–149.

57 Creed RS, Denny-Brown D, Eccles JC, Liddell EGT, Sherrington CS. *Reflex Activity of the Spinal Cord*. Oxford: Clarendon Press; 1932; 37–60.

58 Burke RE, Levine DN, Zajac FE, et al. Mammalian motor units: pathological-histochemical correlation in three type of cat gastrocnemius muscle. *Science* 1971; **174**:709.

59 Brooke MH, Engel WK. The histographic analysis of human muscle biopsies with regard to fiber types. 1. Adult male and female. *Neurology* 1969; **19**:221–33.

60 Brooke MH, Engel WK. The histographic changes in fiber types in disease. 2. Diseases of upper and lower motor neuron. *Neurology* 1969; **19**:378.

61 Brooke MH, Engel WK. The histographic analysis of human muscle biopsies with regard to fiber types. 3. Myotonias, myasthenia gravis and hypokalemic paralysis. *Neurology* 1969; **19**:469.

62 Brooke MH, Engel WK. The histographic analysis of human biopsies with regard to fiber types. 4. Children's biopsies. *Neurology* 1969; **19**:591.

63 Brooke MH, Kaiser KK. Some comments on the histochemical characterization of muscle adenosine triphosphatase. *ArchNeurol* 1970; **23**:369.

64 Drews GA, Engel WK. Reversal of the ATPase reaction in muscle fibres by EDTA. *Nature* 1966; **212**:1551–1553.

65 Dubowitz V. Cross-innervated mammalian skeletal muscle: histochemical, physiological and biochemical observations. *J Physiol (London)* 1967; **193**:481.

66 Romanul FCA, van der Meulen JP. Slow and fast muscles after cross-innervation. *Arch Neurol* 1967; **17**:387–402.

67 Johnson MA, Polgar J, Weghtman D, Appleton D. Data on the distribution of fibre types in thirty-six human muscles. An autopsy study. *J Neurol Sci* 1973; **18**:111–29.

68 Brain WR, Henson RA. Neurological syndromes associated with cancer; the carcinomatous neuromyopathies. *Lancet* 1958; **ii**:971–4.

69 Wagner E. Fall einer seltnen muskelkrankheit. *Arch Heilk* 1863; **4**:282–3.

70 Walton JN, Adams RD. *Polymyositis*. Edinburgh: E & S Livingstone; 1958; 1–270.

71 Pearson CM, Bohan A. The spectrum of polymyositis and dermatomyositis. *Med Clin North Am* 1977; **61**:439–57.

72 Banker BQ, Victor M. Dermatomyositis (systemic angiopathy) of childhood. *Medicine (Baltimore)* 1966; **45**:189–261.

73 Callen JP. Malignancy in polymyositis/dermatomyositis. *Clin Dermatol* 1988; **2**:55–63.

74 Needham M, Mastaglia FL. Inclusion body myositis: current pathogenetic concepts and diagnostic and therapeutic approaches. *Lancet Neurol* 2007; **6**:620–31.

75 Dalakas MC, Karpati G. Inflammatory myopathies. In: Karpati G, Hilton-Jones D, Bushby K, Griggs RC (eds). *Disorders of Voluntary Muscle*, 8th ed. Cambridge: Cambridge University Press; 2010; (Chapter 22) 427–52.

76 Mokri B, Engel AG. Duchenne dystrophy: electron microscopic findings pointing to a basic or early abnormality in the plasma membrane of the muscle fiber. *Neurology* 1975; **25**:1111–20.

77 **Lotz BP, Engel AG.** Are hypercontracted muscle fibers artifacts and do they cause rupture of the plasma membrane?*Neurology* 1987; **37**:1466–75.

78 **Roses AD.** Erythrocytes in dystrophies. In: Rowland LP (ed). *Pathogenesis of Human Muscular Dystrophies*. Amsterdam: Excerpta Medica; 1977; 648–55.

79 **Swash M, Schwartz MS, Carter ND, Heath R, Leak M, Rogers KL.** Benign x-linked myopathy with acanthocytes (McLeod syndrome)—its relationship to x-linked muscular dystrophy. *Brain* 1983; **106**:717–36.

80 **Davies KE, Pearson PL, Harper PS, et al.** Linkage analysis of two cloned DNA sequences flanking the Duchenne muscular dystrophy locus on the short arm of the human X chromosome. *Nucleic Acids Research* 1983; **11**:2303–13.

81 **Monaco AP, Bertelson CJ, Middlesworth W, et al.** Detection of deletions spanning the Duchenne muscular dystrophy locus using a tightly linked DNA segment. *Nature* 1985; **316**:842–5.

82 **Koenig M, Hoffman EP, Bertelson CJ, Monaco RG, Ray C, Kunkel LM.** Complete cloning of the Duchenne muscular dystrophy (DMD) cDNA and preliminary genomic organization of the DMD gene in normal and affected individuals. *Cell* 1987; **50**:509–17.

83 **Hoffman EP, Brown RH, Kunkel LM.** Dystrophin: the protein product of the Duchenne muscular dystrophy locus. *Cell* 1987; **51**:919–28.

84 **Beggs AH, Kunkel LM.** Improved diagnosis of Duchenne/Becker muscular dystrophy. *J clin Invest* 1990; **85**:613–9.

85 **Monaco AP, Bertelson CJ, Liechti-Gallati S, Moser H, Kunkel LM.** An explanation for the phenotypic differences between patients bearing partial deletions of the DMD locus. *Genomics* 1988; **2**:90–5.

86 **Campbell KP, Kahn SD.** Association of dystrophin and an integral membrane glycoprotein. *Nature* 1989; **338**:259–62.

87 **Matsumara K, Campbell KP.** Dystrophin-glycoprotein complex; its role in the molecular pathogenesis of muscular dystrophies. *Muscle Nerve* 1994; **17**:2–15.

88 **Griggs RC, Moxley RT, Mendell JR, et al.** Duchenne dystrophy: randomized controlled trial of prednisone (18 months) and azathioprine (12 months). *Neurology* 1993; **43**:520–7.

89 **Brook JD, McCurrah ME, Harley HG, et al.** Molecular basis of myotonic dystrophy: expansion of a trinucleotide (CTG) repeat at the 3^l end of a transcript encoding a protein kinase family member. *Cell* 1992; **68**:799–808.

90 **Fu YH, Pizzuti A, Fewick RG, et al.** An unstable triplet repeat in a gene related to myotonic muscular dystrophy. *Science* 1992; **255**:1256–8.

91 **Batten F, Gibb H.** Myotonia atrophica. *Brain* 1909; **32**:187–202.

92 **Harper PS.** Congenital myotonic dystrophy in Britain: clinical aspects. *Arch Dis Child* 1975; **50**:505–13.

93 **Swash M.** The morphology and innervation of the muscle spindle in dystrophia myotonica. *Brain* 1972; **95**:357–68.

94 **Day J, Thornton CA.** Myotonic dystrophy. In: Karpati G, Hilton-Jones D, Bushby K, Griggs RC (eds). *Disorders of Voluntary Muscle*, 8th ed. Cambridge: Cambridge University Press; 2010; (Chapter 18) 347–62.

95 **Fournier E, Arzel M, Sternberg D, et al.** Electromyography guides toward subgroups of mutations in muscle channelopathies. *Ann Neurol* 2004; **56**:650–61.

96 **Hoffman EP, Lehmann-Horn PF, Rudel R.** Overexcited or inactive: ion channels in muscle disease. *Cell* 1995; **80**:681–6.

97 **Michel P, Sternberg PY, Jeannet PY, et al.** Comparative efficacy of repetitive nerve stimulation, exercise, and cold in differentiating myotonic disorders. *Muscle Nerve* 2007; **36**:643–50.

98 **Muntoni F, Brockington M, Blake DJ, Torelli S, Brown SC.** Defective glycosylation in muscular dystrophy. *Lancet* 2002; **360**:1419–21.

99 **Bushby KMD, Beckmann JS.** Report of the 30th and 31st ENMC sponsored international workshop—the limb-girdle muscular dystrophies, and proposal for a new classification. *Neuro Dis* 1995; **5**:337–44.

100 **Bushby K, Norwood F, Straub V.** The limb-girdle muscular dystrophies—diagnostic strategies. *Biochim Biophysic Acta* 2007; **1772**:238–42.

101 **Ben Othmane K, Ben Hamida M, Pericak-Vance MA, et al.** Linkage of Tunisian autosomal recessive muscular dystrophy to the pericentromeris region of chromosome 13q. *Nature Genet* 1992; **2**:315–7.

102 **Fardeau M, Hillaire D, Mignard C, et al.** Juvenile limb-girdle muscular dystrophy. Clinical, histopathological and genetic data on a small community living in the Réunion Island. *Brain* 1996; **119**:295–308.

103 **Brockington M, Yuva Y, Prandini P, et al.** Mutations in the fukutin-related protein gene (FKRP) identify limb-girdle muscular dystrophy 2I as a milder allelic variant of congenital muscular dystrophy: MDC1C. *Hum Mol Genet* 2001; **10**:2851–9.

Chapter 13

Peripheral neuropathy

David R. Cornblath and Richard A.C. Hughes

13.0 **Introduction**

Disorders of peripheral nerves are one of the most common neurological problems today. The number of people in the world with symptomatic diabetic polyneuropathy alone is over 40,000,000. In fact, most of the world's 350,000,000 people with diabetes will have neuropathy if tested in detail. In addition to diabetes, the overall number with neuropathy includes those with hereditary neuropathy (estimated as 1 in 2500 live births in the USA), toxic neuropathy (especially from chemotherapy and alcohol), carpal tunnel syndrome, inflammatory neuropathies, radiculopathies, and, increasingly, traumatic injuries. Neuropathic pain is a growing problem without a solution. Discoveries about fundamentals in peripheral neurobiology, especially concerning nerve repair and regeneration, lag in proportion to the number affected. In this Chapter, 10 landmark papers in peripheral nerve disorders have been selected to show where we have been and to raise a series of unanswered questions for the future. Many other papers could have been chosen as landmarks, some of which are referenced in the individual sections. Stimulating new ideas and directions should lead to new advances.

13.1 **Bell's palsy**

Main paper: Bell C. On the nerves; giving an account of some experiments on their structure and functions, which lead to a new arrangement of the system. *Phil Trans R Soc Lond* 1821; 111:398–424.

Background

Ancient Egyptian, Greek, Roman, and subsequent cultures all depicted facial palsy in statues and pictures. Even the Mona Lisa's asymmetrical smile may have been caused by facial palsy [1]. The first description of idiopathic facial palsy is probably that of Nicolaus A. Friedreich, Würzburg, Germany, in 1798, nearly a quarter of a century before Scottish anatomist, Charles Bell (1774–1842). German pathologist, Friedreich (1825–1882), described three patients with unilateral flaccid paralysis of the whole of one side of the face with no apparent cause and eventual recovery [2, 3]. Hearing and sensation were preserved. Friedreich contrasted his cases with facial paralysis occurring in stroke and suggested that the cause was rheumatic affection of the dural portion of the facial nerve triggered by having sat in a draught of cold air. He applied electrical treatment repeatedly and noted eventual recovery in all his cases. Bell may have known of Friedreich's paper because it was summarized in English, in 1800, in the *Annals of Medicine* in Edinburgh, where Bell had recently completed his training. Soon afterwards Bell, later Sir Charles, moved to London and took up the Chair of Anatomy and Surgery in the Royal College of Surgeons. In 1821, he gave his paper on the facial and other cranial nerves to the Royal Society [4] where he was introduced by its famous President and chemist, Sir Humphry Davy (1778–1829), discoverer of potassium, sodium, and calcium and inventor of the Davy safety lamp.

Methods

Bell expertly dissected and himself illustrated the nerves of the face and neck (Fig. 13.1). He used comparative anatomy of different species, operations on live animals, and clinical examples to deduce the functions of the nerves.

Results

Cutting the facial nerve of an ass caused no pain but produced facial paralysis. Cutting the maxillary nerve did cause pain and also difficulty feeding with the upper lip. He found the same in the dog and monkey and reported facial paralysis in a man whose facial nerve had been damaged by 'suppuration'. He removed a tumour from in front of the ear of a coachman, damaging the nerve to the corner of his mouth in doing so. The coachman was grateful for having the tumour removed but complained that he could not whistle for his dogs. On the other hand, dividing the supraorbital branch of the trigeminal nerve for tic douloureux caused no paralysis. Towards the end of his lecture, he writes of a common condition 'vulgarly called a blight' in which young people have a partial facial palsy due sometimes to inflammation of the glands behind the angle of the jaw. In a subsequent case demonstration, Bell showed a man who had been tossed by a bull: its horn pierced his cheek and divided the facial nerve where it exits from the stylomastoid foramen. Facial movement was entirely paralysed on the affected side. However, not only was sensation in the face preserved but the eyeball turned upwards on attempted eye closure [5].

Conclusions

Bell deduced that if a structure is supplied by more than one nerve, each nerve will have a different function. In particular, he reasoned that the function of the facial nerve is motor and the trigeminal nerve, sensory. He predicted that this separation of function would apply to other systems of nerves and contribute to a better understanding of the nervous system.

Critique

Although the animal operations and survival will have been brief, Bell's surgical experiments make uncomfortable reading today because of the lack of anaesthesia. Other times, other customs. The gain in knowledge was considerable. He clarified the function of the confusing network of nerves which anatomists had revealed in the face and neck, in particular, the facial motor and trigeminal sensory nerve fibres. In the light of subsequent knowledge, his observations were incomplete. For instance, he did not include the motor branch of the mandibular division of the trigeminal nerve or know about the taste function of the facial nerve. His description of facial asymmetry in young people due to the 'blight' may have been a reference to what we now call Bell's palsy, but Friedreich had already given a much clearer description in 1798. Nevertheless, Bell's skills as an anatomist, clinician, experimenter, and artist earned the eponymous title of Bell's palsy. His description of Bell's phenomenon has no rival.

Peitersen (from Denmark) has published the largest series of cases, just over 2500, of Bell's palsy: 30% were partial and 70% complete; eventual recovery occurred in 71% and severe sequelae in 4% [1]. The annual incidence of Bell's palsy has been estimated as about 20 per 100,000 in the United Kingdom, in the same ball park as estimates from other countries [6].

Bell did not speculate on the cause of what he called 'the blight'. The passage of two centuries has not advanced on Friedreich's proposition that it is a rheumatic condition. The possibility has been explored that reactivation of latent herpes simplex type 1 infection in the geniculate ganglion might cause Bell's palsy. However, viral DNA can be detected in the ganglia of control subjects and randomized controlled trials have not shown benefit from antiviral agents [7, 8]. Bell did not propose any treatment for facial palsy but Friedreich did try repeated electrical stimulation, a treatment which has been pursued empirically. The evidence from randomized trials of electrotherapy, largely limited to one probably underpowered trial with 86 participants, did not show significant benefit [9]. Evidence from randomized controlled trials has eventually made a convincing case that oral corticosteroids reduce the number of people left with residual facial weakness by one third from 32.5% to 23.2% [10].

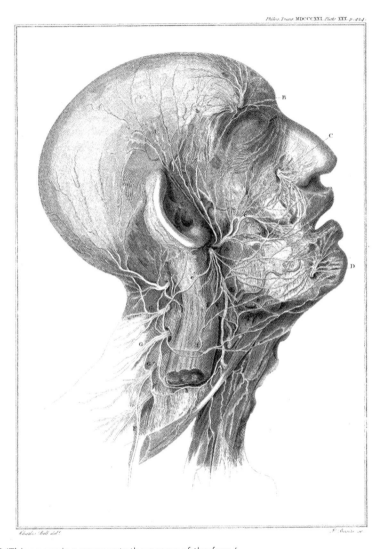

Philos. Trans. MDCCCXXI. *Plate* XXX. *p. 424.*

Fig. 13.1 'This engraving represents the nerves of the face.'
Reproduced from Bell, C., On the nerves; giving an account of some experiments on their structure and functions, which lead to a new arrangement of the system, p. 398–424, (1821), *Phil. Trans. R. Soc. Lond.*

13.2 **Charcot-Marie-Tooth disease**

Main papers: Charcot J, Marie P. Sur une forme particulière d'atrophie musculaire progressive souvent familiale débutant par les pieds et les jambes et atteignant plus tard les mains. *Revue de Médecine* 1886; 6: 97–138.

Background

During most of the nineteenth century, different diseases causing muscle wasting could not be distinguished, although amyotrophic lateral sclerosis, neurosyphilis, and muscle disease were all recognized. The idea that peripheral nerve disease or 'multiple neuritis' might cause paralysis was slow to emerge.

Methods

Legendary French physicians, Jean-Martin Charcot (1825–1893) and Pierre Marie (1853–1940), reviewed the literature and described five patients of their own with a particular type of progressive muscular atrophy [11]. Later the same year, British physician, Howard Henry Tooth (1856–1925), made a similar review of the literature, quoted Charcot and Marie's paper, and developed the concept further in his Cambridge MD thesis [12].

Results

Charcot and Marie described how the symptoms of this new form of progressive muscular atrophy began in the feet and legs and later spread to the hands, but spared the trunk, shoulders, and face. Onset was during childhood and progression was slow. Sensory loss was sometimes present. The knee reflexes were often absent. The ankle reflexes were not reported, not having been described at that time. Tooth summarized the new clinical entity as progressive muscular atrophy beginning in the distal lower extremities, especially the peronei; involving the hand and forearm muscles; starting in childhood; hereditary; causing 'fibrillatory' muscle contractions; producing 'early electrical degenerative changes'; and being slightly more common in males. His thesis included five patients, but only two conformed to this description.

Conclusions

Charcot and Marie considered that the cause was more likely to be a myelopathy. However, Tooth found four post-mortem reports in the literature, of which two showed degenerative changes in the peripheral nerves. From these reports and the clinical picture, he correctly deduced that the pathology was a 'multiple neuritis', as generalized peripheral neuropathy was then described.

Critique

Together, these two papers allowed hereditary motor and sensory neuropathy to be distinguished from amyotrophic lateral sclerosis, muscle disease, and other causes of wasting, and set the stage on which future research was based.

More descriptions of affected families followed. By 1927, Davidenkow was able to review 264 cases from the literature and his own practice. Writing in German, from Moscow, he distinguished 12 subtypes including typical cases and cases with unusual features such as upper limb onset, thickening of the nerves, optic nerve involvement, pyramidal signs, cold paralysis of the hands, and a scapuloperoneal pattern with additional sensory impairment [13, 14]. It was not until 1968 that Dyck and Lambert (Mayo Clinic, Rochester, USA) brought order to clinical understanding by classifying families according to clinical, neurophysiological, and pathological criteria. They described the two main subtypes, one with markedly slowed nerve conduction velocities and one with normal nerve conduction velocities, and a variety of others with additional neurological features such as optic atrophy or spasticity [15, 16].

In 1974, Skre applied genetic techniques to a defined and relatively static population in west Norway and identified three patterns of inheritance [17]. He estimated the prevalence of autosomal dominant cases as 36/100,000, x-linked recessive cases as 3.6/100,000, and autosomal recessive cases as 1.4/100,000. In 1980, London neurologists, Anita Harding (1952–1995) and Peter Kynaston 'PK' Thomas (1926–2008), performed clinical and genetic studies of two groups of cases with autosomal dominant inheritance: these could be separated by measuring the median nerve maximum motor conduction velocity, with a watershed at 38 m/sec, lower values defining hereditary motor and sensory neuropathy Type I and higher values Type II [18, 19]. In later publications, the nomenclature of these groups has been changed to Charcot-Marie-Tooth disease Type 1 (demyelinating) and Type 2 (axonal), with suffixed letters to indicate subgroups caused by different mutations.

These refined clinical and neurophysiological descriptions were needed to define homogeneous entities for genetic studies. The first genetic cause to be identified in detail was a duplication of the gene coding for a minor peripheral myelin protein with a molecular weight of 22 kd, PMP22, in patients with the autosomal dominant demyelinating form of the disease, hereditary motor and sensory neuropathy Type I [20, 21]. This is the most common cause of Charcot-Marie-Tooth (CMT) disease, accounting for about two-thirds of cases worldwide, and is now known as CMT1A. Deletion of one copy of the same gene was shown to cause autosomal dominant hereditary neuropathy with liability to pressure palsies [22]. The phenotype of CMT1 is genetically heterogeneous. Mutations of the gene for the major myelin glycoprotein, P0, were soon found to be an alternative cause of CMT1, and others, including mutations of the PMP22 gene which is duplicated in CMT1A, soon followed. Similarly, CMT2 is genetically heterogeneous. Mutations of the gene for a mitochondrial protein, mitofusin 2, are the most common cause, accounting for about 20% of all cases of CMT2.

Mutations of PMP22, P0, and other genes cause severe early-onset demyelinating neuropathy with hypertrophic changes in the nerves. Autosomal recessive cases of CMT may be demyelinating or axonal and are caused by mutations in a wide variety of genes. Mutations of genes for axonal proteins, such as neurofilament light chain, cause axonal CMT. X-linked inheritance can be caused by mutation of GJB1 (the gene for the gap junction protein, connexin 32) and a few other genes, some as yet unidentified. Conduction velocities are variable and, in *GJB1* mutations, may be intermediate between those of the more purely demyelinating and axonal forms of CMT.

The number of genes causing CMT disease now exceeds 60 and will continue to rise, since about a third of cases in the community still defy genetic diagnosis [23–25]. An up-to-date list is being maintained [26]. It has been a fertile field of research and many more papers have contributed to the understanding of CMT disease than this account can mention. However, the starting line was drawn by Charcot and Marie's delineation of the syndrome and Tooth's recognition that it was caused by peripheral nerve disease. The focus now turns to natural history studies, design of meaningful measures of disease progression, and randomized trials of treatment.

13.3 **Carpal tunnel syndrome**

Main paper: Brain WR, Wright AD, Wilkinson M. Spontaneous compression of both median nerves in the carpal tunnel. Six cases treated surgically. *Lancet* 1947; 1:277–88.

Background

Before the landmark paper by the UK's Lord Brain et al. (1947) [27], there had been much confusion about the cause of the symptoms of carpal tunnel syndrome [28]. In the first clinical description in 1880, US neurology pioneer, James Jackson Putnam (1846–1918) from the Massachusetts General Hospital, described 31 patients, predominantly middle-aged women, with paraesthesiae in their hands, worse at night and relieved by hanging their hands out of bed [29]. Putnam attributed the symptoms to 'alterations of the blood supply to the smaller branches or terminal filaments of the sensitive nerves supplying the affected districts'. For years clinicians, even such British alumni as Sir Edward Farquhar Buzzard (1871–1945; physician to King Edward VII) and Samuel Alexander Kinnier Wilson (1878–1937; of Wilson's disease), misdiagnosed the cause of the symptoms as being due to compression of the brachial plexus by a cervical rib. In 1913, French neurologists, Pierre Marie and Charles Foix (1882–1927), did describe an advanced clinical case in which autopsy showed swelling of the median nerve proximal to and thinning under the transverse carpal ligament [30]. They even wrote that 'perhaps in a case in which the diagnosis is made early enough transection of the ligament could stop development of these phenomena'. However, their prophesy was ignored for more than 30 years. During the 1920s, reports began to appear of operations to decompress the median nerve at the wrist, mostly in cases where it had been compressed by bony deformity as a result of fracture, dislocation, or arthritis [28, 31].

Methods

Brain, Dickson Wright, and Wilkinson described a series of six women with tingling and pain in the fingers and weakness of the thumb which were all relieved by an operation to divide the transverse carpal ligament [27].

Results

The symptoms began in all patients with pain and tingling in the distribution of the median nerve, worse at night and when carrying objects. One or two months or years later, they developed thinning of the thenar eminence and weakness of the thumb. Examination showed wasting of the lateral thenar eminence, weakness of abductor pollicis brevis (and, in most cases, opponens pollicis), and impairment of pinprick, light touch, and, usually, two point discrimination in the median nerve territory. At operation, the surgeon, Dickson Wright, found marked thickening of the median nerve under and proximal to the transverse carpal ligament. He divided the ligament and freed the nerve from adhesions. All six patients had immediate relief of pain and tingling and then a gradual reduction in sensory impairment and weakness. The authors performed experiments on cadavers, showing that the pressure in the carpal tunnel rose on flexion or extension of the wrist, but more on extension.

Conclusions

Since most activities with the hands involve extension of the wrist, using the hands will, in susceptible persons, increase the pressure on the median nerve in the carpal tunnel and cause ischaemia of the nerve, resulting in the characteristic symptoms. The previous attribution of the symptoms to compression of the brachial plexus was incorrect because it would not cause sensory impairment in the median nerve territory. Dividing the transverse carpal tunnel ligament is curative.

Critique

With this series of cases, the authors described what we now call carpal tunnel syndrome, one of the most common neurological disorders affecting 3.8% of the population at any one time [32], and introduced surgical division of the transverse carpal ligament, one of the most common operations worldwide, as a curative treatment. The success of this treatment unequivocally overturned the previous prevailing view that acroparaesthesiae, the name given to this form of tingling of the fingers, were due to compression of the brachial plexus. In 1949, M.J. McArdle, consultant neurologist at Guy's and the National Hospitals in London, suggested and, in 1951, reported to the Association of British Neurologists that acroparaesthesiae alone were due to compression of the median nerve in the carpal tunnel and might be relieved by decompression [32]. Kremer et al. followed up McArdle's suggestion and reported relief of symptoms in 37 out of the 40 patients on whom they operated [33].

Despite the introduction of electrophysiological techniques for measuring delayed conduction across the carpal tunnel in motor nerve fibres [34] and, later, in sensory nerve fibres, clinical history and neurological examination remain the mainstay of diagnosis [33]. The value of surgery has been confirmed in clinical trials [35], but not all patients are satisfied with the outcome; 25% of 4000 patients surveyed did not regard their operation as an unqualified success and 8% thought they were worse [33]. Attempts have been made to improve on the standard operation by endoscopic release through smaller incisions or by additional procedures such as neurolysis. A Cochrane systematic review concluded that such modifications have not produced significant extra benefit [36]. Other treatments are available. Splinting the wrist gives short-term aid, but its long-term benefits are uncertain [37]. In 1957, Phalen and Kendrick reported improvement of carpal tunnel syndrome symptoms in 16 out of 20 patients following injections of corticosteroids, usually repeated, into the carpal tunnel [38]. A Cochrane systematic review of randomized controlled trials confirmed that corticosteroid injection is more effective than placebo after one month, but the evidence was inadequate to decide whether the benefit from steroids lasts longer [39].

13.4 **Paraneoplastic neuropathies**

Main paper: Denny-Brown D. Primary sensory neuropathy with muscular changes associated with carcinoma. *J Neurol Neurosurg Psychiatry* 1948; 11:73–87.

Background

In 1948, the literature on neuropathy was relatively sparse. Most neuropathies at that time were described as sensory and motor, starting distally with proximal progression, and symmetrical. As New Zealand-born neurologist, Derek Ernest Denny-Brown (1901–1981), pointed out in this paper [40], sensory neuropathies were uncommon and usually attributed to tabes or to rare cases of Guillain-Barré syndrome. In experimental animals, deficiencies of select vitamins were known to cause a similar syndrome. However, Denny-Brown had only recently described nutritional neuropathy in man and felt that the sensory neuropathies from nutritional deficiency were different from those in this paper as they had less pain and also had retrobulbar optic neuropathy [41].

Methods and results

The two cases in this landmark paper were collected over a number of years, but publishing was held up due to the loss, during the Second World War, of additional hospital records. Both cases involved men with rapidly progressive, painful, sensory ataxic syndromes involving the entire body. Both had reduced or absent reflexes but normal strength. Both died within 8 months. Post-mortem examination showed severe loss of dorsal root ganglion cells with replacement by residual nodules of Nageotte [42] without inflammation and an unsuspected myositis in association with bronchogenic carcinoma [40].

Conclusions

Denny-Brown concluded that 'the most remarkable change in the two patients presented was the severe loss of nerve cells in the dorsal root ganglia, without corresponding change in the ventral roots' and that 'the close similarity of the condition in the two patients suggests that the coincidence of carcinoma was more than a chance association'.

Critique

On 7 February 1948, Wyburn-Mason published three cases in the *Lancet*, in an article entitled 'Bronchial carcinoma presenting as polyneuritis [43]. For the report, he thanked 'Dr Gordon Holmes, Dr Carmichael, and Dr Denny-Brown for permission to publish the case reports, and Dr Greenfield for the autopsy findings in cases 2 and 3'. Wyburn-Mason considered the possible causes of these neuropathies and discussed tumour invasion into the lymphatics of the peripheral nerves, tumour invasion of the intrathecal portions of the spinal nerves, and a toxic-metabolic neuropathy similar to others known at the time. However, he ended by stating: 'The aetiology of the polyneuritis is discussed, and it is concluded that this is the result of a nervous reflex from the lung.' Apparently unbeknown to each other, Denny-Brown had submitted two of the same cases, in much greater detail, to the

Journal of Neurology, Neurosurgery, and Psychiatry on 12 December 1947, to be published in the following June issue. In a footnote, Denny-Brown wrote:

> The two cases presented here are included with one other in a paper by R. Wyburn-Mason on 'Bronchial Carcinoma presenting as Polyneuritis' in the *Lancet* of Feb. 7, 1948, p. 203, which has appeared since the present paper went to press. The detailed pathological analysis reported here does not support the theory of 'reflex' production of peripheral neuritic symptoms (in analogy with pulmonary osteo-arthropathy) proposed by Wyburn-Mason.

Thus, Denny-Brown concluded: 'The presence of a metabolic disorder related to the tumour cells is presumed, for the neuromuscular condition reproduced changes that have been seen in pantothenic acid and in vitamin E deficiency in animals.' So, both authors proposed the wrong solution, but Denny-Brown ended with: 'The close similarity of the condition in the two patients suggests that the coincidence of carcinoma was more than a chance association.' This last statement proved most prescient and earned Denny-Brown credit for reporting the syndrome we now know as the sensory ganglionopathy associated with cancer caused by a circulating auto-antibody directed to an intracellular antigen in dorsal root ganglion cells, named anti-Hu [44] or anti-neuronal nuclear antibody 1 (ANNA-1).

This report sparked intense interest in the neurological syndromes associated with cancer, and there have been numerous reports over the subsequent decades. Many of these were from London and the group of Brain, Wilkinson, Henson, and Ulrich [45]. Subsequent work by Posner, Lennon, Newsom-Davis, Vincent, Dalmau, and Graus, among others, has greatly expanded our understanding of these syndromes [46]. An expanding number of clear-cut neurological syndromes, both of the peripheral and central nervous system, are now known [46]. While most still think of the sensory ganglionopathy syndrome as the main paraneoplastic neuropathy, the neuropathies associated with monoclonal gammopathies are, in fact, much more frequent [47]. Autonomic neuropathies are also known but rare [48].

The unifying feature of all these syndromes is their immune-mediated pathogenesis [49–51]. The distinct antigens have led to a classification of these, not only by clinical syndrome and auto-antibody, but also by the location of the antigen as either intracellular or extracellular. Additionally, there is overlap in syndromes with and without cancer, as the mechanisms are so similar. In those with auto-antibodies targeting intracellular antigens, cancer is almost always associated. These diseases are mainly related to neuronal death with rare responses to therapy. In these, cellular immunity appears to play a major role. Patients with auto-antibodies targeting membrane antigens such as receptors, channels, or receptor- associated proteins only rarely have cancer. But since the neurological disorders are related to a reversible membrane dysfunction, immunomodulatory treatments are frequently successful. In these, humoral immunity and auto-antibodies play an important role.

13.5 **Neurophysiology of peripheral nerve disease**

Main paper: Dawson GD, Scott JW. The recording of nerve action potentials through skin in man. *J Neurol Neurosurg Psychiat* 1949; 12:259–67.

Background

In 1870, Helmholtz and Baxt [52] recorded motor nerve conduction in humans. In 1929, Adrian and Bronk [53] developed the concentric needle electrode and furthered the field of peripheral nerve physiology. These two papers could also be considered landmarks. Subsequently, using the two techniques of motor nerve conduction and needle electromyography together, a number of clinician-scientists, such as Hodes, Larrabee and German [54], Buchthal and Rosenfalck [55], Lambert [56], and Henrickson [57], made substantial advances in understanding both basic neurobiology and human disease.

Methods

In this landmark paper, Dawson and Scott showed that, with proper techniques, sensory nerve action potentials (SNAPs) could be recorded through the skin in a reliable fashion [58].

Results

In 1949, Dawson and Scott overcame the technical difficulties of recording the small amplitude sensory nerve action potentials in man [58]. Their paper starts by describing, in the most clear and proper scientific language, why a prior report of this technique was incorrect. They then describe their methods in great detail, as this was the critical advance. They showed that the SNAP from both the median and ulnar nerves stimulating at the wrist could be recorded, at or above the elbow, at distances of 25–30 cm (Fig. 13.2). Two of their 15 subjects had abnormal SNAP amplitudes compared to the others—one had had an obvious ulnar nerve injury, with surgical repair years before, but also had a reduced median SNAP amplitude. Dawson and Scott discovered that he had participated in blood pressure cuff experiments in which his median nerve likely sustained a subclinical injury, as the subject no longer had symptoms.

Conclusions

Dawson and Scott concluded: 'In fifteen healthy subjects action potentials have been recorded from electrodes on the skin over the course of the median or ulnar nerve after electrical stimulation of the nerve at the wrist.' Because of the observations on the two with injured nerves, they presciently stated: 'It is suggested that the method may have use in the study of minor degrees of nerve injury.'

Critique

The importance of this paper to the field of peripheral neuropathy cannot be underestimated. It allowed another entire window into the understanding of peripheral nerves in

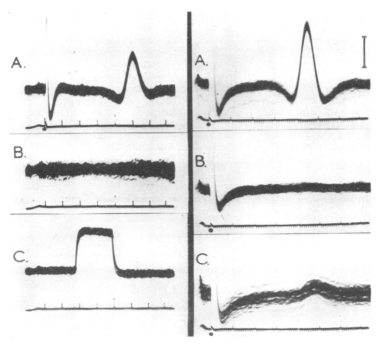

Fig. 13.2 (**A, B, C, left**): The records show the potential differences between a pair of electrodes on the skin over the median nerve above the elbow. In (A), electrical stimuli were applied to the nerve at the wrist at the point indicated by the black dot below the timescale. In (B), the conditions were identical except that no stimuli were applied. Record (C) shows the response of the recording system to a rectangular pulse of 20 μV amplitude delivered from a source of 500 ohms impedance. The timescales show intervals of 1 msec. In these and in all succeeding records, 50 traces were superimposed. (**A, B, C, right**): The records show the effects of movements of the stimulating or recording electrodes. Record (A) shows the responses recorded when the stimulating cathode was over the median nerve at the wrist and the recording electrodes, over the nerve above the elbow. (B) shows the result of moving the stimulating cathode from over the nerve, to the radial styloid, keeping the other conditions as in (A). (C) shows the result of leaving the cathode over the nerve at the wrist but moving the recording electrodes medially off the nerve on to the belly of the biceps muscle. The timescales show 0.1 and 1 msec. intervals.

health and disease. Readers of the paper today, who take the computerized recording of SNAPs as routine, will be amazed at what was required to record a SNAP in those days. The paper was followed by another important paper from the UK's National Hospital for Neurology and Neurosurgery, London, in which Gilliatt and Sears [59] studied a range of disorders including median neuropathy at the wrist (studied previously with motor nerve conduction by Simpson, who made an important contribution to the understanding of conduction block in carpal tunnel syndrome [60]), ulnar neuropathy at the elbow, brachial plexus injury, and polyneuropathy, both acquired and genetic. In all cases, the recording of SNAPs provided information to complement that from the other two techniques, all three of which are so common today. Presciently, Gilliatt and Sears made the reservation that 'these potentials provide no information about the small myelinated and non-myelinated fibres which are thought to be concerned with pain and temperature sensation'. [59] This concept has been rediscovered in the last 15 years with the emphasis on 'small fibre' neuropathy [61].

Papers that built upon the power of the combined techniques are too numerous to mention. We now take all these techniques for granted as, daily, we carry out both sensory and motor nerve conduction tests and electromyography to investigate our patients' symptoms.

13.6 **Familial amyloid polyneuropathy**

Main paper: Andrade C. Peculiar form of peripheral neuropathy: familiar atypical generalized amyloidosis with special involvement of the peripheral nerves. *Brain* 1952; 75:408–27.

Background

Familial polyneuropathies and amyloidosis were known by the time of this paper but a familial amyloid polyneuropathy (FAP) was not.

Methods

Starting in 1939, Portuguese neurologist, Mário Corino da Costa Andrade (1906–2005), investigated a familial polyneuropathy seen in northern Portugal [62, 63]. A breakthrough came in 1942 when an autopsy of one of his patients showed amyloid.

Results

Andrade described all the important features of this unusual 'mal dos pesinhos' including the autosomal dominant genetics, onset in the legs with small fibre and autonomic dysfunction between the age of 20 and 30 years, and death 7 to 10 years later.

Conclusions

Andrade concluded:

> Though the aetiological and pathogenic factors are as yet unknown, we think that the evidence presented in this study allows us to set apart from the group of the known peripheral neuropathies this entity with its peculiar anatomical and clinical picture.

Critique

After his retirement in 1976, the extended natural history of the disease was described, forming the basis of clinical studies since [64]. The Andrade type of FAP initially observed in those from the northern coastal provinces of Portugal and in their Brazilian relatives was found in Japan, Sweden, and elsewhere [65, 66].

Kanda and colleagues determined the complete sequence of plasma thyroxine-binding pre-albumin, later more appropriately named transthyretin (TTR) [67]. Saraiva and colleagues showed the molecular basis of the disorder in these Portuguese kindreds as a valine to methionine substitution at residue 30 of the transthyretin gene (V30M) [68]. This is now known as the most common mutation in FAP. Realizing that most of the TTR is produced in the liver, Holmgren and colleagues performed the first liver transplant as treatment [69], and this remains the standard of care today [70].

With increased understanding of the biology of TTR, three additional approaches to treatment have been studied. Tafamidis is a small molecule that occupies the thyroxine-binding sites with negative co-operativity and kinetically stabilizes the tetrameric TTR molecule. It has been approved by the European regulatory authorities for treatment of stage 1 FAP [71]. Two other agents are currently undergoing clinical trials—an antisense oligonucleotide targeting hepatic mRNA TTR, ISIS-TTRRx [72], and a small interfering RNA targeting wild-type and all mutant forms of TTR, ALN-TTR01 [73]. This entire saga, from the first clinical description in 1952 to approved treatment and active clinical research today, is a great story.

13.7 **Chronic inflammatory demyelinating polyradiculoneuropathy**

Main paper: Austin JH. Recurrent polyneuropathies and their corticosteroid treatment. *Brain* 1958; 81:157–92.

Background

The notion of a chronic inflammatory neuropathy was slow to emerge compared with that of acute polyneuritis which had been heralded by French physician, Jean Baptiste Octave Landry de Thézillat (1826–1865), in 1859, and acknowledged by numerous authors before the famous description by Georges Guillain, Jean Alexandre Barré, and André Strohl in 1916. The first clear description of a recurrent symmetrical polyneuropathy was by Targowla in 1894 [74].

Methods

In 1958, American neurologist, James H. Austin, reviewed 30 cases of recurrent symmetrical neuropathy from the literature and added two of his own [75]. He rejected cases for which the descriptions were inadequate and those for which a cause such as toxin exposure, diabetes mellitus, porphyria, or 'collagen' disease was apparent. For one of his own cases, he gave a meticulous account of the illness over 5 years, comparing the response to adrenocorticotrophic hormone, cortisone, or prednisone with that to placebo (Fig. 13.3).

Results

Austin summarized the clinical picture as follows:

> . . . a young adult who slowly develops over many weeks or months the progressive symptoms and signs of a symmetrical, chiefly distal, chiefly motor polyradiculoneuropathy involving four limbs. Cranial nerves seven, six, three, nine and ten are occasionally involved; sphincters almost always spared. There is usually no obvious cause, infection, symptoms of systemic illness, or prominence of pain. Spinal fluid protein is usually elevated . . . 22 of the 32 cases are males with an average age at onset of 23 years. No cause for male preponderance is apparent. The peak of disability is slowly reached after five months on an average . . . From a plateau of disability the patient then gradually improves and often completely recovers . . . After months or years without symptoms, second, or more, similar bouts occur. Each recurrence is somewhat variable in severity, duration, and residua. The average interval between bouts is four years.

He considered that the thickened nerves in 11 of the 32 cases were due to interstitial hypertrophy and collagen deposition in two and to oedema in nine. Nine of the reviewed patients had had corticosteroids and five had relapsed after corticosteroids, within one day of treatment withdrawal. Improvement following corticosteroids was common but difficult to assess because of the absence of a placebo control in the cases from the literature. The patient he reported in detail had 20 bouts of polyneuropathy over 5 years and he showed that improvement followed soon after adrenocorticotrophic hormone, cortisone, or prednisone, but not after placebo. He depicted the improvement graphically with an

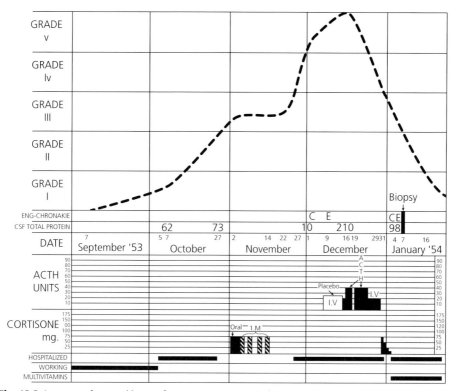

Fig. 13.3 Account of second bout of recurrent symmetrical neuropathy in a patient, during 1953/54. Note the checking of progression during cortisone treatment and the relatively rapid response to adrenocorticotropic hormone (ACTH).

Reproduced from *Brain*, 81, JH Austin, Recurrent polyneuropathies and their corticosteroid treatment, p. 157–192, Copyright (1958), with permission from Oxford University Press.

eight-point scale of his own devising. A nerve biopsy showed interstitial oedema, depletion of myelin with relative preservation of axons and absence of cellular infiltration.

Conclusions

The recovery of function following each bout, the relative preservation of muscle bulk, and the loss of myelin sheaths indicated that the pathology was due to conduction block and not axonal degeneration. Although oedema occurred in the nerves, it could not alone be the cause of the neurological deficit since there was no relationship between nerve oedema and severity of dysfunction. Since improvement followed introduction of corticosteroids in each of the 20 bouts and relapse followed withdrawal, corticosteroids are efficacious. He noted that the dose has to be adjusted according to the needs of the patient at the time. However, corticosteroids are not the 'ultimate treatment' of this disorder because of their serious long-term side-effects. The tempo of the illness is altered by corticosteroids and 'the important point arises as to how far apart . . . these "diseases" [acute and chronic polyneuritis] are'.

Critique

The clinical picture summarized by Austin is instantly recognizable as that of chronic inflammatory demyelinating polyradiculoneuropathy (CIDP) and would fulfil the latest clinical diagnostic criteria promulgated by a joint European Federation of Neurological Societies/Peripheral Nerve Society task force [76]. However, modern criteria now recognize proximal as well as distal weakness as characteristic; accept chronic progressive as well as relapsing–remitting disease courses; and include pain as a not uncommon and sometimes prominent feature [76].

The amount of pathology available to Austin was limited, but Dyck and colleagues and McLeod and Prineas soon demonstrated lymphocytic infiltration and macrophage-associated demyelination in active lesions [77–79]. Neurophysiological demonstration of conduction slowing and partial conduction block subsequently became important in diagnosis, and an elevated cerebrospinal fluid protein with a relatively normal white cell count was recognized as a supportive criterion [76]. Nevertheless, the clinical picture has remained the mainstay of the diagnosis. Although antibodies to gangliosides have emerged as useful biomarkers in some acute inflammatory neuropathies and in multifocal motor neuropathy, there is still a lack of characteristic antibodies or other diagnostic biomarkers in CIDP. While there is evidence of endoneurial and systemic immune activation and impairment of immunoregulatory control in CIDP, the identity of any auto-antigens and detailed pathogenesis are still poorly understood [80].

Austin's use of placebo, albeit single-blinded, was an advance on previous simple observational studies, and his comment that corticosteroids were not the ultimate treatment was prescient. An early randomized but open controlled trial confirmed the efficacy of corticosteroids for CIDP and they have remained a first-line treatment option [81]. Many different corticosteroid regimes are used and one randomized controlled trial showed no significant difference in efficacy between daily oral prednisolone and monthly high-dose dexamethasone [82]. Recognition of the side-effects of corticosteroids led to the introduction of intravenous immunoglobulin [83] and plasma exchange [84], which have both been shown to be efficacious, and of immunosuppressant agents, which have not [85]. The relative advantages of corticosteroids and intravenous immunoglobulin are still debated: a randomized controlled trial showed that response to treatment was faster with intravenous immunoglobulin but longer lasting with monthly high-dose intravenous methylprednisolone [86].

13.8 **Toxic neuropathy**

Main paper: Cavanagh JB. The significance of the 'dying back' process in experimental and human neurological diseases. *Int Rev Exper Pathol* 1964; 3:219–67.

Background

From some of the earliest descriptions of neurological diseases, it was noted that many started distally and progressed proximally. British physician, Sir Seymour John Sharkey (1847–1929), in his paper entitled 'On peripheral neuritis', in 1896, wrote:

> It is a somewhat remarkable thing that in multiple neuritis it is the terminal portions of the nerves are nearly always affected. Why is this? . . . partly perhaps because they are furthest removed from the nerve cells, on the energy radiating from which their health depends. [87]

Experimental work on this topic began in the late nineteenth century. Clinical descriptions of many toxic neuropathies, in the early twentieth century, confirmed this distal to proximal gradient of disease. Spatz made the connection that many inherited and sporadic disorders shared these features (1938 and 1952) [88, 89]. In 1954, pathologist to the UK's National Hospital, J. Godwin Greenfield (1884–1958), published his ground-breaking work, *Spinocerebellar Degenerations* [90], stating 'characteristic of systemic degenerations, whether hereditary or sporadic, that neurons in the systems involved die back gradually from the periphery to the cell body' and, thus, for the first time, really used the concept of 'dying back'. Pathologist, John Cavanagh, studied this problem in a number of experimental systems, culminating in the landmark review paper of 1964 [91].

Methods

Cavanagh reviewed the world literature on both experimental and clinical neurological disease relating to the dying back process. The review cited over 150 references in multiple languages. Credit is clearly given where credit is due.

Results

Cavanagh provided a synthesis of the literature for his thesis of the importance of the dying back process throughout neurology. Starting with an historical overview, he reviewed the literature on the creysl phosphates, aryl phosphates, and the alkyl phosphates. His own work on organophosphates was highly detailed, concentrating on the earliest structural changes in the distal portion of the peripheral and central nervous system then available for study. He identified the differences in single versus cumulative doses (the latter much worse than the former), the differential affectation of sensory and motor fibres (the latter less affected than the former), and the differential affectation of, among sensory fibre populations, small fibres being less affected than large fibres. He then turned his attention to human diseases—amyotrophic lateral sclerosis, spinocerebellar disorders, Werdnig-Hoffman disease, and, lastly, the deficiencies and intoxications (thiamine deficiency, arsenic, acute porphyria neuropathy, and medications).

Conclusions

Cavanagh pointed out a fundamental problem in neurobiology—why do neurodegenerative diseases and toxic neuropathies begin distally and progress proximally? While he outlined the spatial-temporal features of the dying back process in the article, he also raised questions about the metabolic pathogenesis. The idea that the distal axon in all of these conditions depended upon the central neuron for 'nourishment' was clearly stated.

Critique

The clinical features of toxic neuropathies so eloquently outlined by Cavanagh remain tenets of those diseases today: single versus cumulative dosing, selective vulnerability of nerve fibre populations, and the central-peripheral pattern of degeneration that so many of these diseases exhibit which limits recovery [92]. Spencer and Schaumburg added significantly to this literature, summarized in their 1976 paper in which they coined the term 'central-peripheral distal axonopathy' [93]. Toxic neuropathies remain a considerable public health problem today, with no clear solutions. These include neuropathies from chemotherapy agents, other medications such as anti-retrovirals, and industrial toxins.

The neurobiological problem raised in Cavanagh's paper—why does this pattern occur?—continues to defy a clear answer. An entire issue of *Experimental Neurology* is devoted to this problem [94]. With the topics covered in this special issue—amyotrophic lateral sclerosis, Charcot–Marie–Tooth disease, hereditary spastic paraplegia, ischaemic injury, traumatic brain injury, Alzheimer's disease, glaucoma, Huntington's disease, and Parkinson's disease—one could be re-reading Cavanagh. The reader is referred to the issue for further details [94].

Of particular note is the recent interest in distal axonal degeneration in amyotrophic lateral sclerosis (ALS) [95], an area covered by Cavanagh. He noted that the standard dogma was that ALS was a motor neuron cell disorder but did comment on the many studies, even at that time, which showed a distal predominant process pathologically. This has been rediscovered and many additional techniques, including physiological ones, employed to study this [96]. The opportunities for therapy are extensive, as slowing the local process may provide some temporary relief from an otherwise inexorably progressive disease.

One of the most common toxic neuropathies today is that caused by chemotherapy drugs. In fact, it has been stated that chemotherapy-induced peripheral neuropathy (CIPN) is the major dose-limiting side-effect of chemotherapy today [97]. Previously, it was low blood counts, but these have been corrected by the use of growth factors. CIPN has a major impact on cancer therapy by not only causing morbidity, which may be life-long, but also potentially enforcing the use of chemotherapy doses that may not be maximally effective. Much work remains to be done in this area.

A recent collaborative study of oncologists and neurologists have taken a new look at CIPN by asking if physicians are measuring it correctly. So far, the group has completed a cross-sectional study in which they looked at a number of the standard measures of CIPN in order to find those that are valid and reliable [98]. A series of papers have been published, from the same group, suggesting the specific measures that may be used in a longitudinal study to more accurately quantify CIPN [99]. These include data from both the physician and patient perspective. Such a study is critical as it is only with good measures of the disease will we be able to develop interventions that either prevent CIPN or ameliorate it once established. Currently, there are no proven medications or supplements for either purpose [100].

13.9 **Diabetic neuropathies**

Main paper: Eliasson SG. Nerve conduction changes in experimental diabetes. *J Clin Invest* 1964; 43:2353–8.

Background

By 1964, clinically, much was known about diabetic neuropathy, from the earliest description by French physician, Charles-Jacob Marchal de Calvi (1815–1873) [101], to those of Pryce [102] and Martin [103], among others. This knowledge included:

a) the wide spectrum of neuropathies seen, including autonomic neuropathies and acute-onset cranial and limb neuropathies;

b) the common clinical manifestations of distal symmetric polyneuropathy, including frequent absence of ankle reflexes and loss of pin and vibration sense distally, with lesser motor involvement;

c) the understanding that most who developed neuropathy showed long periods of hyperglycaemia and glycosuria preceding the onset of the neuropathy (shown convincingly by Pirart, the following year [104]);

d) the concept that neuropathy could precede the diagnosis of diabetes;

e) the rare appearance of neuropathy precipitated by insulin [105]; and

f) the common occurrence of abnormal nerve conduction studies in those with polyneuropathy [106, 107].

Methods

In this landmark paper, American neurologist, Sven G. Eliasson, showed that nerve conduction changes were present in animals made diabetic either after alloxan injection or pancreatectomy [108].

Results

Eliasson performed nerve conduction studies using *in vitro* preparations from control rats, alloxanized (but not diabetic) rats, alloxanized rats with diabetes, and pancreatectomized rats. Some of the animals were given insulin treatment. Using the techniques then available, he studied sciatic conduction along the length of the nerve and, separately, motor and sensory conduction from the roots out to the sciatic nerve. He showed reduced conduction velocity only in those animals made diabetic. In the insulin-treated animals, insulin was begun 2 or 21 days after the injection of alloxan. In retrospect, he did not measure glucose tightly but, rather, gave a fixed insulin dose.

Conclusions

Eliasson concluded that:

> When a diabetic state was induced in rats after alloxan injection or pancreatectomy, a reduction of conduction velocity of approximately 30% was noted in both sensory and motor fibers of the sciatic nerve. No slowing was observed in vagus nerve fibers.

In his hands:

> Insulin treatment of the diabetic rats or addition of insulin to the in vitro preparation did not affect the reduced conduction velocity.

Critique

The importance of this paper to the field of diabetic neuropathy cannot be understated. Eliasson was the first to show that nerve conduction velocity could be used as a biomarker of experimental diabetic neuropathy and, thus, presumably also of human diabetic neuropathy. At the time of his paper, it was already known that nerve conduction velocity was reduced in human diabetic neuropathy and that greater reductions in velocity were seen in those with long-standing diabetes and severe neuropathy [107, 108]. However, the reversal of the conduction deficit eluded Eliasson. It was not until the papers of Gabbay [109] and Greene and co-workers [110] that it was clear that the conduction abnormality could be reversed with tight glucose control [109, 110] or with myoinositol supplementation [110]. As both these groups were interested in the sorbitol pathway, this began a decade-long pharmaceutical race to find the perfect aldose reductase inhibitor. Company after company fundamentally used the Eliasson paradigm, measuring conduction velocity in experimental diabetic neuropathy rats, to test compound after compound, hoping that reversing the conduction deficit in rats would in fact improve human diabetic neuropathy.

From the perspective of human diabetic neuropathy, many investigators also relied heavily on measurement of motor conduction velocity as a biomarker of human diabetic polyneuropathy. In both cross-sectional and longitudinal studies, Dyck and colleagues showed a close relationship between the changes in motor conduction velocity and other measures of human diabetic polyneuropathy [111, 112]. These then became the standard targets in pharmaceutical trials overseen by the Food and Drug Administration (FDA). Unfortunately, no one yet has been able to meet these criteria [113]. More recently, most likely due to improvements in glucose control over the decades since the original Mayo Clinic studies, it is now thought that these targets may be unattainable in less than 3- to 5-year studies [113, 114]. Thus, the entire field of therapies for diabetic polyneuropathy is undergoing dramatic change.

13.10 **Guillain-Barré syndrome revisited**

Main paper: Feasby TE, Gilbert JJ, Brown WF, et al. An acute axonal form of Guillain-Barré polyneuropathy. *Brain* 1986; 109:1115–26.

Background

Landry's account of acute ascending paralysis, in 1856, heralded a number of papers in the late nineteenth century describing an illness consistent with acute inflammatory neuropathy. In 1916, French neurologists, Georges Guillain (1876–1961) and Jean Alexandre Barré (1880–1967), with physiologist, André Strohl (1887–1977), added to this picture by describing the increased cerebrospinal fluid protein and normal cell count in two soldiers with acute flaccid weakness and absent tendon reflexes [115]. Guillain-Barré(-Strohl) syndrome (GBS) was generally considered to be a homogeneous inflammatory demyelinating process affecting the peripheral nervous system, best illustrated in a post-mortem series by Asbury and colleagues in 1969 [116] and later supported by electrophysiological studies. The pathology of these fatal cases showed prominent lymphocytic infiltration, acute inflammatory demyelinating polyradiculoneuropathy (AIDP) (Fig. 13.4). This resembled experimental autoimmune neuritis induced in rodents by immunization with peripheral nerve myelin and caused by a T-cell-mediated immune response to various myelin proteins. Subsequent research has failed to corroborate similar mechanisms in the human disease.

Methods

In 1986, Feasby et al. published a landmark series of five cases clinically consistent with rapid-onset, very severe GBS but with electrophysiological evidence of inexcitable nerves and pathological evidence of axonal degeneration [117].

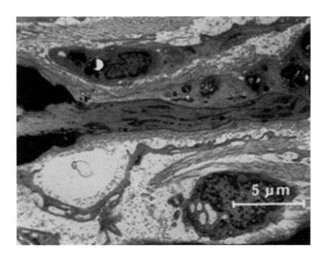

Fig. 13.4 Demyelinated heminode in the AIDP form of GBS.

Reproduced from Hughes RAC, *Guillain-Barre Syndrome*, (1990), Springer Verlag, London.

Results

The five cases came from a total of 60 seen in a 4-year period in London in Ontario, Canada. Recovery was poor and one died. Post-mortem examination of that case showed only axonal degeneration without demyelination in the peripheral nerves and without much in the way of inflammation. Inexcitability could have been due to distal conduction block but widespread fibrillation developed in all cases early and is most consistent with axonal degeneration.

Conclusions

Feasby et al. concluded that:

> . . . the inexcitability of motor nerves, the evidence of severe axonal degeneration and the very poor recovery in these cases set them apart from the usual cases of [GBS] and merit consideration of them as a separate entity of acute axonal neuropathy.

Critique

The paper was not well received initially, and many were sceptical. Confusion arose because patients with very severe GBS of the AIDP type might also have inexcitable nerves as a consequence of axonal degeneration occurring as part of the inflammatory process, and yet the two mechanisms are distinguishable, as addressed in a subsequent paper from this group [118]. However, with the confirming data from a series of papers of an acute paralytic disorder in northern China, the sceptics were won over. In their clinical and electrodiagnostic paper, McKhann et al. distinguished a stereotyped clinical and electrophysiological picture of acute motor axonal neuropathy (AMAN) [119]. Post- mortem studies of the AMAN form of GBS revealed macrophages within the myelin sheath invading the axons and, in severe cases, extensive axonal degeneration. Later studies of the immunopathogenesis showed deposition of complement and immunoglobulin and localization of implicating the nodal axolemma as the target of a presumed autoimmune attack. Conversely in AIDP, complement and immunoglobulin were deposited on the myelin, implicating myelin components as the presumed target of the autoimmune attack [120].

During the 1990s, *Campylobacter jejuni* infection emerged as the most common infection preceding GBS and especially AMAN. The link turned out to be epitopes in the *Campylobacter jejuni* cell wall which resemble the sugar sequences on gangliosides in the axolemma, especially gangliosides GM1 and GD1a [121]. Patients with GBS, especially those with AMAN, have high titres of IgG1 antibodies against ganglioside GM1 or related gangliosides, as first demonstrated by Ilyas and co-workers [122]. Yuki and colleagues produced a model with the same electrophysiological and pathological characteristics as AMAN by immuninizing rabbits with ganglioside GM1 [123]. Willison's group has shown in mutant mice over-expressing gangliosides that complement-fixing antibodies against different gangliosides adhere to and disrupt the distal motor axon terminal and the peri-synaptic Schwann cell [124]. This pathological process could be prevented by treatment with the C5-inhibitor, eculizumab, which raises the hope of introducing this drug for the treatment of AMAN, a possibility which has just moved into clinical trials.

During the 1980s and 1990s, randomized controlled trials showed that plasma exchange or intravenous immunoglobulin, but not corticosteroids, hasten recovery from GBS and reduce the average severity of long-term muscle weakness [125–127]. These trials were largely performed in European and North American patients who are expected to have had AIDP. It is uncertain whether the response of AMAN to treatment is the same. An on-going disease register, the International GBS Outcomes Study, seeks to answer this and many other questions in a larger population.

Key unanswered questions

1 What is the best method of screening for genetic causes of CMT disease?

   Currently, there are over 60 CMT-associated genes, with more discovered each month. For those with CMT1, about 70% worldwide have CMT1A caused by duplication of the gene coding for a minor peripheral myelin protein with a molecular weight of 22 kd, *PMP22*. Thus, testing for those with CMT1 should start with this gene. However, for the rest of CMT1, for CMT2, and for all others with CMT, the best testing algorithm is unclear. Recently, two important techniques have been used—whole exome sequencing and next-generation sequencing. Both have advantages and disadvantages. Papers are available about the impressive results with each of these expensive, but progressively more affordable, techniques. Time and money will sort out a winner.

2 In CIDP, are there other immunosuppressant treatments which are more efficacious than corticosteroids, intravenous immunoglobulin, or plasma exchange and which have acceptable side-effect profiles?

   While the short-term treatment of CIDP is generally good, the long-term situation is more uncertain. Many patients remain on one or more of the aforementioned treatments for decades without seeming hope of a cure or of getting off medication(s). A recent study using pulse dexamethasone has shown that a minority of those treated with that regimen will be cured, when followed for 12 months; however, many relapse more than a year after treatment is stopped. Thus, treatments that cure CIDP are needed. Studies using stronger but potentially more toxic medications, such as fingolimod and alemtuzemab, are underway, and results are eagerly awaited. Whether other immunosuppressant drugs, such as those used for cancer chemotherapy, should be trialled, is an important question.

3 Are there any better treatments than corticosteroids for Bell's palsy?

   Bell's palsy is a common, presumably autoimmune-mediated, acute, monophasic mono-neuropathy. The overall prognosis is good with <10% having significant residua. Corticosteroids are the only effective treatment and are best given early. We know that those with more severe disease will have poorer outcomes. Thus, as with GBS, if we could target treatments towards that subgroup, we would be able to test novel therapies in properly conducted studies.

4 Is carpal tunnel release the best treatment for mild disease?

   Carpal tunnel syndrome is a very common neurological problem. While the exact predisposing factors are debated, many experts recommend avoidance of certain activities, especially those involving repetitive hand activities, for short-term treatment, although this is difficult for many people. Splinting and corticosteroid injections have short-term efficacy. Carpal tunnel release provides more long-lasting relief but is more invasive and expensive. Further studies are needed to discover whether corticosteroid injections or other treatments will avoid the need for an operation, at least in a subgroup of patients.

5 How should GBS patients who do not improve following one course of intravenous immunoglobulin be treated?
   Currently, there are two accepted treatments for patients in the acute stage of GBS—
   plasma exchange and intravenous Ig. In one study, adding intravenous Ig to a completed
   course of plasma exchange did not significantly improve outcome. However, anecdotal
   reports suggest that giving a second course of intravenous Ig may be beneficial. In addition, a retrospective study has suggested that the degree of change in serum Ig concentrations following a course of intravenous Ig in GBS may be important, implying that
   more intravenous Ig may be beneficial in some patients. This question remains a difficult one but is open to study—both a prospective randomized Dutch study, led by P. van
   Doorn, and a prospective collection of clinical cases of GBS, led by B.C. Jacobs, should
   provide answers in the coming years.

References

1 **Peitersen E.** Bell's palsy: the spontaneous course of 2,500 peripheral facial nerve palsies of different etiologies. *Acta Otolaryngol* 2002; **549**(Suppl):4–30.

2 **Bird TD.** Nicolaus A. Friedreich's description of peripheral facial nerve paralysis in 1798. *J Neurol NeurosurgPsychiatry* 1979; **42**(1): 56–8.

3 **Friedreich N.** De paralysi musculorum faciei rheumatica; programma quo ad orationem, die 18° Novembris 1797. *Ann Med* 1800; **5**:214–6.

4 **Bell C.** On the nerves; giving an account of some experiments on their structure and functions, which lead to a new arrangement of the system. *Phil Trans R Soc Lond* 1821; **111**:398–424.

5 **Bell C.** Partial paralysis of the face. *Lond Med Gaz* 1828; **1**(25):747–50. Available from: Bird TD. Nicolaus A. Friedreich's description of peripheral facial nerve paralysis in 1798. *J Neurol Neurosurg. Psychiatry* 1979; 42(1):56–8.

6 **Rowlands S, Hooper R, Hughes RAC, Burney P.** The epidemiology and treatment of Bell's palsy in the UK. *Eur J Neurol* 2002; **9**:63–7.

7 **Lockhart P, Daly F, Pitkethly M, Comerford N, Sullivan F.** Antiviral treatment for Bell's palsy (idiopathic facial paralysis). *Cochrane Data Syst Rev* 2009; (4):CD001869.

8 **Theil D, Arbusow V, Derfuss T, et al.** Prevalence of HSV-1 LAT in human trigeminal, geniculate, and vestibular ganglia and its implication for cranial nerve syndromes. *Brain Pathol* 2001; **11**(4):408–13.

9 **Teixeira LJ, Valbuza JS, Prado GF.** Physical therapy for Bell's palsy (idiopathic facial paralysis). *Cochrane Data Syst Rev* 2011; (12):CD006283.

10 **Salinas RA, Alvarez G, Daly F, Ferreira J.** Corticosteroids for Bell's palsy (idiopathic facial paralysis). *Cochrane Data Syst Rev* 2010; (3):CD001942.

11 **Charcot J, Marie P.** Sur une forme particulière d'atrophie musculaire progressive souvent familiale débutantant par les pieds et les jambes et atteignant plus tard les mains. *Revue Méd* 1886; **6**:97–138.

12 **Tooth HH.** *The Peroneal Type of Progressive Muscular Atrophy*. London: HK Lewis; 1886.

13 **Davidenkow S.** Uber die neurotische muskelatrophie Charcot-Marie: klinisch-genetische studien. II. *Z Neurol* 1927; **108**:344.

14 **Davidenkow S.** Uber die neurotische muskelatrophie Charcot-Marie: klinisch-genetische studien. I. *Z Neurol* 1927; **108**:259.

15 **Dyck PJ, Lambert EH.** Lower motor and primary sensory neuron diseases with peroneal muscular atrophy. I. Neurologic, genetic, and electrophysiologic findings in hereditary polyneuropathies. *Arch Neurol* 1968; **18**:603–18.

16 **Dyck PJ, Lambert EH.** Lower motor and primary sensory neuron diseases with peroneal muscular atrophy. II. Neurologic, genetic, and electrophysiologic findings in various neuronal degenerations. *Arch Neurol* 1968; **18**:619–25.

17 **Skre H.** Genetic and clinical aspects of Charcot-Marie-Tooth's disease. *Clin Genet* 1974; **6**:98–118.

18 **Harding AE, Thomas PK.** Genetic aspects of hereditary motor and sensory neuropathy (types I and II). *J Med Genet* 1980; **17**:329–36.

19 **Harding AE, Thomas PK.** The clinical features of hereditary motor and sensory neuropathy types I and II. *Brain* 1980; **103**:259–80.

20 **Lupski JR, de Oca-Luna RM, Slaugenhaupt S, et al.** DNA duplication associated with Charcot-Marie-Tooth disease type 1A. *Cell* 1991; **66**:219–32.

21 **Raeymaekers P, Timmerman V, Nelis E, et al.** Duplication in chromosome 17p11.2 in Charcot-Marie-Tooth neuropathy type 1a (CMT 1a). The HMSN Collaborative Research Group. *Neuromuscul Disord* 1991; **1**:93–7.

22 **Chance PF, Alderson MK, Leppig KA, et al.** DNA deletion associated with hereditary neuropathy with liability to pressure palsies. *Cell* 1993; **72**:143–51.

23 **Reilly MM, Murphy SM, Laura M.** Charcot-Marie-Tooth disease. *J Peripher Nerv Syst* 2011; **16**:1–14.

24 **Saporta AS, Sottile SL, Miller LJ, Feely SM, Siskind CE, Shy ME.** Charcot-Marie-Tooth disease subtypes and genetic testing strategies. *Ann Neurol* 2011; **69**:22–33.

25 **Murphy SM, Laura M, Fawcett K, et al.** Charcot-Marie-Tooth disease: frequency of genetic subtypes and guidelines for genetic testing. *J Neurol Neurosurg Psychiatry* 2012; **83**:706–10.

26 **Kaplan JC.** The 2012 version of the gene table of monogenic neuromuscular disorders. *Neuromuscul Disord* 2011; **21**:833–61.

27 **Brain WR, Wright AD, Wilkinson M.** Spontaneous compression of both median nerves in the carpal tunnel. Six cases treated surgically. *Lancet* 1947; **1**:277–88.

28 **Pfeffer GB, Gelberman RH, Boyes JH, Rydevik B.** The history of carpal tunnel syndrome. *J Hand Surg (Br)* 1988; **13**:28–34.

29 **Putnam JJ.** A series of cases of paraesthesia, mainly of the hand, of periodical recurrence, and possibly of vaso-motor origin. *Archiv Med (New York)* 1880; **4**:147–62.

30 **Marie P, Foix C.** Atrophie isolé de l'éminence thénar d'origine névritque: rôle du ligament annulaire antérieur du carpe dans le pathogénie de la lésion. *Rev Neurolog* 1913; **26**:647–9.

31 **Amadio PC.** The Mayo Clinic and carpal tunnel syndrome. *Mayo Clin Proc* 1992; **67**:42–8.

32 **Bland JD.** Carpal tunnel syndrome. *BMJ* 2007; **335**:343–6.

33 **Kremer M, Gilliatt RW, Golding JSR, Wilson TG.** Acroparaesthesiae in the carpal tunnel syndrome. *Lancet* 1953; **2**:590–5.

34 **Simpson JA.** Electrical signs in the diagnosis of carpal tunnel and related syndromes. *J Neurol Neurosurg Psychiatry* 1956; **19**:275–80.

35 **Verdugo RJ, Salinas RA, Castillo JL, Cea JG.** Surgical versus non-surgical treatment for carpal tunnel syndrome. *Cochrane Data Syst Rev* 2008, Issue 4. Art. No.: CD001552. DOI: 10.1002/14651858.CD001552.pub2.

36 **Scholten RJPM, Mink van der Molen A, Uitdehaag BMJ, Bouter LM, de Vet HCW.** Surgical treatment options for carpal tunnel syndrome. *Cochrane Data Syst Rev* 2007, Issue 4. Art. No.: CD003905. DOI: 10.1002/14651858.CD003905.pub3.

37 **Page MJ, Massy-Westropp N, O'Connor D, Pitt V.** Splinting for carpal tunnel syndrome. *Cochrane Dat Syst Rev* 2012; **7**:CD010003.

38 **Phalen GS, Kendrick JI.** Compression neuropathy of the median nerve in the carpal tunnel. *JAMA* 1957; **164**:524–30.

39 **Marshall SC, Tardif G, Ashworth NL.** Local corticosteroid injection for carpal tunnel syndrome. *Cochrane Data Syst Rev* 2007, Issue 2. Art. No.: CD001554. DOI: 10.1002/14651858.CD001554. pub2.

40 **Denny-Brown D.** Primary sensory neuropathy with muscular changes associated with carcinoma. *J Neurol Neurosurg Psychiatry* 1948; **11**:73–87.

41 **Denny-Brown D.** Neurological conditions resulting from prolonged and severe dietary restriction. *Medicine* 1947; **26**:41–116.

42 **Nageotte, J.** Neurophages in transplants of spinal ganglion. REVUE NEUROL 1907; **15**:933–944.

43 **Wyburn-Mason R.** Bronchial carcinoma presenting as polyneuritis. *Lancet* 1948; **1**:203–7.

44 **Graus F, Cordon-Cardo C, Posner JB.** Neuronal antinuclear antibody in sensory neuronopathy from lung cancer. *Neurology* 1985; **35**:538–43.

45 **Brain WR, Norris FH Jr (eds).** *The Remote Effects of Cancer on the Nervous System*. New York: Grune & Stratton; 1965.

46 Darnell RB, Posner JB. *Paraneoplastic Syndromes (Contemporary Neurology Series)*. Oxford University Press, USA. 2011.

47 Nobile-Orazio E. Update on neuropathies associated with monoclonal gammopathy of undetermined significance (2008–10). *J Peripher Nerv Syst* 2010; **15**:302–6.

48 Chinn JS, Schuffler MD. Paraneoplastic visceral neuropathy as a cause of severe gastrointestinal motor dysfunction. *Gastroenterology* 1988; **95**:1279–86.

49 Maverakis E, Goodarzi H, Wehrli LN, Ono Y, Garcia MS. The etiology of paraneoplastic autoimmunity. *Clinic Rev Allerg Immunol* 2012; **42**:135–44.

50 Antoine J-C, Camdessanché J-P. Paraneoplastic disorders of the peripheral nervous system. *Presse Med* 2013; 42(6):e235–e244. Available at: <http://dx.doi.org/10.1016/j.lpm.2013.01.059>.

51 Graus F, Dalmau J. Paraneoplastic neuropathies. *Curr Opin Neurol* 2013; **26**:489–95.

52 Helmholtz H, Baxt N. *Neue Versuche uber die Fortpflanzungsgeschwindigkeit der Reizung in Motorischen Nerven des Menschen*. Wissenschaften (Berlin): M ber Kgl Preuss Akad; 1870; 184–91.

53 Adrian ED, Bronk DW. The discharge of impulses in motor nerve fibres: part II. The frequency of discharge in reflex and voluntary contractions. *J Physiol* 1929; **67**:119–51.

54 Hodes R, Larrabee MG, German W. The human EMG in response to nerve stimulation and the conduction velocity of motor axons. *Arch Neurol Psychiat* 1948; **60**:340–65.

55 Buchthal F, Rosenfalck A. Evoked action potentials and conduction velocities in human sensory nerves. *Brain Res* 1966; **3**:1–119.

56 Lambert EH. Electromyography and electric stimulation of peripheral nerves and muscle. In: *Clinical Examinations in Neurology (Mayo Clinic)*. Philadelphia: Saunders; 1956; 287–317.

57 Henrikson JD. Conduction velocity of nerves in normal subjects and patients with neuromuscular disorders. Thesis (M.S.Phys.Med.) University of Minnesota; 1956.

58 Dawson GD, Scott JW. The recording of nerve action potentials through skin in man. *J Neurol Neurosurg Psychiatry* 1949; **12**:259–67.

59 Gilliatt RW, Sears TA. Sensory nerve action potentials in patients with peripheral nerve lesions. *J Neurol Neurosurg Psychiatry* 1958; **21**:109–18.

60 Simpson JA. Electrical signs in the diagnosis of carpal tunnel and related syndromes. *J Neurol Neurosurg Psychiatry* 1956; **19**:275–80.

61 Holland NR, Crawford TO, Hauer P, Cornblath DR, Griffin JW, McArthur JC. Small-fiber sensory neuropathies: clinical course and neuropathology of idiopathic cases. *Ann Neurol* 1998; **44**:47–59.

62 Andrade C. Peculiar form of peripheral neuropathy: familiar atypical generalized amyloidosis with special involvement of the peripheral nerves. *Brain* 1952; **75**:408–27.

63 Villanueva T. Corino de Andrade: neurologist who discovered and gave his name to a hereditary form of amyloidosis. *BMJ* 2005; **331**:163.

64 Coutinho P, Martins da Silva A, Lopes Lima J, Resende Barbosa A. Forty years of experience with type I amyloid neuropathy. Review of 483 cases. In: Glenner G, Costa P, de Freitas, A (eds). *Amyloid and Amyloidosis*. Amsterdam: Execerpta Medica; 1980; 88–98.

65 Tawara S, Nakazato M, Kangawa K, Matsuo H, Araki S. Identification of amyloid prealbumin variant in familial amyloidotic polyneuropathy (Japanese type). *Biochem Biophys Res Commun* 1983; **116**:880–8.

66 Dwulet FE, Benson MD. Primary structure of an amyloid prealbumin and its plasma precursor in a heredofamilial polyneuropathy of Swedish origin. *Proc Nat Acad Sci* 1984; **81**: 694–8.

67 Kanda Y, Goodman DS, Canfield RE, Morgan FJ. The amino acid sequence of human plasma pre-albumin. *J Biol Chem* 1974; **249**:6796–805.

68 Saraiva MJM, Birken S, Costa PP, Goodman DS. Family studies of the genetic abnormality in transthyretin (prealbumin) in Portuguese patients with familial amyloidotic polyneuropathy. *Ann NY Acad Sci* 1984; **435**:86–100.

69 Holmgren G, Steen L, Ekstedt J, et al. Biochemical effect of liver transplantation in two Swedish patients with familial amyloidotic polyneuropathy (FAP-met30). *Clin Genet* 1991; **40**:242–6.

70 Benson MD. Liver transplantation and transthyretin amyloidosis. *Muscle Nerve* 2013; **47**:157–62.

71 Coelho T, Maia LF, Martins da Silva A, et al. Tafamidis for transthyretin familial amyloid polyneuropathy: a randomized, controlled trial. *Neurology* 2012; **79**:785–92.

72 Benson MD, Kluve-Beckerman B, Zeldenrust SR, et al. Targeted suppression of an amyloidogenic transthyretin with antisense oligonucleotides. *Muscle Nerve* 2006; **33**:609–18.

73 Coelho T, Adams D, Silva A, Lozeron P, Hawkins PN, Mant T. Safety and efficacy of RNAi therapy for transthyretin amyloidosis. *N Engl J Med* 2013; **369**:819–29.

74 Targowla J. Polynevrite recidivante, envahissement des nerfs craniens et diplegie faciale. *Rev Neurolog* 1894; **2**:465–72.

75 Austin JH. Recurrent polyneuropathies and their corticosteroid treatment. *Brain* 1958; **81**:157–92.

76 Van Den Bergh PY, Hadden RD, Bouche P, et al. European Federation of Neurological Societies/ Peripheral Nerve Society guideline on management of chronic inflammatory demyelinating polyradiculoneuropathy: report of a joint task force of the European Federation of Neurological Societies and the Peripheral Nerve Society—first revision. *Eur J Neurol* 2010; **17**:356–63.

77 Dyck PJ, Lais AC, Ohta M, Bastron JA, Okazaki H, Groover RV. Chronic inflammatory polyradiculoneuropathy. *Mayo Clin Proc* 1975; **50**:621–51.

78 Prineas JW, McLeod JG. Chronic relapsing polyneuritis. *J Neurol Sci* 1976; **27**:427–58.

79 Prineas JW. Demyelination and remyelination in recurrent idiopathic polyneuropathy. An electron microscope study. *Acta Neuropathol* 1971; **18**:34–57.

80 Vallat J-M, Sommer C, Magy L. Chronic inflammatory demyelinating polyradiculoneuropathy: diagnostic and therapeutic challenges for a treatable condition. *Lancet Neurol* 2010; **9**:402–12.

81 Dyck PJ, O'Brien PC, Oviatt KF, et al. Prednisone improves chronic inflammatory demyelinating polyradiculoneuropathy more than no treatment. *Ann Neurol* 1982; **11**:136–41.

82 Eftimov F, Vermeulen M, van Doorn PA, Brusse E, van Schaik IN, PREDICT. Long-term remission of CIDP after pulsed dexamethasone or short-term prednisolone treatment. *Neurology* 2012; **78**:1079–84.

83 Vermeulen M, van der Meché FG, Speelman JD, Weber A, Busch HF. Plasma and gamma-globulin infusion in chronic inflammatory polyneuropathy. *J Neurol Sci* 1985; **70**:317–26.

84 Dyck PJ, Daube J, O'Brien P, et al. Plasma exchange in chronic inflammatory demyelinating polyradiculoneuropathy. *N Engl J Med* 1986; **314**:461–5.

85 Mahdi-Rogers M, van Doorn PA, Hughes RAC. Immunomodulatory treatment other than corticosteroids, immunoglobulin and plasma exchange for chronic inflammatory demyelinating polyradiculoneuropathy. *Cochrane Data Syst Rev* 2013, Issue 6. Art. No.: CD003280. DOI: 10.1002/14651858.CD003280.pub4.

86 Nobile-Orazio E, Cocito D, Jann S, et al. Intravenous immunoglobulin versus intravenous methylprednisolone for chronic inflammatory demyelinating polyradiculoneuropathy: a randomised controlled trial. *Lancet Neurol* 2012; **11**:493–502.

87 Sharkey SJ. On peripheral neuritis. *BMJ* 1896; **1**:456–8.

88 Spatz H. Die 'systematischen atrophien.' Eine wohlgekennzeichnete gruppe der erbkrankheiten des nervesnsystems. *Arch Psych Nervenkrankj* 1938; **108**:1–18.

89 Spatz H. *La maladie de Pick, les atrophies systematisées progressives et al senescence cérébrale pre-maturée localisée*. First International Congress of Neuropathology, Rome, 1952; 2:375.

90 Greenfield JG. *The Spinocerebellar Degenerations*. Oxford: Blackwell; 1954.

91 Cavanagh JB. The significance of the 'dying back' process in experimental and human neurological diseases. *Int Rev Exper Pathol* 1964; **3**:219–67.

92 Spencer PS, Schaumburg HH, Ludolph AC. *Experimental and Clinical Neurotoxicology*, 2nd ed. New York: Oxford University Press; 2000.

93 Spencer PS, Schaumbug HH. Central–peripheral distal axonopathy the pathology of dying-back polyneuropathies. *Prog Neuropathol* 1976; **3**:253–95.

94 Coleman MP. The challenges of axon survival: introduction to the special issue on axonal degeneration. *Exp Neurol* 2013; **246**:1–5.

95 Fischer-Hayes LR, et al. Axonal degeneration in the peripheral nervous system: implications for the pathogenesis of amyotrophic lateral sclerosis. *Exp Neurol* 2013; **246**:6–13.

96 Kanai K, Kuwabara S, Misawa S, et al. Altered axonal excitability properties in amyotrophic lateral sclerosis: impaired potassium channel function related to disease stage. *Brain* 2006; **129**:953–62.

97 Argyriou AA, Bruna J, Marmiroli P, Cavaletti G. Chemotherapy-induced peripheral neurotoxicity (CIPN): an update. *Crit Rev Oncol Hematol* 2012; **82**:51–77.

98 Cavaletti G, et al. The chemotherapy-induced peripheral neuropathy outcome measures standardization study: from consensus to the first validity and reliability findings. *Ann Oncol* 2013; **24**:454–62.

99 Binda D, et al. Rasch-built Overall Disability Scale for patients with chemotherapy-induced peripheral neuropathy (CIPN-R-ODS). *Eur J Cancer* 2013; **49**:2910–8.

100 Albers JW, Chaudhry V, Cavaletti G, Donehower RC. Interventions for preventing neuropathy caused by cisplatin and related compounds. *Cochrane Data Syst Rev* 2011; (2):CD005228. doi: 10.1002/14651858.CD005228.pub3.

101 Marchal de Calvi C-J. *Recherches sur les Accidents Diabétiques et Essai d'une Théorie Générale du Diabète*. Paris: P. Asselin; 1864.

102 Pryce TD. On diabetic neuritis, with a clinical and pathological description of three cases of diabetic pseudo-tabes. *Brain* 1893; **16**:416–24.

103 Martin MM. Diabetic neuropathy. A clinical study of 150 cases. *Brain* 1953; **76**:594–624.

104 Pirart J. Diabetic neuropathy: a metabolic or a vascular disease? *Diabetes* 1965; **14**:1–9.

105 Caravati CM. Insulin neuritis: a case report. *Va Med Mon* 1933; **59**:745–56.

106 Mulder DW, Lambert EH, Bastron JA, Sprague RG. The neuropathies associated with diabetes mellitus. A clinical and elctromyographic study of 103 unselected diabetic outpatients. *Neurology* 1962; **11**:275–84.

107 Liberson WT. Determination of conduction velocities in the sensory nerve fibres. *Electroenceph Clin Neurophysiol* 1961; **13**:319.

108 Eliasson SG. Nerve conduction changes in experimental diabetes. *J Clin Invest* 1964; **43**:2353–8.

109 Gabbay KH. Role of sorbitol pathway in neuropathy. *Adv Metab Dis* 1973; **2**(suppl 2):417–24.

110 Greene DA, De Jesus PV, Winegrad AI. Effects of insulin and dietary myoinositol on impaired peripheral motor nerve conduction velocity in acute streptozotocin diabetes. *J Clin Invest* 1975; **55**:1326–36.

111 Dyck PJ, Karnes JI, Daube J, O'Brien PC, Service FJ. Clinical and neuropathological criteria for the diagnosis and staging of diabetic polyneuropathy. *Brain* 1985; **108**:861–80.

112 Dyck PJ, Davies JL, Litchy WJ, O'Brien PC. Longitudinal assessment of diabetic polyneuropathy using a composite score in the Rochester Diabetic Neuropathy Study cohort. *Neurology* 1997; **49**:229–39.

113 Obrosova IG. Diabetic painful and insensate neuropathy: pathogenesis and potential treatments. *Neurotherapeutics* 2009; **6**:638–47.

114 **Gibbons CH, Freeman R, Tecilazich F, et al.** The evolving natural history of neurophysiologic function in patients with well-controlled diabetes. *J Peripher Nerv Syst* 2013; **18**:153–61.

115 **Guillain G, Barré JA, Strohl A.** Sur un syndrome de radiculo-névrite avec hyperalbuminose du liquide céphalo-rachidien sans réaction cellulaire. Remarques sur les caractéres cliniques et graphiques des réflexes tendineux. *Bull Soc Méd Hôp Paris* 1916; **40**:1462–70.

116 **Asbury AK, Arnason BG, Adams RD.** The inflammatory lesion in idiopathic polyneuritis. Its role in pathogenesis. *Medicine* 1969; **48**:173–215.

117 **Feasby TE, Gilbert JJ, Brown WF, et al.** An acute axonal form of Guillain-Barré polyneuropathy. *Brain* 1986; **109**:1115–26.

118 **Feasby TE, Hahn AF, Brown WF, Bolton CF, Gilbert JJ, Koopman WJ.** Severe axonal degeneration in acute Guillain-Barre syndrome: evidence of two different mechanisms? *J Neurol Sci* 1993; **116**:185–92.

119 **McKhann GM, Cornblath DR, Ho TW, Li CY, Bai AY, Wu HS.** Clinical and electrophysiological aspects of acute paralytic disease of children and young adults in northern China. *Lancet* 1991; **338**:593–7.

120 **Griffin JW, Li CY, Ho TW, et al.** Guillain-Barré syndrome in northern China. The spectrum of neuropathological changes in clinically defined cases. *Brain* 1995; **118**:577–95.

121 **Yuki N, Hartung HP.** Guillain-Barré syndrome. *N Engl J Med* 2012; **366**:2294–304.

122 **Ilyas AA, Willison HJ, Quarles RH, et al.** Serum antibodies to gangliosides in Guillain-Barré syndrome. *Ann Neurol* 1988; **23**:440–7.

123 **Yuki N, Yamada M, Koga M, et al.** Animal model of axonal Guillain-Barre syndrome induced by sensitization with GM1 ganglioside. *Ann Neurol* 2001; **49**:712–20.

124 **McGonigal R, Rowan EG, Greenshields KN, et al.** Anti-GD1a antibodies activate complement and calpain to injure distal motor nodes of Ranvier in mice. *Brain* 2010; **133**:1944–60.

125 **Hughes RA, Swan AV, van Doorn PA.** Intravenous immunoglobulin for Guillain-Barre syndrome. *Cochrane Data Syst Rev* 2012;7:CD002063.

126 **Hughes RA, van Doorn PA.** Corticosteroids for Guillain-Barre syndrome. *Cochrane Data Syst Rev* 2012; **8**:CD001446.

127 **Raphael JC, Chevret S, Hughes RA, Annane D.** Plasma exchange for Guillain-Barre syndrome. *Cochrane Data Syst Rev* 2012; 7:CD001798.

Chapter 14

Neuromuscular junction disorders

Satoshi Kuwabara

14.0 **Introduction**

The neuromuscular junction is a specialized synapse with a complex structural and functional organization. The blood–nerve barrier is deficient in the neuromuscular junction and, therefore, it is a target for a variety of antibody-mediated immunological disorders. The understanding of the immunological basis of myasthenia gravis (MG), the most common neuromuscular junction disorder, has expanded in the recent years. Whereas most patients have antibodies to the acetylcholine receptor, novel antibodies against muscle-specific tyrosine kinase were identified, and the antibodies define a different subgroup of MG.

The early descriptions of MG date back to the seventeenth century, by Thomas Willis, and the disorder acquired its name at the end of the nineteenth century; 'gravis' is Latin for grievous or serious, although more development of modern immune-modulating treatments has resulted in significant improvement in the prognosis. Myasthenic crises can now be successfully managed by plasma exchange or intravenous immunoglobulin therapy with modern ventilatory support systems, and for refractory MG, calcineurin inhibitors such as tacrolimus and cyclosporin are frequently used and, most recently, anti-CD20 (B cell marker) monoclonal antibody is being assessed. Thymectomy has been recommended for early-onset MG, but the positive effects of thymectomy for patients without thymoma has not been established by controlled trials. To solve this issue, an international multi-centre randomized trial (thymectomy and MG clinical challenge: MGTX study) is currently underway.

In this chapter, 10 papers on the three representative disorders of the neuromuscular junction— MG, Lambert-Eaton myasthenic syndrome, and congenital myasthenic syndrome—are described. Some deal with historical perspectives on the concept of the disease, and others, with recent advances on immunological, molecular–biological, and genetic researches. I hope that the selected papers will be of both clinical and scientific interest, and lead to further discussion for readers.

14.1 **The first recognition of myasthenia gravis as a clinical entity**

Main paper: Willis T. *De Anima Brutorum Quae Hominis Vitalis ac Sensitiva est*. Oxford: Ric Davis; 1672.

Background

The clinical picture of MG is usually distinctive, with muscle weakness and associated fatigability. The early clinical descriptions date back to the seventeenth century, by physicians who carefully enquired into the clinical history. MG was first recognized as a disease entity by Thomas Willis, in 1672, in his monograph. However, it was written in Latin, and therefore largely went unnoticed until his work was later re-introduced by Guthrie, in the *Lancet*, in 1903 [1].

Methods

Thomas Willis (1621–1674) is well-known as an anatomist, and described the 'Circle of Willis'. He occupied the Chair of Natural Philosophy at Oxford, and gave a series of lectures—not on philosophy though, but on anatomy, physiology, and pathology. These lectures and his notes were published as textbooks, all in Latin; one of them was published as *De Anime Brutorum* ('on function of the brain' in English) in 1672. Willis appeared to be familiar with MG, and described patients with clinical presentations consistent with MG.

Results

In the chapter, 'On the palsy' (translated), Willis described 'patients who in the morning are able to walk firmly, to fling their arms, or to take up any heavy things, but before noon they are scarce able to move hand or foot'. He also described 'a woman, who for many years have been obnoxious bulbar palsy and limb weakness; she can speak freely and readily enough, but after she has spoken long, or hastily, or eagerly, she is not able to speak a word, but becomes mute as a fish'. Willis had traced peripheral nerves to their destination in muscles. He also believed that there was a substance circulating in the blood, which he called the 'explosive copula', and that it was fluctuation of the amount of this substance that caused the 'palsy' [2].

Conclusions and critique

Willis was writing Latin and inventing new words to explain his teaching. In anatomical terms, his findings were clear, but in respect to physiology and the more general theories about the disease, his meaning remains somewhat obscure. However, he certainly described cases of MG probably for the first time as a clinical disease entity.

14.2 **The first clinical descriptions of myasthenia gravis**

Main paper: Wilks S. Cerebritis, hysteria, and bulbar paralysis, as illustrative of arrest of function of the cerebrospinal centres. *Guy's Hosp Rep* 1877; 22:7–55.

Background and methods

Over 200 years since the early descriptions of MG, the next report was undertaken by Sir Samuel Wilks (1824–1911), writing in English. Wilks was not a neurologist, and was for many years a consultant physician at Guy's Hospital, London. He published many papers in pathology, appearing in *Guy's Hospital Reports*, a journal which he edited [2]. The 1877 issue included a paper entitled 'Cerebritis, hysteria, and bulbar paralysis, as illustrative of arrest of function of the cerebrospinal centres' in which his MG patient was described (Fig. 14.1).

Results

His case of MG was described as 'bulbar paralysis; fatal; no disease was found'. A stout girl had strabismus, bulbar palsy, and limb weakness, fluctuating in course. Her house physician was inclined to regard the case as one of hysteria. She died of respiratory failure, presumably due to myasthenic crisis. Autopsy findings did not show any abnormality in the central nervous system.

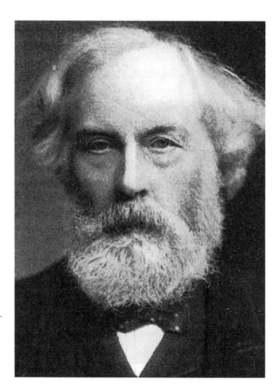

Fig. 14.1(a) Sir Samuel Wilks.
Reproduced from *J Neuromuscular Disorders*, 15, Hughes T, The early history of myasthenia gravis, p. 878–886, Copyright (2005), with permission from Elsevier.

ON

CEREBRITIES, HYSTERIA, AND BULBAR
PARALYSIS,

AS ILLUSTRATIVE OF

ARREST OF FUNCTION OF THE CEREBRO-SPINAL CENTRES.

————

By SAMUEL WILKS, M.D.

Fig. (b) Wilks's paper on myasthenia gravis.
Reproduced from *Guy's Hosp Rep*, 22, p. 7–55, (1877).

Conclusions and critique

Wilks was a pathologist and familiar with the bulbar palsy of motor neuron disease and findings of the neuronal loss and gliosis in the cranial nuclei. He discussed hysteria, and dismissed it as an explanation of the weakness. Although there was no clear statement that the patient suffered from MG, this was considered the first case in English literature. In 1879, German neurologist, Wilhelm Erb (1840–1921), described three cases of MG in the first paper dealing entirely with this disorder [3]. Erb distinguished these cases from 'progressive bulbar palsy' (bulbar-onset amyotrophic lateral sclerosis) because they did not follow the inexorable downhill course.

14.3 **How myasthenia gravis acquired its name**

Main paper: Jolly F. Ueber myasthenia gravis pseudoparalytica. *Berlin Klin Wochenschr* 1895; 32:1–4.

Background and results

Several attempts were made to name the new disease. In German literature, it was called Erb's disease (it has never been called Willis's disease). In 1895, Friedrich Jolly (1844–1904) presented two cases at a meeting of the Berlin Society, under the title 'myasthenia gravis pseudo-paralytica', the first two words of which have persisted to this day. Myasthenia comes from the Greek words for 'muscle' and 'weakness', and gravis is Latin for 'grievous' or 'serious'.

Conclusions and critique

For the name of MG, the mixture of Greek and Latin appears regrettable. Furthermore, gravis is currently inappropriate for the mild cases, particularly ocular myasthenia. It is understandable that at the time of Jolly's description, myasthenic crisis certainly meant death due to respiratory failure, but in contemporary usage, the terminology should reflect modern treatments and the fact that over 60% of patients have long-lasting remission or only ocular symptoms, with death due to MG being very rare [4]. Moreover, 'gravis' gives an unnecessary fear for MG patients, and neurologists require additional time to explain this condition. In the future, 'gravis' should ideally be removed, and a more appropriate term should be considered by an international advisory board.

14.4 **The first symptomatic treatment for myasthenia gravis: the miracle of St Alfege's**

Main paper: Walker MB. Treatment of myasthenia gravis with physostigmine. *Lancet* 1934; i:1200–1. (As seen in '1935 prostigmin demonstration for MG', YouTube, http://video.search.yahoo.co.jp/search?ei=UTF-8&fr=top_ga1_sa&p=mary+walker+mg)

Background

As medical treatments for MG, strychnine, arsenic, and iodides were tried, up to the 1930s, without clinical benefit. In 1934, a brief but remarkable letter was published in the *Lancet* describing the beneficial effect of physostigmine on the symptoms of MG. The author was Mary Broadfoot Walker (1888–1974). She described that 'the abnormal fatigability in MG has been thought to be due to curare-like poisoning of the motor nerve-endings or of the myoneural junctions in the affected muscles'. In the same year, Sir Henry Dale's Nobel Prize winning work showed acetylcholine as a neurotransmitter at the neuromuscular junction [5].

Results

Dr Mary Walker, a house physician at St Alfege's Hospital, Greenwich, London, had in her care a 56-year-old woman with MG. In April 1934, this patient was seen by the visiting neurologist, Derek Denny-Brown (1901–1981). The diagnosis was probably not in doubt, but the neurologist explained to Dr Walker that the syndrome resembled the effect of curare poisoning. Dr Walker, reading that the effect of curare could be reversed by injecting physostigmine, tried this drug on her patient, with remarkable improvement of the paresis (Fig. 14.2).

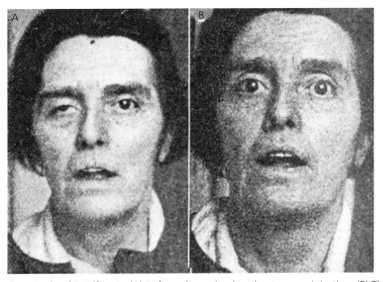

Fig. 14.2 The miracle of St Alfege's. (A) Before physostigmin subcutaneous injection. (B) Thirty minutes after injection, the eye was fully open.
Reproduced from *Lancet*, i, Walker MB, Treatment of myasthenia gravis with physostigmine, p. 1200–1201, Copyright (1934), with permission from Elsevier.

Subsequently, Dr Walker treated a second case, a 40-year-old woman. On this occasion, she used prostigmine, recommended to her by Philip Hamil, a pharmacology colleague at St Alfeges's [6]. Prostigmine had recently been synthesized, and was marketed by Roche. This case was described at a meeting of the Royal Society of Medicine in December 1934, and, in the following year, published in the Proceedings [6].

Conclusions and critique

It is interesting how Mary Walker came up with the idea of using physostigmine. The story was written up in a letter by Derek Denny-Brown (consultant at St Alfege's Hospital) to Daniel B. Drachman, in which he described his conversation with Mary Walker about the MG patient [7]:

> Denny-Brown (D-B): "This is myasthenia gravis." Mary Walker (MW): "What's that?"
>
> D-B: "It is a muscular disorder of unknown aetiology."
>
> MW: "What is the cause?"
>
> D-B told her arrow poisoning and some patients at Queen Square.
>
> MW: "Where did my patient get curare?"
>
> D-B: "This is not curare poisoning, only resembling it."
>
> Somewhat later . . .
>
> MW: "May I have permission to give that patient with myasthenia some physostigmine?"
>
> D-W: "Go ahead."

The detailed story is described in a review article by John C. Keesey [7]. After 'the miracle of St Alfege's', the many drugs used to treat myasthenia take the subject beyond this review. First in 1947, and more effectively in 1954, pyridostigmine (Mestinon) was tried [2]. Cholinesterase inhibitors were then set to become the mainstay of symptomatic treatment of MG.

14.5 **Thymic abnormalities and thymectomy for myasthenia gravis**

Main paper: Blalock A, Mason MF, Morgan HJ, Riven SS. Myasthenia and tumours of the thymus gland, report of a case in which the tumour was removed. *Ann Surg* 1939; 110:554–61.

Related paper: Blalock A. Thymectomy in the treatment of myasthenia gravis, report of 20 cases. *Thoracic Surg* 1944; 13:316–39.

Background

In 1901, Leopold Laquer (1857–1915) from Frankfurt presented an autopsy case of MG at a German meeting: a 55-year-old female patient showed a malignant lymphoma in the anterior mediastinum. The association of MG and the thymus then drew attention. In 1917, Elexious Thompson Bell (1880–1963) found that the thymus was abnormal in at least half of MG cases [8]. Gordon Holmes (1876–1965; National Hospital, Queen Square, London), in 1923, reported tumour or hyperplasia of the thymus in six out of eight MG patients [9]. These findings aroused interest in thymectomy as a treatment of MG.

Results

In 1936, Alfred Blalock (1899–1964), the pioneer heart surgeon at Johns Hopkins Hospital, Baltimore, performed a thymectomy on a girl of 19 years with severe generalized myasthenia. X-rays showed a dense shadow in the thymus. He operated during a remission, and the myasthenia disappeared. Twenty-one years later, the patient was well. She had suffered only a few mild remissions of myasthenia, related to other illnesses. In 1941, Blalock operated on six myasthenic patients, removing the entire thymus, which, in all cases, was grossly normal. All recovered well from the operation and, a month later, required no medication. In 1944, Blalock reported successful operations on 20 patients, of which two had thymus tumours.

Conclusions and critique

Since Blalock's report, many MG patients have undergone thymectomy, initially at Queen Square and, since the 1940s, the Mayo Clinic [2]. Thymectomy, with or without the presence of thymoma, has gained widespread acceptance as a form of treatment for MG. However, a randomized controlled study of the effectiveness of thymectomy has never been done, and the role of thymectomy in the management of MG remains uncertain, particularly for patients without thymoma. Nevertheless, physicians have to advise their patients regarding the benefits of thymectomy based on the existing literature. In 2000, a meta analysis by the Subcommittee of the American Academy of Neurology showed that the benefit of thymectomy in non-thymomatous autoimmune MG has not been firmly established. The conclusion is that 'for patients with nonthymomatous autoimmune MG, thymectomy is recommended as an option to increase the probability of remission or improvement' [10]. This report was somewhat shocking for neurologists, and the subject is still controversial. To solve the issue, an international multi-centre randomized trial (thymectomy and myasthenia gravis clinical challenge: MGTX study) is ongoing [11].

The current rationale for thymectomy in MG is supported by experimental evidence. Available data suggest that MG may begin in the thymus by, as yet, enigmatic triggers, and is maintained there by an ongoing pathological immune reaction. This pathological immune reaction involves peptides derived from acethylcholine receptor subunits that are expressed by medullary thymic epithelial cells and, likely, prime autoreactive T cells [12, 13]. In this regard, thymectomy is a fundamental treatment for MG, at least theoretically, but it is possible that sensitized T cells have already moved to peripheral lymph nodes during the disease. Currently, many neuroimmunologists are eagerly waiting for the conclusive results of the international MGTX study.

14.6 **An autoimmune hypothesis in myasthenia gravis**

Main paper: Simpson JA. Myasthenia gravis: a new hypothesis. *Scottish Med J* 1960; 5:419–36.

Background

The accumulation of thymectomized MG cases proved a fertile area of research. In 1960, John Simpson proposed that MG is caused by an autoimmune action directed against the motor end plates.

Results

John Alexander Simpson (1922–2009) was a neurologist at the Northern General Hospital, Edinburgh and, later, Editor in Chief of the *Journal of Neurology, Neurosurgery and Psychiatry*. In 1960, he proposed that MG is an autoimmune response of muscle in which an antibody to end-plate protein may be formed (Fig. 14.3). His assumption was based on a detailed analysis of 440 cases and of the literature, in which he identified several common factors:

1 female dominancy

2 peak of onset age in the 20s

3 frequent association of established autoimmune diseases such as pure red cell dysplasia, rheumatoid arthritis, and immune-mediated thyroid diseases

4 pathological evidence of lymphocytic infiltration in the skeletal muscles

5 association of thymoma or thymic hyperplasia

6 electrophysiological evidence of impaired neuromuscular transmission.

He mentioned that no other theory could explain all the phenomena, clinical and experimental.

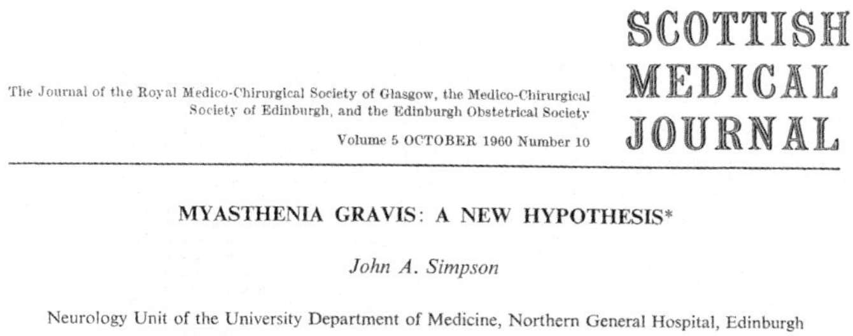

SCOTTISH
MEDICAL
JOURNAL

The Journal of the Royal Medico-Chirurgical Society of Glasgow, the Medico-Chirurgical Society of Edinburgh, and the Edinburgh Obstetrical Society

Volume 5 OCTOBER 1960 Number 10

MYASTHENIA GRAVIS: A NEW HYPOTHESIS*

John A. Simpson

Neurology Unit of the University Department of Medicine, Northern General Hospital, Edinburgh

Fig. 14.3 Myasthenia gravis: a new hypothesis.

Reproduced from *Scottish Medical Journal*, 5, John A Simpson, Myasthenia gravis: a new hypothesis, p. 419–36, Copyright (1960), with permission from SAGE.

Conclusions and critique

Simpson had a keen and prescient insight into the pathogenesis of MG. The autoimmune hypothesis has been proved by the discovery of anti-acetylcholine receptor antibodies and their blocking effect on neuromuscular transmission, by development of animal models immunized with acetylcholine receptor proteins [14], and by the effects of immune-modulating treatments with corticosteroids, immunosuppressants, plasma exchange, and immunoglobulin infusion [15, 16].

14.7 **Establishment of anti-acetylcholine receptor antibody assay in myasthenia gravis**

Main paper: Lindstrom JM, Seybold ME, Lennon VA, Whittingham S, Duane DD. Antibody to acetylcholine receptor in myasthenia gravis. Prevalence, clinical correlates, and diagnostic value. *Neurology* 1976; 26:1054–9.

Background

Since Simpson's autoimmune hypothesis for MG, many researchers looked for antibodies against a neuromuscular junction structure, particularly acetylcholine receptors (AChR). MG patients' sera were first assayed for AChR antibodies by inhibition of a-bungarotoxin binding to AChR from denervated rat muscle or by complement fixation using purified receptor from the Pacific electric ray, *Torpedo californica* [17]. Soon after, a radio-immunoprecipitation assay was developed using receptor from denervated human muscle, which expresses mainly the fetal isoform [18]. In 1976, Lindstrom and colleagues firstly showed the high specificity and sensitivity of a radio-immunoprecipitation assay in a sufficient number of patients and controls.

Results

Anti-AChR antibodies were measured in 69 patients with MG, 100 neurological controls, 54 autoimmune disease controls, and 19 normal controls. The antibodies were positive in 87% of MG patients, and in none of the control groups. The sensitivity was 87% and specificity 100% (Fig. 14.4).

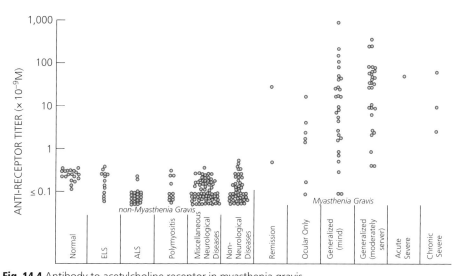

Fig. 14.4 Antibody to acetylcholine receptor in myasthenia gravis.

Reproduced from *Neurology*, 26, Lindstrorm JM, et al., Antibody to acetylcholine receptor in myasthenia gravis, p. 1054–1059, Copyright (1976), with permission from Lippincott Williams & Wilkins.

Conclusions and critique

Nine years later, in 1985, Angela Vincent and John Newsom-Davis (Oxford University, UK) reported results of 153 validated cases and 2967 diagnostic assays [19]. Currently, the routine detection and measurement of serum AChR auto-antibodies is widely performed on ^{125}I-α-bangarotoxin-labelled AChR [20]. The sensitivity is usually 80–85% in generalized MG, and the specificity is very high, although false positives may occur in patients with thymoma. At present, the AChR antibody assay is commercially available, and the antibody is used as a useful diagnostic biomarker in routine clinical practice.

In addition, one of the authors of the main paper, Vanda Lennon (Mayo Clinic, Rochester, Minnesota, USA), later identified anti-calcium channel antibodies in her husband Edward Lambert's eponymous myasthenic syndrome [21] (see section 14.9), as well as anti-aquaporin-4 antibodies in neuromyelitis optica, in 2005 [22]. All three antibodies have been subsequently shown to be directly associated with the pathogenesis of the respective disorders.

14.8 **Anti-MuSK antibodies in myasthenia gravis**

Main paper: Hoch W, McConville J, Helms S, Newsom-Davis J, Melms A, Vincent A. Auto-antibodies to the receptor tyrosine kinase MuSK in patients with myasthenia gravis without acetylcholine receptor antibodies. *Nat Med* 2001; 7:365–8.

Background

After the discovery and establishment of the anti-AChR antibody assay in MG, it was found that 15–20% of generalized MG patients do not have detectable anti-AChR antibodies, termed 'seronegative' MG. Searches for new antibodies in such patients led to the discovery of new antibodies against muscle-specific tyrosine kinase (MuSK) in 2001, and low-density lipoprotein receptor-related protein 4 (Lrp4) in 2011 [23].

Results

Samples were obtained from 24 patients (18 female, 6 male) with moderate or severe generalized MG in whom the standard radio-immunoprecipitation assay for anti-AChR antibodies was negative. All had typical fatigable muscle weakness. The diagnosis was confirmed by electromyographic evidence of a defect in neuromuscular transmission. The authors showed that 70% of AChR-Ab–seronegative MG patients, but not AChR-Ab–seropositive MG patients, had serum auto-antibodies against MuSK. The anti-MuSK antibodies were specific for the extracellular domains of MuSK expressed in transfected COS7 cells and strongly inhibited MuSK function in cultured myotubes.

Conclusions and critique

After the discovery of anti-MuSK antibody, MG is currently classified into three categories according to the antibody profile:

1 AChR-positive MG (80%)

2 MuSK-positive MG (10%)

3 Dual-seronegative MG (10%).

MuSK mediates the agrin-induced clustering of AChRs during synapse formation, and is also expressed at the mature neuromuscular junction. The exact pathophysiology of MuSK-MG is not fully understood, but measurement of MuSK antibodies aids diagnosis and clinical management. In 2011, the third antibody against low-density lipoprotein receptor-related protein 4 (Lrp4) was reported [19], but currently, this antibody is found only rarely among AChR-seronegative MG patients. Figure 14.5 shows localization of the major target molecules—voltage-gated calcium channel (VGCC), acetylcholine receptor (AChR), and muscle-specific tyrosine kinase (MuSK).

Clinically, MuSK-MG has a somewhat different phenotype from AChR-MG and the remaining seronegative MG [24–26]. MG with anti-MuSK antibodies was characterized by a striking prevalence of females (approximately 7.5:1); severe, predominantly facial and bulbar weakness (80%); and more frequent occurrence of atrophy of facial muscles and tongue [27]. Thymus pathology is less common in this subgroup of MG patients and, therefore, thymectomy may not be indicated. Repetitive nerve stimulation testing shows a low sensitivity [28]. The specific clinical presentation, the thymus pathology, and the therapeutic response implicate that MuSK-MG is a specific subgroup of MG. Recognizing these features is important in clinical practice.

In my experience, some MuSK-MG patients show prominent bulbar weakness without daily fluctuation and response to choline-esterase inhibitors, resembling bulbar-type amyotrophic lateral sclerosis. In such patients, jitter measurements, with single-fibre electromyography, may be normal in limb muscles but show prominent jitter in facial muscles [29, 30]. Assuming that MuSK protein is similarly expressed in limb and facial muscles, future studies will be required to elucidate mechanisms for predominant involvement of bulbar/facial muscles in MuSK-MG, and recognition of such a peculiar clinical phenotype is clinically important.

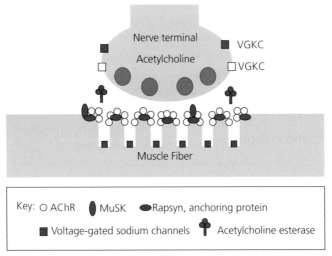

Fig. 14.5 Diagrammatic representation of the neuromuscular junction (NMJ) with the ion channels, muscle-specific kinase (MuSK), and acetylcholinesterase (AChE) that are essential for normal function. The cytoskeletal protein, rapsyn, helps to anchor the AChR. (VGKC: voltage-gated potassium channels; VGCC: voltage-gated calcium channels; MuSK: muscle-specific kinase; AChR: acetylcholine receptors.)

Reproduced from *Drug Discovery Today*, 4, Vincent A, Mechanisms in myasthenia gravis, p. 401–408, Copyright (2005), with permission from Elsevier.

14.9 **Lambert-Eaton myasthenic syndrome**

Main paper: Lambert EH, Eaton LM, Rooke ED. Defect of neuromuscular conduction associated with malignant neoplasms. *Am J Physiol* 1956; 187:612–3.

Related paper: Lennon VA, Kryzer TJ, Griesmann GE, et al. Calcium-channel antibodies in the Lambert-Eaton syndrome and other paraneoplastic syndromes. *N Engl J Med* 1995; 332:1467–74.

Background

In 1953, Anderson and colleagues described a 47-year-old man with progressive muscle weakness and diminished tendon reflexes [31]. After a small-cell lung carcinoma (SCLC) was surgically removed, the patient's improvement was striking. In 1956, Edward Lambert, Lee Eaton, and Edward Rooke, at the Mayo Clinic, described six similar cases. This syndrome has become known as Lambert–Eaton myasthenic syndrome (LEMS).

Results

Lambert and colleagues described six patients with a distinctive electrophysiological pattern seen by repetitive nerve stimulation (well-known as waxing). The report was in the abstract form and surprisingly short, described in only a half of a page. Forty years later, Vanda Lennon (Lambert's wife) identified the responsible antibodies [21]. The discovery of pathogenic auto-antibodies to VGCC has facilitated diagnosis and improved the understanding of the pathophysiological mechanisms leading to LEMS. The finding of functional VGCC on the SCLC provided an aetiological basis for the disorder, at least in those with an underlying carcinoma.

Conclusions and critique

LEMS is a neuromuscular autoimmune disease that has served as a model for autoimmunity and tumour immunology. Later studies have improved our diagnostic skills and knowledge of the pathophysiological mechanisms and association of LEMS with SCLC, and have aided early tumour detection.

However, not all LEMS patients have carcinoma. In the largest series including 50 patients with LEMS, 25 (50%) had carcinoma (of whom 21 had SCLC), but in the remaining 50%, no carcinoma was found after follow-up for years, indicating a subgroup of patients with autoimmune LEMS not triggered by neoplasm [32]. The presence or absence of carcinoma significantly affects treatment strategy for LEMS. For example, in LEMS patients with carcinoma, a single treatment of removal of anti-VGCC antibodies by plasma exchange would induce expansion of the tumour because the antibodies are primarily produced against antigens expressed on tumour cells.

14.10 **Congenital myasthenic syndromes**

Main paper: Engel AG, Lambert EH, Gomez MR. A new myasthenic syndrome with end-plate acetylcholinesterase deficiency, small nerve terminals, and reduced acetylcholine release. *Ann Neurol* 1977; 1:315–30.

Background

Congenital myasthenic syndromes (CMS) are genetic disorders of neuromuscular transmission that should be considered in the differential diagnosis of neuromuscular disorders. They are present at birth but may not manifest until childhood or adult life. CMS are heterogeneous disorders arising from pre-synaptic, synaptic, or post-synaptic defects. In each CMS, the specific defect compromises the safety margin of neuromuscular transmission by one or more mechanisms. In 1977, the first case of CMS due to acetylcholine esterase deficiency was described by Andrew Engel and colleagues (Mayo Clinic, Rochester, Minnesota, USA).

Results

Engel and colleagues described a patient whose symptoms began soon after birth and included generalized weakness increased by exertion, easy fatiguability, hyporeflexia, and refractoriness to anti-cholinesterase drugs. Electromyography showed a decremental response at all frequencies of stimulation and a repetitive response to single nerve stimulation. Acetylcholinesterase (AChE) was absent from the motor end plates by histochemical and electron cytochemical criteria. Biochemical studies indicated total absence of the endplate-specific 16 S species of AChE and marked decrease in total muscle AChE.

Conclusions and critique

In the present case, a congenital defect in the molecular assembly of AChE represents the basic abnormality and physiological alteration. After this report, the authors' group extensively examined many types of CMS, identifying pre-synaptic, synaptic, and post-synaptic defects, and ascertained the molecular bases underlying defects of AChR, rapsyn, Nav1.4, collagen Q, and choline acetyltransferase [33]. A classification system of CMS based on molecular genetics is under evolution. Clinical and neurophysiological correlations with molecular studies have defined diagnostic criteria that assist the clinician in identifying specific clinical subtypes of CMS [34]. Table 14.1 shows currently identified subtypes of CMS.

Table 14.1 Congenital neuromuscular junction disorders

---

1. Pre-synaptic defects
  Congenital MG + episodic apnoea (familial infantile): ChAT; 10q11
  Paucity of synaptic vesicles & reduced quantal release
  Congenital Lambert-Eaton-like
  Episodic ataxia 2: CACNA1A; 19p13
  Reduced quantal release

Table 14.1 (continued) Congenital neuromuscular junction disorders

2. Synaptic basal lamina defects
Acetylcholinesterase (AChE) deficiency at NMJs: ColQ; 3p25
Laminin β2 (LAMB2) deficiency: 3p21

3. Post-synaptic defects: AChR disorders; α, β, δ, e subunits
Kinetic abnormalities in AChR function
Reduced numbers of AChRs at NMJs
Slow AChR channel syndromes: increased response to ACh
Delayed channel closure: AChR mutations
Repeated channel re-openings: AChR mutations
Fast-channel syndromes: reduced response to ACh
Mode-switching kinetics disorder: AChR e subunit
Gating abnormality: AChR α or e subunit
Low ACh affinity: AChR δ or e subunit
Reduced expression & fast channel: AChR δ
Arthrogryposis: AChR δ subunit
Normal numbers of AChRs at NMJs: reduced response to ACh
Fast-channel syndrome: low ACh-affinity of AChR; AChR e subunit
Fast-channel syndrome: reduced channel openings; AChR α subunit
High conductance & fast closure of AChRs
Increased numbers of AChRs at NMJs
Slow AChR channel syndrome: AChR subunit βL262M
No kinetic abnormalities in AChR function
Reduced numbers of AChRs at NMJs
AChR mutations
Usually: e subunit; 17p13
Rarely, other subunits: α; 2q24, β; 17p12, δ; 2q33
Arthrogryposis syndromes
Recurrent congenital MG: maternal antibodies vs. fetal AChRs
Multiple pterygium syndrome (escobar): AChR γ-subunit mutations

4. Post-synaptic defects: other
Agrin: 1pter
MuSK: 9q31
Plectin deficiency: plectin; 8q24
Rapsyn: 11p11
Weakness + episodic apnoea & bulbar dysfunction: SCN4A; 17q35
Lethal congenital myopathy: contactin-1; 12q11
Limb-girdle MG + tubular aggregates 2: DPAGT1; 11q23

5. Pre-synaptic + Post-synaptic defects
Centro-nuclear myopathies
Limb-girdle MG; familial: Dok-7; 4p16
Limb-girdle MG + tubular aggregates: GFPT1; 2p13

6. Other hereditary MG syndromes
Congenital MG
Benign congenital MG & facial malformations: rapsyn
Congenital + acquired MG
Other
Familial immune
TPM3

Data from: Neuromuscular Disease Center, Washington University, USA. 2015. Myasthenia Gravis & Neuromuscular Junction (NMJ) Disorders. Available at: <http://neuromuscular.wustl.edu/synmg.html>

Key unanswered questions

As described in this chapter, our understanding of the immunological or genetic basis on the neuromuscular junction disorders has been extended and immune-modulating treatments and adequate management of myasthenic crisis have resulted in significant improvement in the prognosis. However, several issues remain unresolved or controversial.

1 Why is there a need for more effective treatment?

    An observational study involving 470 MG patients showed that 30% were in clinical remission (no symptoms with/without medication), 34% had only ocular symptoms, and the remaining 35% still had weakness of bulbar or limb muscles. The prognosis of MG is now generally favourable, but despite the frequent use of thymectomy and immunosuppressive treatments, approximately one-third of patients still have generalized weakness [4]. More effective or intensive treatments are required to improve the prognosis.

2 How effective is thymectomy as a treatment?

    If the trigger of antibody production in MG is an acethylcholine receptor subunit-like structure expressed by medullary thymic epithelial cells, theoretically, thymectomy is fundamental treatment for MG. However, there are no controlled randomized trials on the effects of thymectomy. An ongoing international multi-centre randomized trial (thymectomy and myasthenia gravis clinical challenge: MGTX study) will reach its conclusion in the near future.

3 Are there controlled randomized trials for MG and LEMS?

    Because of the relative rarity of the disorders, there are few controlled trials of immune-modulating therapy for MG and LEMS. Therefore, evidence-based data on treatment are limited. Future studies should be randomized controlled trials.

4 What is the best treatment for patients with anti-MuSK antibody?

    The antibody against MuSK defines a particular subgroup of MG. Thymectomy is not generally recommended, and responses to choline-esterase inhibitor may be poor in this subgroup. Optimal treatment for MuSK-MG should be established.

5 Why is it important to identify the underlying genetic defect in CMS?

    CMS are caused by genetic defects, leading to pre-synaptic, synaptic, and post-synaptic dysfunction. Phenotypes may vary widely and symptoms can be unspecific, therefore they are often missed. Most patients are eligible for drug therapy with esterase inhibitors, 3,4-diaminopyridine, ephedrine, fluoxetine, or quinidine, but the effect of these drugs differs depending on the underlying genetic defect. Currently, diagnostic work-up and care, including pharmacological treatments, should be improved.

References

1 **Guthrie L.** 'Myasthenia gravis' in the seventeenth century. *Lancet* 1903; **1**:330–1.

2 **Hughes T.** The early history of myasthenia gravis. *Neuromusc Disord* 2005; **15**:878–86.

3 **Erb W.** Zur casuistic der bulbaren lahmungen. (3) Uber einen neuen wahrscheinlich bulbaren symptomcomplex. *Archiv Psychiat Nervenkrank* 1899; **9**:336–50.

4 **Kawaguchi N, Kuwabara S, Nemoto Y, et al.**; Study Group for Myasthenia Gravis in Japan. Treatment and outcome of myasthenia gravis: retrospective multi-center analysis of 470 Japanese patients, 1999–2000. *J Neurol Sci* 2004; **224**: 43–7.

5 **Pearce JMS.** Mary Broadfoot Walker (1888–974): an historic discovery in myasthenia gravis. *Eur Neurol* 2005; **53**:51–3.

6 **Walker MB.** Case showing the effect of prostigmin on myasthenia gravis. *Proc Roy Soc Med* 1935; **28**:759–61.

7 **Keesey JC.** Historical neurology. Contemporary opinions about Mary Walker: a shy pioneer of therapeutic neurology. *Neurology* 1998; **51**:1433–9.

8 **Bell EJ.** Tumours of the thymus gland in myasthenia gravis. *J Nerv Ment Dis* 1917; **45**:130–43.

9 **Holmes G.** Discussion of a case presented to the Royal Society of Medicine. *Brain* 1923; **46**:237–41.

10 **Gronseth GS, Barohn RJ.** Practice parameter: thymectomy for autoimmune myasthenia gravis (an evidence-based review): report of the Quality Standards Subcommittee of the American Academy of Neurology. *Neurology* 2000; **55**:7–15.

11 **Aban IB, Wolfe GI, Cutter GR, et al; MGTX Advisory Committee.** The MGTX experience: challenges in planning and executing an international, multicenter clinical trial. *J Neuroimmunol* 2008; **201–2**:80–4.

12 **Link H, Xu ZY, Melms A, et al.** The T-cell repertoire in myasthenia gravis involves multiple cholinergic receptor epitopes. *Scand J Immunol* 1992; **36**:405–14.

13 **Melms A, Malcherek G, Gern U, et al.** T cells from normal and myasthenic individuals recognize the human acetylcholine receptor: heterogeneity of antigenic sites on the alpha-subunit. *Ann Neurol* 1992; **31**:311–8.

14 **Lennon VA, Lindstrom JM, Seybold ME.** Experimental autoimmune myasthenia: a model of myasthenia gravis in rats and guinea pigs. *J Exp Med* 1975; **141**:1365–75.

15. **Farrugia ME, Vincent A.** Autoimmune mediated neuromuscular junction defects. *Curr Opin Neurol* 2010; **23**:489–95.

16 **Benatar M, Kaminski H.** Medical and surgical treatment for ocular myasthenia. *Cochrane Database Syst Rev* 2012; **12**:CD005081.

17 **Almon RR, Andrew CG, Appel SH.** Serum globulin in myasthenia gravis: inhibition of alpha-bungarotoxin binding to acetylcholine receptors. *Science* 1974; **186**:55–7.

18 **Leite MI, Waters P, Vincent A.** Diagnostic use of autoantibodies in myasthenia gravis. *Autoimmunity* 2010; **43**:371–9.

19 **Vincent A, Newsom-Davis J.** Acetylcholine receptor antibody as a diagnostic test for myasthenia gravis: results in 153 validated cases and 2967 diagnostic assays. *J Neurol Neurosurg Psychiatry* 1985; **48**:1246–52.

20 **Vincent A.** Impact commentaries. Acetylcholine receptor antibody as a diagnostic test for myasthenia gravis: results in 153 validated cases and 2967 diagnostic assays. *J Neurol Neurosurg Psychiatry* 2012; **83**: 237–8.

21 **Lennon VA, Kryzer TJ, Griesmann GE, et al.** Calcium-channel antibodies in the Lambert-Eaton syndrome and other paraneoplastic syndromes. *N Engl J Med* 1995; **332**:1467–74.

22 Lennon VA, Kryzer TJ, Pittock SJ, Verkman AS, Hinson SR. IgG marker of optic-spinal multiple sclerosis binds to the aquaporin-4 water channel. *J Exp Med* 2005; **15**(202):473–7.

23 Higuchi O, Hamuro J, Motomura M, Yamanashi Y. Autoantibodies to low-density lipoprotein receptor-related protein 4 in myasthenia gravis. *Ann Neurol* 2011; **69**:418–22.

24 Lavrnic D, Losen M, Vujic A, et al. The features of myasthenia gravis with autoantibodies to MuSK. *J Neurol Neurosurg Psychiatry* 2005; **76**:1099–102.

25 Vincent A, Leite MI. Neuromuscular junction autoimmune disease: muscle specific kinase antibodies and treatments for myasthenia gravis. *Curr Opin Neurol* 2005; **18**:519–25.

26 Vincent A, McConville J, Farrugia ME, Newsom-Davis J. Seronegative myasthenia gravis. *Semin Neurol* 2004; **24**:125–33.

27 Takahashi H, Kawaguchi N, Ito S, Nemoto Y, Hattori T, Kuwabara S. Is tongue atrophy reversible in anti-MuSK myasthenia gravis? Six-year observation. *J Neurol Neurosurg Psychiatry* 2010; **81**:701–2.

28 Nemoto Y, Kuwabara S, Misawa S, et al. Patterns and severity of neuromuscular transmission failure in seronegative myasthenia gravis. *J Neurol Neurosurg Psychiatry* 2005; **76**:714–8.

29 Kuwabara S, Nemoto Y, Misawa S, Takahashi H, Kawaguchi N, Hattori T. Anti-MuSK-positive myasthenia gravis: neuromuscular transmission failure in facial and limb muscles. *Acta Neurol Scand* 2007; **115**:126–8.

30 Farrugia ME, Kennett RP, Newsom-Davis J, Hilton-Jones D, Vincent A. Single-fiber electromyography in limb and facial muscles in muscle-specific kinase antibody and acetylcholine receptor antibody myasthenia gravis. *Muscle Nerve* 2006; **33**:568–70.

31 Anderson HJ, Churchill-Davidson HC, Richardson AT. Bronchial neoplasm with myasthenia— prolonged apnoea after administration of succinylcholine. *Lancet* 1953; **265**:1291–3.

32 O'Neill JH, Murray NM, Newsom-Davis J. The Lambert-Eaton myasthenic syndrome. A review of 50 cases. *Brain* 1988; **111**:577–96.

33 Engel AG, Ohno K, Sine SM. Congenital myasthenic syndromes: recent advances. *Arch Neurol* 1999; **56**:163–7.

34 Palace J, Beeson D. The congenital myasthenic syndromes. *J Neuroimmunol* 2008; 201/2:2–5.

Chapter 15

Neuroimmunology

Angela Vincent

15.0 **Introduction**

My career has been so serendipitous that it has been difficult to think of a coherent manner in which to present these papers; the best method appears to be the order in which they came to inform and enhance my understanding of neuroscience and neurology, which is how they appear, rather than the chronological order. This partly reflects my strong preference, initially, for basic science and complete ignorance of the history of neurology until forced, by very good fortune, to start working on rare, fascinating diseases, most of which appear to have been described in detail—to some extent or another—by clinicians in the past.

The chapter falls into two sections, neuromuscular and central diseases, and I start by illustrating how the ingenuity of basic scientists, often not working in well-funded laboratories, can help to answer questions that they thought worthwhile, and which turn out to have much wider relevance.

15.1 **Discovery of neuromuscular toxins**

Main paper: Chang CC, Lee CY. Isolation of neurotoxins from the venom of bungarus multicinctus and their modes of neuromuscular blocking action. *Arch Int Pharmacodyn Ther* 1963;144:241–57.

Background

Dr Chuan-Chiung Chang was a pharmacologist working in Taiwan in the 1950s (Fig. 15.1), and this paper summarizes one aspect of the work that he painstakingly undertook at the College of Medicine in the National Taiwan University over 49 years. He started as the

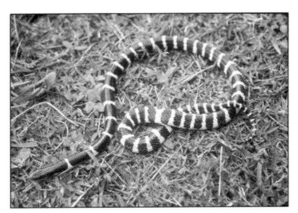

Fig. 15.1 (a) Bungarus multicinctus, the Taiwan banded krait.

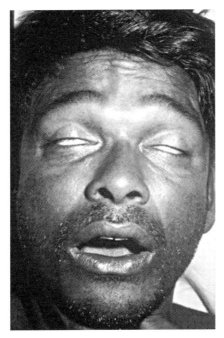

Fig. (b) A patients suffering from krait envenomation. Notice the ptosis and extraocular muscle paralysis, the floppy jaw and tongue, but the furrowed brow as he attempts to open his eyes. Snake toxins frequently target muscle groups that are also affected in myasthenia
Image courtesy of Professor David Warrell.

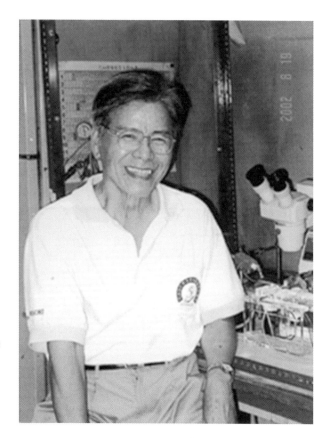

Fig. (c) Professor Chang in his laboratory where he was the first to fractionate bungarus multicinctus venom and demonstrate the post-synaptic binding to putative acetylcholine receptors.
Image courtesy of Professor Chang.

postdoc of Dr C.Y. Lee and, together, they described one of the most important developments of 1963, the identification and characterization of alpha-bungarotoxin [1]. In the introduction to this paper, he reminds us that 'the history of science abounds with examples of milestone discoveries that are made in not-well-funded laboratories'. The discovery and analysis of the effects of alpha- bungarotoxin illustrates this to perfection.

Methods

Snake toxin envenoming is a substantial clinical problem in Taiwan and many other countries, and the mechanisms involved needed to be understood. Chang realized that the venom had both pre- and post-synaptic effects on neuromuscular transmission (the method used was a rat or frog phrenic nerve-hemidiaphram preparation) and that he would need to separate the venom into its constituents in order to define which of the two effects was the most harmful and how to prevent it in envenomed patients. In order to do this, and without the benefits of modern ready-made columns and high-performance liquid chromatography (HPLC) machines, he devised a paper electrophoresis method to show that some separation into different constituents could be obtained. In order to prepare enough material for classical experiments, however, he needed a much larger-scale approach:

> I designed a starch zone electrophoresis apparatus made of a glass half-cylinder trough (2–4 cm diameter x 40 cm length) according to the knowledge obtained from paper electrophoresis and the space in my refrigerator. A rectifier removed from a discarded machine provided power supply. It was a slow and tedious process that took almost one week to complete one run.

Results

Thus, he separated the venom into four main fractions, so that he could analyse the actions of each on the physiological preparation. The most important result from the neurologist's point of view, and the most highly cited, was the effects of bungarotoxin on the post-synaptic acetylcholine receptors (AChRs)—although it is important to realize that, at that time, no one knew for sure what an AChR was. He found that bungarotoxin blocked the nerve-evoked muscle response and its action could be prevented by high concentrations of d-tubocurarine—a drug whose post-synaptic action in blocking the 'receptors' for ACh was already well studied. This suggested that the bungarotoxin and d-tubocurarine competed for binding to the putative receptors, and this was supported by subsequent experiments using radiolabelled 3H-acetyl-bungarotoxin that bound specifically to the post-synaptic 'end plate' regions of the muscle.

Conclusions

Alpha-bungarotoxin binds to the membrane entity that responds to ACh and initiates muscle activity. The paper was submitted to the *Journal of Physiology* but rejected because they did not publish on venom toxins! It was subsequently accepted by *Archive Internationale de Pharmacodynamie et de Thérapie* and published in 1963 [1], but even then its significance was not recognized by the much larger community of scientists interested in understanding synaptic transmission at a molecular level. In fact, Chang relates how only after visiting him in Paris, did the famous French molecular neuroscientist and biologist, Jean-Pierre Changeux, take up the offer of using the toxin to try to identify the receptor for ACh, leading to another landmark paper—the first to characterize the binding of the toxin to AChRs in detergent extracts of *E electrocus* electric organ membranes [2]. This was followed, shortly after, by several other related publications, the first only three months later [3].

Critique

The influence of this work has been enormous. Alpha-bungarotoxin was taken up by many of the leading neuroscientists of the time as a tool for isolating the putative AChR protein by affinity purification (successfully), which subsequently led to the separation of the four main subunits. N-terminal sequencing of the alpha subunit, and cloning of each AChR subunit DNA, was performed, mainly by the outstanding Japanese scientist, Shosaku Numa and his extraordinarily talented team, and subsequently by others, including David Beeson in Oxford, UK.

Meanwhile, radioactive bungarotoxin—produced independently (initially by this author, on the open laboratory bench, although subsequently in a fume cupboard) and then by Amersham UK—was used to identify the number and distribution of AChRs in all species (with a few exceptions such as the mongoose, whose AChRs are resistant to the action of snake toxins [4]) including humans with myasthenia gravis [5], and, of course, as a probe for AChRs in radio-immunoprecipitation assays for antibodies in myasthenia [6]. This assay is used worldwide to this day. Finally, fluorescent bungarotoxin has provided an excellent probe for studying AChR development, localization, and turnover in normal and diseased muscle.

Despite the relatively modest background to this work, the original paper has been cited more than 500 times.

15.2 **Passive transfer of antibody-mediated diseases**

Main paper: Toyka KV, Drachman DB, Griffin DE, et al. Myasthenia gravis. Study of humoral immune mechanisms by passive transfer to mice. *N Engl J Med* 1977; 296(3):125–31.

Background

By 1975, it was known that AChR numbers were reduced at myasthenia gravis (MG) end plates [5] and that immunization against electroplax AChR, purified using affinity-chromatography based on binding of the AChR to certain snake toxins, led to striking signs of anticholinesterase-responsive MG in rabbits [7]. Over the next two years, several groups began to demonstrate serum IgG antibodies that bound to or interfered with bungarotoxin binding to mammalian, including human, AChRs. All of these findings were first presented at the International Conference on Myasthenia Gravis in New York in 1975, a very exciting gathering of everyone in the field and my introduction to many of the leading players [8]. One of the highlights of the meeting was the first report of passive transfer of the disease to mice by injection of a crude immunoglobulin fraction, published later that year in *Science* [9]. This landmark paper, in 1977, described the results in more detail [10].

Methods

Sixteen patients were studied. Crude immunoglobulins, purified IgG, protein-A adsorbed IgG, complement-inactivation of the preparations, and complement C3 depletion of the mice were all tested. The purified IgG was injected daily at 10 mg per day for 1–14 days. C5 complement-deficient mice were also tested to assess further the role of complement in the pathogenic effect. Clinical features, miniature end-plate potentials, and AChR numbers were the main outcome measures in the mice.

Results

There were striking reductions in the amplitude of miniature end-plate potentials in the injected mice, which were absent when IgM fraction or pre-adsorbed IgG was injected instead of whole IgG. These physiological effects were accompanied by reduced AChR numbers at the endplates, very similar to the reductions shown in patients [5]. Some of the mice showed marked clinical weakness beginning 2-7 days after the first injection, and some demonstrated decrements in muscle responses to nerve stimulation. Interestingly, the effects of complement depletion were not very striking and the results of injection into complement-deficient mice were not significantly different from those of the control mice.

Conclusions

This was a major study, extending the earlier one [9] and establishing just how useful the passive transfer approach can be in demonstrating the role of antibodies in disease. In fact, the effectiveness of the approach for transferring MG would not necessarily have been anticipated since we know now, and were beginning to appreciate then, that there are differences in the sequences and particularly the antigenicity between rodent and human AChRs. Nevertheless, the results were real and important and have led to the approach being applied in other peripheral nerve and muscle conditions.

Critique

Most of their conclusions were valid but one aspect deserves comment. The effect of depleting complement C3 was not very striking in some experiments, and injecting mice that were C5 deficient did not appear to alter the response. They interpreted this as suggesting that only the early part of the complement cascade was involved, rather than the latter part which leads to the cytolytic effects via C5–9. Thus, they would not have predicted the C5–9 membrane attack complex activation which was clearly shown later by Andrew Engel and his colleagues [11] in the muscle of myasthenic patients. Why was this? In fact, human IgG antibodies do not always activate mouse complement effectively and to demonstrate an effect of complement activation, it is often helpful to inject human fresh serum or complement components in parallel (e.g. [12]).

15.3 **Plasma exchange therapy in acquired myasthenia gravis**

Main paper: Pinching AJ, Peters DK, Davis JN. Remission of myasthenia gravis following plasma-exchange. *Lancet* 1976; 2(8000):1373–6.

Background

For a number of years, plasmapheresis had had a variety of uses including red cell exchange, leukophoresis, plasma exchange, and thrombopheresis [13]. John 'Jack' Hobbs (1929–2008) was a very well-known immunologist at Westminster Hospital Medical School (where I was a medical student), but although we all recognized his scientific excellence, it was somewhat later that he became internationally famous for his bone marrow transplantation work. He and Oon indicated that plasmapheresis could be used to collect antibodies (for instance, for anti-tumour use) but they did not specifically mention the treatment of putative autoantibody-mediated diseases. However, Goodpasture's disease was already known to be caused by antibodies and Lockwood et al. [14] performed plasmapheresis in a cyclophosphamide-resistant case, demonstrating graphically the fall in antibody and creatinine levels that occurred following the treatment. It was probably another member of the team, Tony (A.J.) Pinching, who suggested that the same treatment might be applied to patients with myasthenia gravis, following the newly published evidence for antibodies to the AChRs that the paper succinctly summarizes [15].

Methods

Three patients with myasthenia were treated, including one male who had had the disease since childhood and was considered to have a congenital (later hereditary) form of disease, rather than autoimmune. Nevertheless, all three had been thymectomized and had proved relatively unresponsive to surgery or steroid therapy. Two litres were exchanged each day and the results monitored by use of the Medical Research Council strength scales. Fatigability was assessed simply by the time for which the patient could hold their leg or arm horizontally. Anticholinesterase medication was carefully timed in order not to confound the functional results.

Results

The first patient was a 51-year-old woman who had presented 20 years before and had had a thymoma removed. Weakness and respiratory infections were common and she had just begun to do better on alternate-day prednisolone but had developed bone disease. AChR antibodies were highly raised. Her condition was stable over the preceding 2 weeks. About 2–3 days after starting the exchange, 1 litre for 4 days and then 2 litres for the next 5 days, she began to improve, with marked changes in her functional measurements (the vital capacity increasing from 1.3 litres to 2.0 litres in the first 18 days, and arm outstretched time from 10 sec to 30 sec); the improvement was maintained with azathioprine and a reducing prednisolone regime. The second patient also showed a striking response to the exchanges, but the improvement was not sustained and she deteriorated within a few weeks of stopping the exchanges without change in medication. The third patient was a male with consanguineous parents and had been floppy from birth. Four exchanges of 2 litres had no consistent effect on symptoms or muscle strength.

Conclusions

This paper, although short, proved unequivocally that a plasma factor was involved in acquired myasthenia and that even patients with very long-standing and severe disease could improve substantially, a possibility that was likely not appreciated until that time. They commented that this invasive treatment would likely only be used as an adjunct to immunosuppressive therapy, and would be most useful in the initial control of fulminating disease, as it is generally used to this day. Finally, the results also demonstrated that the congenital form of myasthenia, occurring at or shortly after birth, was very unlikely to be autoimmune since that patient made no improvement, paving the way for the many family and genetic studies that followed.

Critique

One suspects that there was a certain pressure to publish as soon as possible (a similar study was performed by Peter Dau et al. [16]) and so some of the data mentioned— immunoglobulin levels, complement C3—were not reported until the subsequent paper, in 1978, which also included antibody levels [17]. Perhaps the greatest omission in the discussion was not to appreciate the extent to which plasma exchange was going to prove an essential step in confirming the antibody basis of, as well as in the treatment for, further autoimmune diseases; John Newsom-Davis and colleagues subsequently used the response to plasmapheresis as a guide to determining the antibody basis for AChR-antibody-negative forms of myasthenia, Lambert-Eaton myasthenic syndrome, and acquired neuromyotonia.

15.4 **The discovery of muscle-specific kinase**

Main paper: Valenzuela DM, Stitt TN, Distefano PS, et al. Receptor tyrosine kinase specific for the skeletal muscle lineage—expression in embryonic muscle, at the neuromuscular junction and after injury. *Neuron* 1995; 3:573–84.

Background

By the 1990s, much was known about the structure of the neuromuscular junction from many detailed electron microscopic and experimental studies [18]. The motor nerve terminal bouton formed a synapse with the muscle membrane; the synapse was quite wide compared with a central nervous system synapse, and there was a clearly visible basal lamina present which was a collagen-based extracellular matrix that anchors acetylcholine esterase. The motor endplate was made up of the multiple folds of post-synaptic membrane; on the nerve-facing aspect and down the sides of each fold, there was a high density of protein—the AChRs themselves—as shown by autoradiographic studies using radioactive bungarotoxin [19]. The aggregation or clustering of the AChRs was due to their tethering to an intracellular scaffold of which the most specific component was receptor aggregating protein at the synapse, now known as rapsyn. Below the post-synaptic folds, a nucleus could be seen which was thought to be responsible for transcription of the endplate-specific proteins, including AChR and rapsyn.

However, it was still not clear quite how the whole structure was formed. In particular, although it was thought that agrin, a protein released from the motor nerve during development, was important in clustering the AChRs, it was also beginning to be understood that even in the absence of agrin, clusters could form in developing myotubes. Additionally, no specific growth factor receptor had been identified at the neuromuscular junction. This very informative paper [20], and many others led by George D. Yancopoulos and D.J. Glass, illustrates how much could be achieved with the resources available; of the 12 authors (from four different institutions), eight, including the two senior authors, were from Regeneron Pharmaceuticals Inc.

Methods

The authors searched in a denervated muscle cDNA preparation for sequences shared with receptor tyrosine kinases, the most ubiquitous growth factor receptors. They used denervated muscle because that leads to upregulation of genes and proteins (e.g. the AChR) that are expressed at low levels at the neuromuscular junction in mature muscle. They identified a sequence that expressed a protein they named muscle-specific kinase (MuSK). They then characterized the distribution and expression of both the RNA and protein using *in situ* hybridization and antibodies raised against peptides of the ectodomain of MuSK.

Results

They found expression of the MuSK transcripts was very low in innervated skeletal muscle, as well as in other tissues such as the spleen and retina, but very high at early stages of muscle development, at times when no other tissue appeared to express the gene. MuSK was a typical receptor tyrosine kinase with a kinase domain that was highly homologous to other signalling molecules of this type, although the ectodomain, with its four Ig-like domains, also shared homology with a related gene sequence previously isolated from the electric organ of Torpedo. MuSK gene expression and protein expression were increased dramatically in denervated muscles of all fibre types, and also when muscles were immobilized (ankle joint fixation), indicating that muscle activity regulated MuSK expression. In addition, crucially, they demonstrated, unequivocally, that in adult muscle, MuSK (both cDNA and protein) was expressed predominantly or exclusively at the neuromuscular junction, and co-localized with AChRs. Finally, they mapped the gene to Chromosome 4 in the mouse and 9q31.3–32 in humans.

Conclusions

The main conclusion was that MuSK is a highly specific receptor tyrosine kinase that appeared to be important during development and, subsequently, localized to the adult neuromuscular junction. They proposed that MuSK could be involved in agrin-mediated aggregation of AChRs, particularly since AChR aggregation involves phosphorylation and MuSK is a tyrosine kinase. They also proposed that MuSK might be involved in signalling to the sub-synaptic nuclei, and could feed back signals to the nerve terminal, although how this might take place was not clear. They suggested that MuSK might be the gene defective in Fukuyama muscular dystrophy, as the genetic loci mapped very close.

Critique

This is one of the landmark papers in understanding the neuromuscular junction. In providing the description of a membrane protein that in adult muscle was essentially restricted to the neuromuscular junction, it also led to the subsequent identification of MuSK antibodies in a proportion of patients with MG [21]. Some of the conclusions were a little premature, since MuSK expression has now been reported in a number of tissues including the central nervous system, and it may play roles in these tissues too. Moreover, the only genetic disorders of MuSK in humans are very rare congenital myasthenic syndromes and, perhaps because MuSK is so essential during development (as shown in another paper by the same group [22]), mutations in patients are very rare indeed [23]. Finally, they proposed, very reasonably, that MuSK might be the receptor for agrin. However, it soon became clear that agrin does not bind directly to MuSK but, rather, to another membrane protein now called low-density lipoprotein receptor (LDLR)-related protein 4 (LRP4). Interestingly, LRP4 not only mediates agrin-induced MuSK activation, resulting in rapsyn and AChR phosphorylation and clustering, but has been shown to be a target for antibodies in a very small proportion of MG patients and may act as a retrograde signal to the motor nerve terminal. This may begin to explain clinical aspects of disease in MG patients with both MuSK and LRP4 antibodies.

15.5 **Molecular understanding of the neuromuscular synapse**

Main paper: Gautam M, Noakes PG, Moscoso L, et al. Defective neuromuscular synaptogenesis in agrin-deficient mutant mice. *Cell* 1996; 85(4):525–35.

Background

The Yancopoulos group went on to study mice in which MuSK had been knocked out, demonstrating the importance of that molecule in neuromuscular junction formation. Meanwhile, the other major group at the time, led by American neuroscientist, Josh Sanes, had already published on the knock-out of rapsyn, and here described the agrin-deficient mutant mouse. It was clear that the nerve released a substance that induced post-synaptic differentiation including AChR clustering, and that agrin, a proteoglycan, was one of the main factors that had this property. Agrin was released from the motor nerve terminal and retained in the basal lamina within the synaptic cleft. Agrin is a large molecule but the protein core is around 200 kDa and undergoes alternative splicing with different functional activities—z-agrin is neuron-specific and the most active in inducing AChR clustering, but other factors had been shown to have some activity and it was not clear whether agrin was crucial for neuromuscular junction formation, since some agrin-independent AChR clustering could occur in agrin-deficient mice, as mentioned in 15.4.

Methods

They engineered an agrin-deficient mouse by replacing the z-agrin-specific domains with a neomycin-resistance gene and using homologous recombination to create cell lines to generate germ-line chimeras. Heterozygotes were normal and could be bred to produce homozygote agrin-deficient progeny. Antibodies to agrin, synaptophysin, AChR, rapsyn, and other molecules were used to localize the pre- and post-synaptic components.

Results

The mice had dramatically reduced levels of all agrin isoforms, not just the z-agrin, probably due to interference in transcription resulting from the inserted gene. The embryos failed to move but survived until day 18 *in utero*, when they died or were stillborn. The striking result was the reduced size and reduced AChR expression in the neuromuscular junctions that were distributed, multiply, along the length of the muscle fibres, instead of concentrated at the end-plate region. Total AChR levels were normal, so the defect had not reduced receptor expression overall; rather, they were able to show that nerve endings terminated blindly with no post-synaptic AChR cluster, and some clusters existed without motor nerve terminals. Nevertheless, where there was apposition of the nerve to the AChR cluster, this appeared relatively normal, confirming that even agrin-deficient axons can induce AChR clusters and form neuromuscular junctions. On further examination, AChR gene expression was still mainly localized in the end-plate region of the muscle, although somewhat reduced compared with unaffected mice, and that post-synaptic differentiation, as indicated by rapsyn and laminin beta2 expression, was also fairly normal. By contrast, the patterns of neurite outgrowth in the embryos was disturbed, with many axons ending in undifferentiated terminals, and electron microscopy demonstrated substantial loss of synaptic vesicles in many, but not all, of the terminals.

Conclusions

Overall, it appeared from this study [24] that z-agrin is a critical organizer of post-synaptic differentiation, with agrin deficiency being lethal in the mutant mouse, although some degree of differentiation can occur even when agrin is absent, suggesting that there must be additional signalling molecule(s). The mixture of pre- and post-synaptic defects was somewhat unexpected and the discussion includes a very comprehensive and carefully considered assessment of the relevance of both axonal and post-synaptic factors, including muscle activity, in the formation of the junctional synapse.

Critique

This was one of a series of excellent papers detailing the phenotypes of mice defective in neuromuscular junction proteins, and helping to build a better understanding of synapse formation. Agrin proved to be rather less easy to characterize than some proteins, but the results raised important questions regarding axon guidance and retrograde signalling that we need to understand better when considering the pathophysiology of disorders of neuromuscular transmission, both genetic and autoimmune, and how they might be treated.

15.6 **Limbic encephalitis**

Main paper: Corsellis JAN, Goldberg GJ, Norton AR. Limbic encephalitis and its association with carcinoma. *Brain* 1968; 91(3):481–96.

Background

In the 1960s, a series of papers was published dealing with what we now call paraneoplastic disorders, many of them from Lord Brain and colleagues in London, UK. Although in some of the patients, there was evidence of cortical inflammation, most had brainstem or more caudal inflammation, and there was still some discussion regarding whether these changes were related to the associated carcinomas and whether the brain pathology was viral, inflammatory, or degenerative. John Corsellis (1915–1994) was a neuropathologist, based in Essex and the Institute of Psychiatry in London, who provided the first detailed morphological studies of dementias, schizophrenia, and psychoses, as well as epilepsies, hippocampal sclerosis, and limbic encephalitis. His many attributes and contributions have been reviewed [25]. This paper [26] describes, carefully, the pathology of different brain areas associated with cancer, in what we now call paraneoplastic limbic encephalitis.

Methods

Three patients, two males and one female, who presented with severe memory defects and disorientation are described. All three had probable oat-cell (small-cell) carcinoma, although in one, the tumour was undifferentiated. The neuropathology is described and illustrated and the discussion refers to all relevant previous reports.

Results

The three patients had disturbance of recent memory with some retrograde loss but preserved earlier memories. Seizures were variable. One had an enlarged testis but, on orchidectomy, no tumour tissue was found and, at post-mortem, enlarged mediastinal lymph nodes appeared to be infiltrated with oat-cell bronchial carcinoma. The nature of the defect in recent memory is clearly recorded, with about one minute retention of new information and retrograde amnesia of several years; this same patient also exhibited disorientation and some generalized epileptic attacks. The main pathology was in the leptomeninges, with mild lymphocytic infiltrates and occasional cuffing. Similar findings were seen in the cortex and white matter, with no apparent neuronal loss. However, in the medial temporal lobes, there was extensive loss of nerve cells and astrocytosis with gliosis, and perivascular infiltration. Similar changes were seen in the amygdalae, together with a patch of necrosis on the right side and in the fimbriae, fornices, and anterior columns. There were also some changes in the hypothalamus and thalamus but, otherwise, the abnormalities were few and neuronal loss was not evident.

The second case had mainly memory problems and disorientation. He had an undifferentiated carcinoma of the lung and a neuromyopathy causing wasting of the hands. The histological changes were similar to those of the other male, with particular involvement of the amygdalae, parahippocampal gyri, and substantia nigrae.

The third case, a woman, was older, and a bronchial oat-cell carcinoma was found at necropsy. Her brain showed substantial gliosis, astrocytosis, and neuronal loss in the amygdalae, hippocampus, subiculum, and parahippocampal gyri. The brown discoloration on visual inspection of the brain was a feature that related to underlying inflammation.

Conclusions

The discussion begins with a detailed review of other case reports in which inflammatory brain disease was associated with tumours. These included one by Brierly, Corsellis, and others [27] in which they concluded that it was unlikely that the finding of carcinomatous lymph nodes was related to the encephalitis. Some of the other authors thought similarly, or they tended towards the view that the inflammatory changes were more likely to be secondary to degeneration rather than the primary pathology. However, when they come to the discussion of their own cases, it is clear that they had changed their minds, and considered the evidence to support an inflammatory disease, mainly of the limbic system, that was in some way related to the carcinomas.

Critique

This is a very clear, comprehensive, and carefully argued paper which ends by relating the memory defects in particular, and the dementia to some extent, to the predominance of limbic grey matter damage. It does not come out strongly in favour of a mechanism by which the association with carcinoma occurs, although it is clear that the authors now thought that the relationship was no coincidence. The importance of this study is the striking clinical picture in which recent memory loss dominates, with relatively preserved retrograde memories, and its relationship with inflammatory changes and neuronal loss in the limbic system. The role of the carcinomas, although evident in these three cases, was not found in every patient reviewed even then, predicting the now common experience that many patients with limbic encephalitis do not have tumours and are likely to have an antibody-mediated disease that responds to immunotherapies (e.g. [28]). Paraneoplastic diseases, in general, although very important to consider in the differential diagnosis of many neurological diseases, are not very frequent [29], but are often indistinguishable from the non-paraneoplastic counterparts.

15.7 **Autoantibodies to neuronal receptors**

Main paper: Rogers SW, Andrews PI, Gahring LC, et al. Autoantibodies to glutamate receptor GluR3 in Rasmussen's encephalitis. *Science* 1994; 265:648–51.

Background

In the 1990s, it became possible to use cDNA clones to express many hitherto unpurified proteins as fusion constructs in *E coli*. The main reason was often to make large amounts of the polypeptide chains that formed the protein structure for crystallization studies. Another was to be able to raise antibodies in experimental animals in order to provide high-affinity reagents for use in further cellular, histological, and functional studies. An American group, led by James McNamara, were particularly interested in epilepsy and they wanted to induce antibodies to glutamate receptors, the main excitatory central nervous system receptors.

Methods

They immunized rabbits with gene fusion proteins representing the extracellular domains (ecds) of the glutamate receptors (including what we would now call AMPAR1, 2, and 3). They observed the rabbits for clinical signs and looked at the histology of their brains. They tested the sera of four children with Rasmussen's encephalitis for antibodies to the relevant fusion proteins, using western blotting, and also by binding to human embryonic kidney (HEK) cells expressing the full-length cDNAs (without the fusion protein). The final method, with one patient, was plasma exchange.

Results

Two of the three rabbits immunized with GluR3ecd fusion protein developed seizure-like episodes, including tongue biting in one, while none of the other 48 animals immunized against GluR 1, 2, 5, or 6, exhibited any abnormal behaviours. The pathology of the affected animals showed meningeal and perivascular lymphocytic infiltrates and microglial nodules, mainly in the cortex and highly reminiscent of Rasmussen's encephalitis [30]. Three of the patients showed reactivity with the GluR3ecd fusion protein on western blotting, particularly strong in one patient, whilst none of the controls tested demonstrated such a response. Finally, and importantly, they also detected binding to full-length GlyR3 in HEK cells expressing the cDNA; three patients with active disease were positive, whereas the one who had undergone previous hemispherectomy, and was seizure free, was negative. As a test of whether these antibodies were pathogenic, they plasma exchanged one of the children, demonstrating a remarkable seizure improvement over the first seven, weekly exchanges, with discernible improvements in drawing and writing skills (Fig. 15.2).

Conclusions

They concluded, reasonably, that GluR3 antibodies are present in patients with active Rasmussen's encephalitis and that the transient improvement following plasma exchange

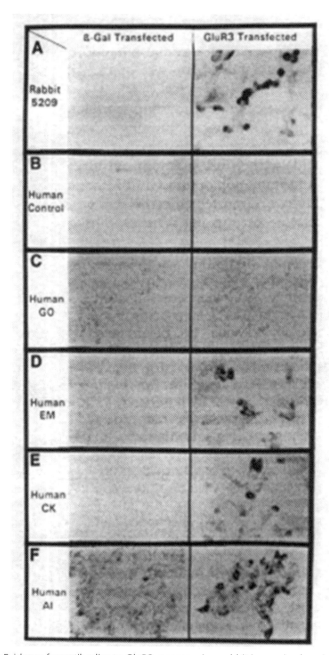

Fig. 15.2 (a) Evidence for antibodies to GluR3 receptors in a rabbit immunized against recombinant GluR3 (A), and lack of antibodies in a human control serum (B). Four patients (C-F) with Rasmussen's encephalitis were strongly positive for binding to the GluR3 transfected, but not the Gal-transfected (control), cells.

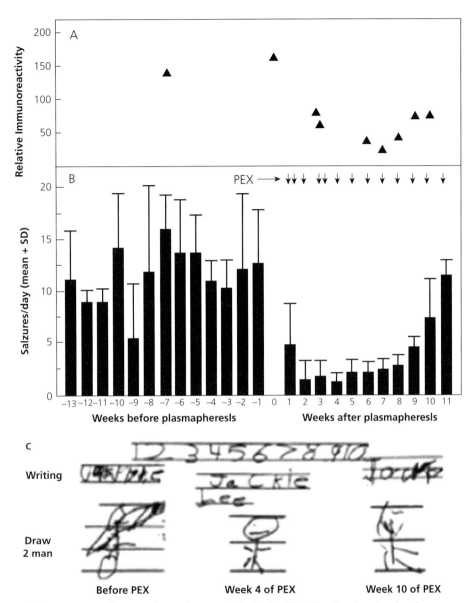

Fig. (b) Response to plasma exchange in one child with GluR3 antibodies showing the changes in detectable antibody (A) and the reduction in seizure frequency (B) before and after plasma exchange was commenced. The child's drawing showed a marked improvement (C) but as the antibodies rose following exchanges, the seizures returned and the drawing deteriorated.

All images reproduced from *Science*, 265(5172), Rogers SW, Andrews PI, Gahring LC, Whisenand T, Cauley K, Crain B, et al., Autoantibodies to glutamate receptor GluR3 in Rasmussen's encephalitis, p. 648–51, Copyright (1994), with permission from the American Association for the Advancement of Science.

(as in myasthenia) suggests that these antibodies could contribute to the pathogenesis [31]. They then hypothesized as to how the circulating antibodies could get into the brain through focal disruption of the blood–brain barrier, perhaps sometimes associated with head injury which was known to occasionally precede the condition, and how this might explain the marked unilaterality of the pathology in the majority of patients. They drew attention to the fact that other epilepsies might have similar causes.

Critique

This was really the first demonstration that antibodies to central nervous system (CNS) receptors or other neuronal surfaces, rather than intracellular proteins, could be present in patients, and that these were likely to be pathogenic. From the point of view of this volume, it was a little disappointing that they did not draw attention to the (probable) serendipity of their findings and the analogy with myasthenia gravis induction in rabbits immunized against purified (not fusion protein) acetylcholine receptors which had been demonstrated 21 years previously in the same journal [7]! Moreover, although they ex-pressed the full-length GluR3 in HEK cells to reproduce the 'native' protein, they did not look specifically at the binding of the antibodies to the surface of intact live cells in order to confirm that the antibodies could bind to extracellular domains of the native membrane protein; at that time, it is likely that neither the expression constructs nor the microscopy were ideal for doing that crucial experiment. They did not appear to question whether there were antibodies detectable in the cerebrospinal fluid (CSF), and if so, whether there was intrathecal synthesis of the specific antibodies. However, they did discuss, quite rea-sonably, the possible scenarios by which peripheral autoantibodies could gain entry and contribute to, even if not be the main cause of, the CNS condition.

This was a definite landmark paper at the time and attracted much attention for the fol-lowing decade or so. Unfortunately, however, it did not lead quite as far as it could have done. This may have been because the authors subsequently showed that a peptide epitope was the main target of the antibodies to GluR3, and many less technically advanced la-boratories thought that measuring antibodies by binding to peptides on enzyme-linked immunosorbent assay plates was much easier than using the expression techniques that Rogers and colleagues had established. As a result, many likely misleading reports claimed the presence of GluR3 peptide antibodies in different types of epilepsy, whereas some failed to find them at all (e.g. [32]), depending on the stringency of the assays or the inter-pretation of the results.

Techniques have moved on and now it is standard practice to look for potentially patho-genic antibodies using live cells expressing the full (as far as one is able to determine) native protein structure of the receptor or ion channel, often involving co-expression of several different subunits. These approaches are backed up with immunostaining of rodent tissue sections and binding of the patients' antibodies to the surface of primary neuronal cultures. With these methods, antibodies to the voltage-gated potassium channel (VGKC)-complex associated proteins, LGI1 and CASPR2, or to NMDA, AMPA1/2, GABA (a and b forms), and glycine receptors can be detected in patients, both adults and children, with different clinical syndromes that are thought to be autoantibody-mediated disorders [33, 34] and often show very good immunotherapy responses. In addition, it is now becoming clear that there are some patients with other forms of epilepsy, of previously unknown cause, who may have these antibodies (e.g. [35, 36]), although prospective studies are needed to demonstrate their relevance to diagnosis and management. Whether there are truly pathogenic antibodies in Rasmussen's encephalitis, or only cyotoxic T cells [30], still remains a major question.

15.8 **Morvan's syndrome**

Main paper: Morvan AM. De la choree fibrillaire per de Dr Morvan de Lannills. *Gazette Hebdomadaire de Medicine et de Chirurgie* 1890; 15:173–17:200.

Background

French physician, Augustin Marie Morvan (1819–1897), was a very gifted clinician, working at much the same time as Charcot. He practiced in Brittany, contributed greatly to the local community of his town, and, as a result, eschewed more widespread recognition. He described at least three previously unrecognized conditions: myxoedema, syringomyelia, and what we now often call acquired neuromyotonia or peripheral nerve hyperexcitability [37]. The latter, particularly when associated with CNS involvement, is usually called Morvan's syndrome. His life and work have recently been reviewed by Walusinski and Honnorat [38].

Methods

This is a sequence of five very carefully described case reports and relevant discussion, published in three sections on the 12th, 19th, and 26th of April 1890. These papers also describe some heroic attempts to identify the source of excessive sweating by dissection, under anaesthetic, of two horses 'past their prime'.

Results

The first case is described with typical modesty: 'I have once again been favoured by chance . . .' The patient was a local farmer with an eight-day history of fibrillary contractions in his calf muscles and posterior muscles of the thighs. Within a few days, these had extended to reach other regions of the body and was visible as raised points along the surface of the muscles, transiently appearing and disappearing. These movements decreased during voluntary contraction and were accompanied by shooting pains throughout the body, mainly in the twitching muscles, and frequently disturbing the patient's sleep. Excessive sweating was noticed and the man's condition deteriorated rapidly within a few weeks, as he became delirious and went into a coma, dying after less than one month of illness. Insomnia was evident in the last few days. The other cases were less serious but the four patients variously complained of the muscle contractions, fatigue and lassitude, shooting pain, agitation, and excessive perspiration.

Conclusions

Morvan himself suggested that the anterior horn cells were involved in the pathology and that the posterior columns of the spinal cord were implicated in what we would call autonomic disturbance of sweating and cardiac rhythm, which he had noted. He distinguished the condition from Sydenham's chorea, but acknowledged similarities with paramyoclonus multiplex as previously described in Germany. These and other apparently related conditions were all reviewed by Edouard Krebs, an intern of Joseph Babinski, in his thesis of

1922, where he also discussed the condition in relation to the recently described agrypnic forms of encephalitis lethargica (see 15.10). All of these aspects are reviewed briefly by Walunsinski and Honnorat [38].

Critique

There were a number of patients with this and related syndromes reported in the French literature over the following century, but remarkably few in the English literature, and the condition has always been thought to be very rare. Why then would Morvan have identified five patients in his sleepy little Brittany town? Do they frequently go unreported, unrecognized, or was there a mini-epidemic following an infectious or perhaps toxic event in rural Lannilis? Should he have looked for a unifying precipitant? None were thought to have a thymoma—at least one might have been expected from current knowledge of the syndrome. Over the last 10 years, several more cases have been described [39] but Morvan's syndrome, defined as a combination of peripheral nerve hyperexcitability, autonomic disturbance, and CNS symptoms dominated by insomnia, is still thought to be rare.

But did he really describe what we think of as Morvan's syndrome? It is not clear that any of his patients had insomnia as a major feature; the only patient for whom the term was used was delirious and terminally ill at the time. Thus, the term 'Morvan's fibrillary chorea' should properly be used to describe neuromyotonia, and those of us who have used the term for patients who have coincident insomnia and other CNS disturbance are wrong!

One can understand Morvan attempting to produce a unifying theory for the peripheral and central (and autonomic) disease by locating the disease to the spinal cord, but it now seems that Morvan's syndrome, if that is what we are continuing to call it, is a truly multi-localized condition with, in the majority of cases, autoantibodies that bind to components of the voltage-gated potassium channel complex. As will be mentioned in section 15.9, the main identified target in Morvan's syndrome is CASPR2 which is present at multiple peripheral and CNS sites.

15.9 **Autoantibodies to voltage-gated potassium channels**

Main paper: Liguori R, et al. Morvan's syndrome: peripheral and central nervous system and cardiac involvement with antibodies to voltage-gated potassium channels. *Brain* 2001; 124:2417–26.

Background

The evidence of antibodies in Rasmussen's encephalitis did not immediately lead to a changed perception of the ability of antibodies to cause CNS disorders, but about the same time, our group in Oxford, UK, began to move slowly towards the CNS. Neurologist, John Newsom-Davis (1932–2007, see 15.3), had become convinced that neuromyotonia was an autoimmune disease, and he showed that some patients responded clinically to plasma exchange and their serum IgG could transfer evidence of peripheral nerve hyperexcitability to mice [40]. Subsequent studies showed that patients' plasma IgG modestly increased neurotransmitter release at the neuromuscular junction [41] and the serum antibodies immunoprecipitated Kv1, shaker-type, VGKCs [42]. Another interest in the peripheral motor nerve stemmed from a fruitful collaboration with Hugh Willison in Glasgow, UK. Miller-Fisher syndrome sera transiently increased neurotransmitter release from mouse nerve-muscle preparations *in vitro*, which was followed by complete cessation of release [43]; this 'latrotoxin-like' effect and the pathophysiological consequences of many different ganglioside antibodies binding to peripheral nerves have subsequently been studied in detail by Willison and his Dutch collaborators [44].

Although it was clear that the neuromyotonia patients often had subtle CNS disturbance such as psychological changes or sleep disruption [45], the move towards the CNS really came about when a serum was sent for antibody testing from the Institute of Neurology in Bologna, followed not long after by Dr Rocco Liguori carrying a large plasmapheresis sample, and deep-frozen brain tissue in a cold-box. The patient had had Morvan's syndrome.

Methods

This was a clinico-pathological study of one patient. Investigations included electrophysiology, polysomnography, autonomic testing, neurohormone levels, immunochemistry, and post-mortem pathology. Getting the journal, *Brain*, to accept this single-case report required carefully composed arguments addressed to the Deputy Editor, John Rothwell (the Editor, John Newsom-Davis, was conflicted by virtue of the Oxford connection)!

Results

The patient was a 76-year-old man who presented with muscle twitching and weakness, sweating and salivation, joint pain, and itching. Over 12 months, he deteriorated, with confusion, disorientation, visual and auditory hallucinations, and progressive insomnia with complex behaviours during sleep and day-time drowsiness. There was also constipation, increased lacrimation, and urinary incontinence. Wake electroencephalography (EEG) demonstrated striking theta activity with alpha and fast activities; there were typical neuromyotonic discharges in the muscle leads, and cardiac arrhythmia with extrasystoles in the electrocardiogram (ECG) (Fig. 15.3a).

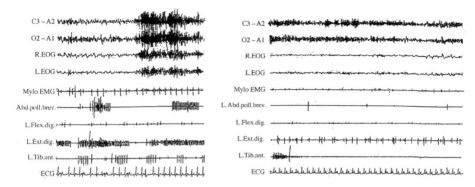

Fig. 15.3 (a) Polysomnography during 'wakefulness' before and after extensive plasma exchanges in the patient with Morvan's syndrome. Most of the abnormal activity in each of the leads was markedly reduced by the treatment, including the cardiac arrhythmia.

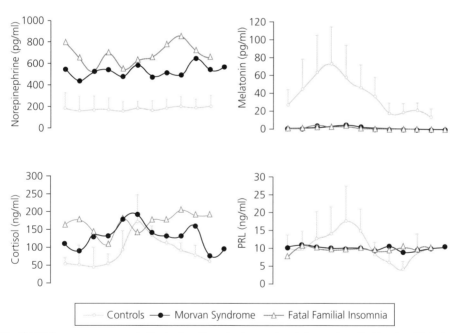

Fig. (b) 24-hour measurements illustrating the raised norepinephrine and cortisol levels with lack of clear diurnal cortisol changes, and the markedly flat melatonin and prolactin levels with absent circadian rhythm. Particularly striking were the similar measurements in patients with the prion disease, fatal familial insomnia.

Fig. 15.3b reproduced from *Brain*, 124, Liguori R, et al., Morvan's syndrome: peripheral and central nervous system and cardiac involvement with antibodies to voltage-gated potassium channels, p. 2417–2426, Copyright (2001), with permission from Oxford University Press.

At various stages in his illness, other investigations were performed. His autonomic disturbance was documented by tilt and sweat tests, and 24-hour hormone estimations showed circadian rhythm abnormalities . These were particularly dramatic in that melatonin and prolactin levels were completely flat, rather than showing a typical diurnal pattern, whereas both norepinephrine and cortisol levels were raised. As demonstrated in the paper (Fig. 15.3b), the hormonal findings were strikingly similar to those of fatal familial insomnia, a well-established genetic condition caused by mutations in the prion protein.

Because of the muscle hyperexcitability, his serum was sent for testing and was highly positive for VGKC antibodies, with a titre of >3000 pM; surprisingly, CSF, a little later in the course of the disease, was not positive (<5 pM). Despite this, the response to plasmapheresis suggested that the antibodies were in some way involved in his syndrome. To try to demonstrate this more clearly, the frozen brain tissue was examined by immunohistochemistry. Frozen sections were either fixed immediately and stained for human IgG to demonstrate any diffusion of IgG from blood vessels into the parenchyma, or washed briefly, before fixing and staining, in the hope of demonstrating IgG bound to the VGKCs. Although not entirely clear, there did appear to be diffusion of IgG into certain parts of the brain, notably the thalamus, but not the cortex. Conventional *post-mortem* pathology did not show any brain changes other than those that might be expected for a man of his age, but revealed a small lung adenocarcinoma.

Conclusions

The relationship between the VGKC antibodies and the clinical findings seemed more than a coincidence, but had the antibodies truly accessed the brain parenchyma to cause the CNS disease? Did this mean that peripheral antibodies really could cause a CNS disease by diffusion through a disrupted blood–brain barrier, which was against all the prevailing dogma? The authors were fairly cautious and suggested an alternative possibility: could it be that the action of the antibodies on secretion of peripheral hormones, such as cortisol and norepinephrine (Fig. 15.3b), indirectly led to the CNS dysfunction?

Critique

The cautious approach was unnecessary since there now seems no doubt that antibodies can cause CNS disease, but what could not be anticipated at the time was how the field would move forward. The same year, Buckley et al. [46] published the first two cases of limbic encephalitis with VGKC antibodies; only one of these had a tumour and the other recovered spontaneously over two years. From then on, further, mostly non-paraneoplastic cases were identified [47]. However, this raised an important question: how was it that neuromyotonia, Morvan's syndrome, and limbic encephalitis were all associated with the same VGKC antibodies?

We now know that the VGKC antibodies are frequently directed at other components of a 'VGKC complex'. So far, the only identified targets for patients' antibodies are CASPR2, LGI1, and contactin-2, each of which is part of the VGKC-complex which exists in situ [48]. CASPR2 antibodies are the most frequent and highest titre in Morvan's syndrome

[39], whereas LGI1 antibodies are typically found in limbic encephalitis [48, 49] and a newly identified form of epilepsy called faciobrachial dsytonic seizures [50]. However, at the time, none of this was anticipated, nor was the number of patients who would subsequently prove to have these antibodies.

One aspect of the condition that has still not been adequately addressed is the neuronal mechanisms involved in Morvan's syndrome and why the features are so similar to fatal familial insomnia [51].

15.10 **Encephalitis lethargica**

Main paper: von Economo C. *Encephalitis Lethargica*. First published Vienna, 1929; translated and adapted by Newman KO, Oxford Medical Publications, 1931.

Background

Constantin von Economo (1876–1931; Fig. 15.4a), of Greek origins but a Romanian by birth, was brought up in Trieste and ended his life working in Vienna, having previously also studied in Paris, Strassbourg, Munich, and Berlin. He was a romantic figure who inherited from his father, the title of Baron, and was the first Austrian to hold a pilot's licence. During World War I, he served as a pilot for the German army. His great achievements were in describing the cytoarchitecture of the brain, mapping the different layers and the different functional regions of the cortex; he was particularly interested in the regulation of sleep and defined a sleep centre in the mesencephalon (see [52]; Fig. 15.4b). This interest stemmed from his observations of the complex sleep disturbances seen in encephalitis lethargica, a condition of epidemic proportions that arose following World War I. In this book, he first describes, with great care, how he recognized and collated the information on this hitherto unclassified condition, defining different subtypes and investigating the aetiology.

The book was translated by Dr K.O. Newman of New College, Oxford, in 1931, with acknowledgements to many distinguished colleagues (e.g. Buzzard and Greenfield), also recognized as contributors to the understanding of the disease by von Economo in his foreward to the English edition. My fascination with this work, and the reason for leaving it until last, stems from the recent development of diseases that share many of the clinical features of encephalitis lethargica but are now thought to be caused by autoantibodies.

Methods

Detailed descriptions of cases, definitions of different forms, the long-term consequences, their morbid anatomy, and histological findings are all described in detail. I cannot possibly do justice to this remarkable work but i have tried to retain some elements of his descriptions of the different patients.

Fig. 15.4 (a) The neuroscientist and neurologist, Constantin von Economo.

Fig. 15.4a reproduced from *Scottish Medical Journal*, 57(4), Demetriades AK, From encephalitis lethargica to cerebral cytoarchitectonics: the polymath talent of Constantin von Economo (1876–1931), pioneer neuroanatomist, neurophysiologist and military aviator, p. 232–6, Copyright (2012), with permission from SAGE.

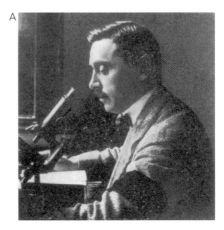

A

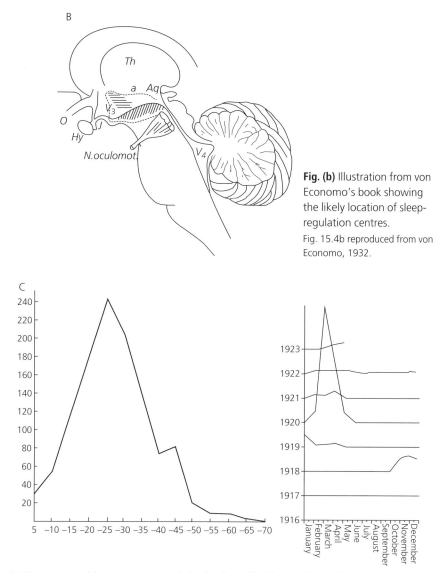

Fig. (b) Illustration from von Economo's book showing the likely location of sleep-regulation centres.

Fig. 15.4b reproduced from von Economo, 1932.

Fig. (c) The age at incidence and seasonal distribution of incidence of encephalitis lethargica cases in the epidemic.

Fig. 15.4c reproduced from von Economo, 1932.

Results

The whole monograph is essentially descriptive and the introductory chapter starts with a certain lack of modesty. Von Economo wanted to make it quite clear from the beginning that he discovered this disease, and each of the subtypes, and that those who claimed otherwise were misguided and had probably not read his papers. He gives a brief historical perspective, referring to accounts of possibly related epidemics in earlier centuries including the Tubingen sleeping sickness of 1712 and the so-called 'nona' epidemic of 1890–1891 in northern Italy. He describes the epidemiology of the 20th century epidemic, starting in 1916 and relatively constant up to 1923, except for a substantial peak during February to April in 1920 (see Fig. 15.4c). The disease appeared to affect all ages but mainly younger adults, peaking between 20 and 35 years old (Fig. 15.4c), and transfer from mother to fetus or newborn child was mentioned, although he did not appear to have observed this himself.

The epidemic nature of the condition, and its existence in different countries at different times, as he reviews, strongly suggested that an infectious agent must be involved, but the fact that the cases were described before the start of the famous Spanish influenza epidemic, appeared, to him, to exclude this virus (subsequently confirmed by viral studies on archived brains; e.g. [53]). Nevertheless, Von Economo performed brain tissue transfer experiments to monkeys to identify an infectious agent and was convinced that a filterable virus was responsible, although its identity was not known then or now; others thought that a toxic agent might be involved and it is striking that he often refers to the 'toxicity' of the infection. Various alternative explanations are considered but discarded in a very detailed and, generally, fair and well-argued manner.

The main forms of encephalitis lethargica are described in Chapter II. Summarizing the very detailed information is near impossible but the main features of the three different subtypes are reasonably clear, although somewhat overlapping, and can be found in modern and informative reviews (e.g. [54]). In most cases, the disease was preceded by a prodromal stage with slight fever and pharyngitis, but he stresses that subsequently, the fever, secretary disturbances, and sleep disruption are caused by brain ('mid-brain') rather than systemic involvement (an interesting comparison with the cautious interpretation of Liguori et al. [55], 15.9). Ultimately, the infectious agent establishes itself, and the ensuing inflammation, in certain parts of the brain, results in the characteristic features of the three forms.

The somnolent-ophthalmoplegic form

A prodromal phase, followed by somnolence, with perhaps some meningism occurring; headache could be intense but the severity was moderate overall. Somnolence then increased but, if woken, the patients were orientated and fully conscious. Spontaneous recovery could take place at that stage but in many patients, deterioration to a comatose condition followed, which could be fatal. Motor disturbance was rare but delirium with hallucinations was particularly common in the Vienna epidemic and yet did not relate to fever. In fact, he stresses that fever is likely to be due to involvement of the diencephalon adjacent to the third ventricle, and not to the infectious agent itself. Simultaneously, various palsies, particularly of the eye muscles, occur; these were frequently asymmetric, partial, and without impairment of accommodation or papillary reactions. Supranuclear palsies were observed less frequently and nystagmus was of varied extents and character. More general hypotonia with reduced reflexes were also common but in some patients, ataxia was evident, whereas in others, a state of rigidity developed—for instance, he cites the London epidemic of 1918 as being less somnolent but with mask-like features. Epilepsy was rare. Mortality was relatively high but about 50% exhibited 'complete recovery'. Sporadic cases occurring after the epidemic(s) were already recognized by the time the book was published in 1929.

The hyperkinetic form

This form was characterized by chorea of various kinds, fascicular and myoclonic twitches, and 'wild jactations'! Some patients exhibited psychomotor restlessness, anxiety, or even frenzy. These features occurred in different individuals within the same epidemic or within the same individual over time. This form appeared in Italy, Austria, and Switzerland, before spreading around Europe. After the prodrome, there was vomiting, pain, fever, and sometimes extensive herpes on the lips, spreading over the face. The neurological features were often violent at onset with mental unrest and continuous motor activities, similar to psychoses, and with hallucinations that terrified the patient. This phase could be followed by a state of sleeplessness/sleep inversion which could continue for months. In the hyperkinetic patients, oculomotor disturbance was uncommon but abnormal papillary reactions were typical.

The choreiform movements occurred generally after the initial, more voluntary, movements that represented the psychomotor disturbance described. The chorea was generalized and often bilateral, and more severe than in typical 'chorea' and absent during sleep. Coarse myoclonic twitches were distinctive and present during sleep, as was twitching of the corner of the mouth or limb that could simulate epilepsy. He suggested that the hyperkinetic movements might be due to removal of the normal inhibitory effect of the cortex on the deeper centres, but the myoclonic and fascicular twitches could originate in the anterior horn cells. The outcomes could be good, within days or longer, although sudden death might occur. Others continued into a more somnolent ophthalmoplegic form, which he assumed involved the brainstem, and a few developed an amyostatic or Parkinson-like state. Interestingly, he states that the hyperkinetic form appeared much more coincident with the influenza outbreak and was less frequently observed subsequently.

Amyostatic-akinetic form

This form was characterized by a relatively mild prodrome followed by a state of akinesia. The patients were conscious and could respond, but only very slowly, to questions. Voluntary movements were very slow and could be arrested without completion, reminiscent of catatonia. The face was mask-like with complete lack of expression. The eyes stared unblinking but the patients were mentally intact, and aware of their condition. Eye movement disorders and bulbar paralytic disturbances were frequent in the English and Hamburg epidemics.

This was then complicated, in many cases, by an extrapyramidal increase in muscle tone which was responsible for the Parkinsonian-like features of stiffness, slowness, bent posture, and festinating gait. Tremor was not uncommon. Increased salivation and retention of urine were also associated. Sleep functions were also disturbed in this form, with stupor during the day and agrypnia (motor movements during sleep). He suggests that this is because the diurnal cycles of 'brain' sleep and 'body' sleep are not synchronized ('dissociation of the sleep-components'), but towards the evening, the two waking states overlap and there are periods when the patient is relatively normal, and conversely, during the later night, the sleep states overlap and the patient's sleep is normal. The existence of formes frustes or mild cases that resolved spontaneously without obvious consequences is clearly stated.

I have only touched on the first 50 of over 150 pages that also include detailed descriptions of other forms of the acute disease, residual features, the sequaelae (particularly the post-encephalitic Parkinsonism), as well as blood and CSF changes and brain histopathology. The latter is particularly detailed, clearly demonstrating inflammatory infiltrates of lymphocytes, including some plasma cells, around vessels in the grey matter, particularly the brainstem, with some loss of neurons but no obvious necrosis.

Conclusions

The final chapter is a general review which returns to the somewhat hubristic attitudes of the first. He claims that the study of encephalitis has provided a breakthrough in understanding the functions of the brain, indicating that many 'functional' syndromes can be organic, that involvement can be partial and reversible rather than total and progressive, and deriving new ideas on the neuro-anatomical relationships. He particularly draws attention to the hypothalamic origin of vegetative symptoms which previously had been assumed to be hormonal, and the striking different types of sleep disorders that can occur, sometimes within the same individual. He emphasizes the importance of the connections between the cortex and the basal ganglia and discusses the implications for understanding the basis for the different types of movement disorders, distinguishing between the intentional (cortical) and impulsive (basal ganglia), and suggesting that the latter dominate in children.

Although very clearly based mainly on his own observations, he does discuss the views of others thoroughly and often states their precedence in terms of a particular theory. He finishes with a discussion of neuroses and even ventures to explain 'self-consciousness'. However, the final sentence is perhaps not so prescient:

> One thing is certain: whoever has observed without bias the many forms of encephalitis lethargica—and this probably includes the majority of medical men of our generation—must of necessity have quite considerably altered his outlook on neurological and psychological phenomena during this last decade. Encephalitis lethargica can scarcely again be forgotten.

Not forgotten perhaps, but surprisingly few cases have been identified since, and the cause of the epidemic is still unknown.

Critique

This monograph raises many issues, of course, and others have already discussed these [54]. Were the epidemics the same or separate conditions? Why were they so frequent at that time and the diseases hardly recognized since? Were they infectious or post-infectious and, therefore, likely to be autoimmune? My understanding is that most data indicate that the influenza virus itself was not the cause, and the historical evidence given by von Economo that many cases preceded the influenza epidemic suggests that it may not have been the only or even the main cause. But does this relate to all forms of the disease? Encephalitis lethargica has been recognized in sporadic forms since the 1930s and is still a diagnosis used occasionally in paediatric neurology. It would thus be tempting to imagine that each form/epidemic of encephalitis lethargica was the result of a post-infectious autoimmune response to a virus or other infection, not necessarily the Spanish influenza.

We now know that there are CNS diseases that are caused by autoantibodies and which respond clinically to immunotherapies. These include Morvan's syndrome and limbic encephalitis, as described above, and both old and newly described disorders. In many cases, they have probably previously been assumed to be infectious or of unknown aetiology, and only retrospective analysis of sera has identified specific autoantibodies in a proportion of cases (e.g. [56]). Now, they are identified relatively commonly. The most frequent antibodies known currently are to the NMDA receptor and the VGKC-complex with its associated proteins LGI1 and CASPR2. Antibodies to glycine, AMPA, GABA (a and b), and dopamine receptors are also reported, but in smaller numbers of patients [33, 34].

None of these antibodies, of course, were linked to encephalitis lethargica at the time of their first reports, but the similarities in some of the clinical features is striking, particularly sleep and movement disorders, both hyperkinetic and hypokinetic. In 2007, Spanish neurologist, Josep Dalmau, and colleagues in Philadelphia, first reported N-methyl-D-aspartate receptor (NMDAR) antibodies in patients with an apparently new form of encephalitis, called anti-NMDAR encephalitis [57.58]. These patients had an encephalopathy with striking hyperkinetic features and many were young females with an ovarian tumour. Two years later, Dale and colleagues identified the NMDAR antibodies in 10 of the 20 children with a previous diagnosis of encephalitis lethargica, mainly hyperkinetic, collected over some years and without tumours. More recently, the same authors have reported antibodies to dopamine receptors in some of the remaining, less hyperkinetic, patients [59]. Whether this distinction holds up with further study remains to be seen.

Another feature of 'von Economo's disease' that may prove of current relevance is the possibilities of overlaps and associations between infectious and autoimmune forms of encephalitis. Von Economo mentioned the exacerbation of facial herpes during the early stages of the hyperkinetic form of his disease. Interestingly, there is emerging recognition of coexistence of viral infections with NMDAR antibodies, and NMDAR antibodies have been reported to be present at high titre during virus negative relapses of herpes simplex virus encephalitis in children [60,61]. The implications of these complex relationships could be substantial.

Key unanswered questions

1 How did neurotoxins evolve and become so useful to man?

There is no doubt that many plant and animal toxins have evolved rapidly, although quite what the evolutionary pressure was is not always clear (e.g. why is it useful for poppy flowers to produce opium?). The neurotoxins are far more diverse than most people are aware; just concentrating on those that are useful in neuroscience, there are toxins from sea anemones, cone snails, scorpions, snakes, and spiders, each of which has specificity for different forms of pre- and post-synaptic ion channels, receptors, or other key functional molecules, particularly the phospholipase As. Although in some cases (e.g. phospholipases), their homology with proteins of known function suggests merely a rather fast 'accelerated' evolution, in other cases, there does not appear to be any homology with naturally useful proteins or other compounds in the particular species—so how did the genes originate?

2 What is the process of retrograde signalling at the neuromuscular junction?

When Elmqvist and colleagues [62] demonstrated the reduced miniature end-plate potentials of myasthenic muscles, they questioned whether it was a pre-synaptic or post-synaptic defect. It was not until bungarotoxin was used to quantify and localize the acetylcholine 'receptors' that it was clear that the defect was post-synaptic (see section 15.1). However, the story was not quite so simple. The antibodies to the AChRs cause not only AChR loss but morphological damage that reduces the numbers of voltage-gated sodium channels which provide the muscle action potential. Why are the patients not completely paralysed with this attack on their end plates? There is compensatory increase in AChR synthesis that tries to restore AChR numbers and, more surprisingly, increased release of ACh from the pre-synaptic motor nerve terminal (the quantal content; [63]). How does the motor nerve terminal sense the post-synaptic defect? This is not only a fundamental question in neurobiology but also of clinical relevance, since MuSK antibodies cause not only post-synaptic changes but reduce, rather than increase, the release of ACh from the nerve terminal. How is MuSK involved in retrograde signalling and could this be a target for treatment?

3 At what point in the disease process does intrathecal synthesis become important?

It was a surprise to many that VGKC-complex and NMDAR antibodies were not predominantly found in the CSF. A common comment was 'there must be intrathecal synthesis of the antibody in the CSF and we ought to be sending CSF for diagnosis' but, in fact, the serum levels are almost always considerably higher than CSF levels of these specific antibodies (at presentation and usually thereafter too). So which is most important for pathogenesis? Many of the patients' problems seem to start in the limbic area, with epilepsy and behavioural and cognitive changes. Is the limbic area somewhat leaky to serum antibodies, and is it diffusion through a leaky blood– brain barrier that begins the disease process? Does intrathecal synthesis then take over, unless the patient is lucky enough to be treated quickly to reduce serum levels and prevent further antibody and B cells reaching the brain parenchyma? These are questions that are proving difficult to address but need to be answered.

4 Causes of antibody-mediated diseases—post-infectious or are they mostly occult paraneoplastic?

Until recently, CNS autoimmune diseases were thought to be paraneoplastic; even if no tumour could be found, it was assumed to be occult and perhaps eliminated by a successful anti-tumour response. This was not an unreasonable assumption in older individuals, perhaps, but is less likely to apply to adults with VGKC-complex antibodies or the children who are being diagnosed with NMDAR-antibody encephalitis. Both these antibodies have a tendency to be monophasic, and many patients can be treated successfully and eventually weaned off immunosuppresssion, and some have even improved spontaneously. Now with the evidence for NMDAR antibodies in some forms of encephalitis lethargica, an apparently epidemic disease, and the presence of these antibodies in children relapsing after proven viral encephalitis, we have to revisit the relationship between infections and autoimmunity.

5 What is the best way to treat these diseases?

As discussed, the antibody-mediated CNS diseases appear to be due to a systemic immune response that somehow gains access to the brain parenchyma, followed in many cases by intrathecal synthesis of the antibodies that may, or may not, take over the main pathogenic role. What are the best treatments for these often severe and potentially disabling diseases? Should they be targeted much more systematically to the CNS? At present, most of the treatments are non-specific, and even the widely used rituximab is supposed to delete the B cells but not the plasma cells that make the antibodies; not surprisingly, therefore, disease-specific antibodies fall slowly or sometimes not at all after this treatment. We need to understand much better how to reduce quickly the level of the antibodies in both serum and CSF, and probably also the pro-inflammatory processes that often accompany the resulting CNS inflammation.

References

1 Chang CC, Lee CY. Isolation of neurotoxins from the venom of bungarus multicinctus and their modes of neuromuscular blocking action. Arch Int Pharmacodyn Ther 1963; **144**:241–57.

2 Changeux JP, Kasai M, Lee CY. Use of a snake venom toxin to characterize the cholinergic receptor protein. Proc Natl Acad Sci USA 1970; **67**(3):1241–7.

3 Miledi R, Molinoff P, Potter LT. Isolation of the cholinergic receptor protein of Torpedo electric tissue. Nature 1971; **229**(5286):554–7.

4 Barchan D, Kachalsky S, Neumann D, et al. How the mongoose can fight the snake: the binding site of the mongoose acetylcholine receptor. Proc Natl Acad Sci USA 1992; **89**(16):7717–21.

5 Fambrough DM, Drachman DB, Satyamurti S. Neuromuscular junction in myasthenia gravis: decreased acetylcholine receptors. Science 1973; **182**(4109):293–5.

6 Lindstrom JM, Seybold ME, Lennon VA, Whittingham S, Duane DD. Antibody to acetylcholine receptor in myasthenia gravis. Prevalence, clinical correlates, and diagnostic value. Neurology 1976; **26**(11):1054–9.

7 Patrick J, Lindstrom J. Autoimmune response to acetylcholine receptor. Science 1973; **180**(4088):871–2.

8 Vincent A. New support for autoimmune basis of myasthenia gravis. Nature 1975; **256**:10–1.

9 Toyka KV, Brachman DB, Pestronk A, Kao I. Myasthenia gravis: passive transfer from man to mouse. Science 1975; **190**(4212):397–9.

10 Toyka KV, Drachman DB, Griffin DE, et al. Myasthenia gravis. Study of humoral immune mechanisms by passive transfer to mice. N Engl J Med 1977; **296**(3):125–31.

11 Engel AG. Myasthenia gravis and myasthenic syndromes. Ann Neurol. 1984 Nov;**16**(5):519–34.

12 Saadoun S, Waters P, Bell BA, Vincent A, Verkman AS, Papadopoulos MC. Intra-cerebral injection of neuromyelitis optica immunoglobulin G and human complement produces neuromyelitis optica lesions in mice. Brain 2010; **133**(Pt 2):349–61.

13 Oon CJ, Hobbs JR. Clinical applications of the continuous flow blood separator machine. Clin Exp Immunol 1975; **20**(1):1–16.

14 Lockwood CM, Boulton-Jones JM, Lowenthal RM, Simpson IJ, Peters DK. Recovery from Goodpasture's syndrome after immunosuppressive treatment and plasmapheresis. BMJ 1975; **2**(5965):252–4.

15 Pinching AJ, Peters DK. Remission of myasthenia gravis following plasma-exchange. Lancet 1976; **2**(8000):1373–6.

16 Dau PC, Lindstrom JM, Cassel CK, Denys EH, Shev EE, Spitler LE. Plasmapheresis and immunosuppressive drug therapy in myasthenia gravis. N Engl J Med 1977; **297**(21):1134–40.

17 Newsom-Davis J, Pinching AJ, Vincent A, Wilson SG. Function of circulating antibody to acetylcholine receptor in myasthenia gravis: investigation by plasma exchange. Neurology 1978; **28**(3):266–72.

18 Hall ZW, Sanes JR. Synaptic structure and development: the neuromuscular junction. Cell. 1993 Jan;**72** Suppl:99–121.

19 Porter CW, Barnard EA, Chiu TH. The ultrastructural localization and quantitation of cholinergic receptors at the mouse motor endplate. J Membr Biol 1973; **14**(4):383–402.

20 Valenzuela DM, Stitt TN, Distefano PS, et al. Receptor tyrosine kinase specific for the skeletal muscle lineage—expression in embryonic muscle, at the neuromuscular junction and after injury. Neuron 1995; **3**:573–84.

21 Hoch W, McConville J, Helms S, Newsom-Davis J, Melms A, Vincent A. Auto-antibodies to the receptor tyrosine kinase MuSK in patients with myasthenia gravis without acetylcholine receptor antibodies. Nat Med 2001; **7**(3):365–8.

22 **DeChiara TM, Bowen DC, Valenzuela DM, Simmons MV, Poueymirou WT, Thomas S, et al.** The receptor tyrosine kinase MuSK is required for neuromuscular junction formation in vivo. Cell 1996; **85**(4):501–12.

23 **Beeson D.** Synaptic dysfunction in congenital myasthenic syndromes. Ann NY Acad Sci 2012; **1275**:63–9.

24 **Gautam M, Noakes PG, Moscoso L, et al.** Defective neuromuscular synaptogenesis in agrin-deficient mutant mice. Cell 1996; **85**(4):525–35.

25 **Kasper BS, Taylor DC, Janz D, et al.** Neuropathology of epilepsy and psychosis: the contributions of J.A.N. Corsellis. Brain 2010; 133(Pt 12):3795–805.

26 **Corsellis JA, Goldberg GJ, Norton AR.** 'Limbic encephalitis' and its association with carcinoma. Brain 1968; **91**(3):481–96.

27 **Brierley JB, Corsellis JAN, Hierons R, et al.** Subacute encephalitis of later adult life mainly affecting the limbic areas. Brain 1960; **83**:357–68.

28 **Bien CG, Schulze-Bonhage A, Deckert M, et al.** Limbic encephalitis not associated with neoplasm as a cause of temporal lobe epilepsy. Neurology 2000; **55**(12):1823–8.

29 **Giometto B, Grisold W, Vitaliani R, Graus F, Honnorat J, Bertolini G; PNS Euronetwork.** Paraneoplastic neurologic syndrome in the PNS Euronetwork database: a European study from 20 centers.Arch Neurol. 2010 Mar;**67**(3):330–5.

30 **Bien CG, Bauer J, Deckwerth TL, et al.** Destruction of neurons by cytotoxic T cells: a new pathogenic mechanism in Rasmussen's encephalitis. Ann Neurol 2002; **51**(3):311–8.

31 **Rogers SW, Andrews PI, Gahring LC, et al.** Autoantibodies to glutamate receptor GluR3 in Rasmussen's encephalitis. Science 1994; **265**(5172):648–51.

32 **Watson R, Jiang Y, Bermudez I, et al.** Absence of antibodies to glutamate receptor type 3 (GluR3) in Rasmussen encephalitis. Neurology 2004; **63**(1):43–50.

33 **Vincent A, Bien CG, Irani SR, Waters P.** Autoantibodies associated with diseases of the CNS: new developments and future challenges. Lancet Neurol 2011; **10**(8):759–72.

34 **Lancaster E, Dalmau J.** Neuronal autoantigens—pathogenesis, associated disorders and antibody testing. Nat Rev Neurol 2012; **8**(7):380–90.

35 **Suleiman J, Brenner T, Gill D, et al.** VGKC antibodies in pediatric encephalitis presenting with status epilepticus. Neurol 2011; **76**(14):1252–5.

36 **Brenner T, Sills GJ, Hart Y, et al.** Prevalence of neurologic autoantibodies in cohorts of patients with new and established epilepsy. Epilepsia 2013 Jun; **54**(6):1028–35.

37 **Newsom-Davis J, Mills KR.** Immunological associations of acquired neuromyotonia (Isaacs' syndrome). Report of five cases and literature review. Brain 1993; **116** (Pt 2):453–69.

38 **Walusinski O, Honnorat J.** Augustin Morvan (1819–97), a little-known rural physician and neurologist. Rev Neurol (Paris) 2013; **169**(1):2–8.

39 **Irani SR, Pettingill P, Kleopa KA, et al.** Morvan syndrome: clinical and serological observations in 29 cases. Ann Neurol 2012; **72**(2):241–55.

40 **Sinha S, Newsom-Davis J, Mills K, Byrne N, Lang B, Vincent A.** Autoimmune aetiology for acquired neuromyotonia (Isaacs' syndrome). Lancet 1991; **338**(8759):75–7.

41 **Shillito P, Molenaar PC, Vincent A, et al.** Acquired neuromyotonia: evidence for autoantibodies directed against K + channels of peripheral nerves. Ann Neurol 1995; **38**(5):714–22.

42 **Hart IK, Waters C, Vincent A, et al.** Autoantibodies detected to expressed K + channels are implicated in neuromyotonia. Ann Neurol 1997; **41**(2):238–46.

43 **Roberts M, Willison H, Vincent A, Newsom-Davis J.** Serum factor in Miller-Fisher variant of Guillain-Barre syndrome and neurotransmitter release. Lancet 1994; **343**(8895):454–5.

44 **Plomp JJ, Willison HJ.** Pathophysiological actions of neuropathy-related anti-ganglioside antibodies at the neuromuscular junction. J Physiol 2009; **587**(Pt 16):3979–99.

45 **Hart IK, Maddison P, Newsom-Davis J, Vincent A, Mills KR.** Phenotypic variants of autoimmune peripheral nerve hyperexcitability. Brain 2002; **125**(Pt 8):1887–95.

46 **Buckley C, Oger J, Clover L, et al.** Potassium channel antibodies in two patients with reversible limbic encephalitis. Ann Neurol 2001; **50**(1):73–8.

47 **Vincent A, Buckley C, Schott JM, et al.** Potassium channel antibody-associated encephalopathy: a potentially immunotherapy-responsive form of limbic encephalitis. Brain 2004; **127**(Pt 3):701–12.

48 **Irani SR, Alexander S, Waters P, et al.** Antibodies to Kv1 potassium channel-complex proteins leucine-rich, glioma inactivated 1 protein and contactin-associated protein-2 in limbic encephalitis, Morvan's syndrome and acquired neuromyotonia. Brain 2010; **133**(9):2734–48.

49 **Lai M, Huijbers MG, Lancaster E, et al.** Investigation of LGI1 as the antigen in limbic encephalitis previously attributed to potassium channels: a case series. Lancet Neurol 2010; **9**(8):776–85.

50 **Irani SR, Michell AW, Lang B, Pettingill P, Waters P, Johnson MR, Schott JM, Armstrong RJ, S Zagami A, Bleasel A, Somerville ER, Smith SM, Vincent A.** Faciobrachial dystonic seizures precede Lgi1 antibody limbic encephalitis. Ann Neurol. 2011 May;**69**(5):892–900

51 **Lugaresi E, Provini F, Cortelli P.** Agrypnia excitata. Sleep Med 2011; **12** Suppl 2:S3–10.

52 **Demetriades AK.** From encephalitis lethargica to cerebral cytoarchitectonics: the polymath talent of Constantin von Economo (1876–1931), pioneer neuroanatomist, neurophysiologist and military aviator. Scott Med J 2012; **57**:232–6.

53 **McCall S, Henry JM, Reid AH, Taubenberger JK.** Influenza RNA not detected in archival brain tissues from acute encephalitis lethargica cases or in postencephalitic Parkinson cases. J Neuropathol Exp Neurol 2001; **60**(7):696–704.

54 **Reid AH, McCall S, Henry JM, Taubenberger JK.** Experimenting on the past: the enigma of von Economo's encephalitis lethargica. J Neuropathol Exp Neurol 2001; **60**(7):663–70.

55 **Liguori R, Vincent A, Clover L, et al.** Morvan's syndrome: peripheral and central nervous system and cardiac involvement with antibodies to voltage-gated potassium channels. Brain 2001; **124**(Pt 12):2417–26.

56 **Granerod J, Ambrose HE, Davies NW, et al.** Causes of encephalitis and differences in their clinical presentations in England: a multicentre, population-based prospective study. Lancet 2010; **10**(12):835–44.

57 **Dalmau J, Tüzün E, Wu HY, Masjuan J, Rossi JE, Voloschin A, Baehring JM, Shimazaki H, Koide R, King D, Mason W, Sansing LH, Dichter MA, Rosenfeld MR, Lynch DR.** Paraneoplastic anti-N-methyl-D-aspartate receptor encephalitis associated with ovarian teratoma. Ann Neurol. 2007 Jan;**61**(1):25–36.

58 **Dalmau J, Gleichman AJ, Hughes EG, et al.** Anti-NMDA-receptor encephalitis: case series and analysis of the effects of antibodies. Lancet Neurol 2008; **7**(12):1091–8.

59 **Dale RC, Merheb V, Pillai S, et al.** Antibodies to surface dopamine-2 receptor in autoimmune movement and psychiatric disorders. Brain 2012; **135**(Pt 11):3453–68.

60 **Armangue T, Titulaer MJ, Malaga I, et al.** Pediatric anti-N-methyl-D-aspartate receptor encephalitis-clinical analysis and novel findings in a series of 20 patients. J Pediat 2013; **162**(4):850–6 e2.

61 **Hacohen Y, Wright S, Waters P, et al.** Paediatric autoimmune encephalopathies: clinical features, laboratory investigations and outcomes in patients with or without antibodies to known central nervous system autoantigens. J Neurol Neurosurg Psychiat 2013; **84**(7):748–55.

62 **Elmqvist D, Hofmann WW, Kugelberg J, Quastel DM.** An electrophysiological investigation of neuromuscular transmission in myasthenia gravis. J Physiol 1964; **174**:417–34.

63 **Plomp JJ, Molenaar PC, O'Hanlon GM, et al.** Miller Fisher anti-GQ1b antibodies: alpha-latrotoxin-like effects on motor end plates. Ann Neurol 1999; 45(2):189–99.

Chapter 16

Multiple sclerosis

Alasdair Coles and Alastair Compston

16.0 **Introduction**

Having been recognized only since the early nineteenth century, there has been just over 175 years of research on multiple sclerosis. Over this time, a picture has emerged of this disease as an inflammatory disorder of the central nervous system, caused by a complex interplay of multiple genetic susceptibility alleles and unknown environmental triggers. We have tried to illustrate this in our choice of landmark papers, at the same time being aware that strong cases could be pressed for other studies to be included. It is clear that many lines of scientific evidence relating on the disease have benefited from increasingly sophisticated technologies. Three of our 'top 10' were authored by Ian McDonald (1933–2006), testimony to his extraordinary contribution to understanding multiple sclerosis [1].

16.1 **Pathological anatomy of multiple sclerosis**

Main paper: Dawson JD. The histology of disseminated sclerosis. *Trans Roy Soc Edinburgh* 1916; 50:517–740.

Background

With this paper, James Dawson (1870–1927) left the greatest pathological account of multiple sclerosis in the English language. First, he summarizes the literature. The issue (then, as now, for some contemporary commentators) is whether the disease is 'inflammatory' or 'developmental' (degenerative). The preliminary vascular, inflammatory doctrine was espoused by Dejerine [2], Williamson [3, 4] and Marie [5], who suggested that infections initiate the changes in blood vessels. Bielschowsky [6] considered that the vascular process is directed primarily at nerve fibres; conversely Strumpell [7] believed that exogenous insults act upon an 'intrinsically weakened' system; and Bramwell [8] also saw multiple sclerosis as primarily a developmental disturbance. Müller [9], the most articulate teacher from the developmental school, proposed that any participation of the blood vessels within the lesion is secondary, and his concept of 'multiple gliosis' as the essential process rehearses the final position taken by Charcot [10] and most of his school. Redlich [11] and Huber [12] also saw the insult as a toxin- or micro-organism-induced primary degeneration of the myelin sheath with secondary inflammation and blood vessel changes. However, as often is the case, the best account was the first: Rindfleisch [13] assigned priority to the blood vessels, proposing a sequence in which a chronic irritative condition of the vessel wall alters the nutrition of nerve elements, leading to atrophy with metamorphosis of the connective tissue producing monster glia (Deiters or Rindfleisch cells).

Methods

Reviewing the histology of nine personal cases (L.W., a kitchen maid, aged 28; C.S., aged 22; Mrs G., aged 30; J.W.; S.S., a nurse aged 44; C.G., a baker's shop-woman, aged 24; J. McN., a cabinet maker, aged 42; M.R., a typist, aged 33; and L.H., aged 30), Dawson devotes the majority of his text to L.W. She was admitted to hospital in Edinburgh under the care of Dr Alexander Bruce on 4th April 1910 with a two-year history of weakness and tremor in all four limbs, dysarthria, and sphincter disturbance. In hospital she has an episode of brainstem demyelination (deafness and tinnitus, right facial palsy, numb left arm, right lateral rectus weakness, tongue deviation to the left, and dysphagia) starting on 29th May. In August, she loses vision in both eyes, develops increasing bulbar failure, and dies from septicaemia on 5th September 1910. Dawson describes the features of early and established lesions in the spinal cord and cerebrum (Fig. 16.1), offering an analysis of their evolution through stages of fat granule cell myelitis (in the cord) to glial hyperplasia. He devotes text to the unusual lesions, including Markschattenherde (shadow plaques), and those appearing in grey matter and around the ventricles, optic nerve, peripheral nerves, and roots (which he considers to be evolving lesions). In addition, he mentions three hyperacute cases with an accelerated clinical pattern of relapses, rapid accumulation of deficits, and characteristic histological features. Curiously, he neglects an important monograph identifying shadow plaques which we now know to be indicative of remyelination, not partial demyelination [14]. Next, Dawson turns to an analysis of the changes to be observed in each cellular element of the nervous system—nerve cells and their axons, neuroglia, blood vessels, and lymphatics. Form, symmetry, and the distribution of lesions are all addressed.

Results

After listing the tragic accumulation of lesions throughout the brain and spinal cord of the unfortunate L.W., Dawson attempts a clinicopathophysiological correlation. Weakness in the legs is consistent with the extensive spinal cord gliosis; intention tremor, with lesions in the superior cerebellar peduncles and red nuclei; disordered eye movements, with the periaqueductal plaques; and the several cranial nerve palsies, with involvement of the pons and medulla. Dawson shows that old (sclerotic) lesions are characterized by complete absence of myelin (Weigert stain), dense fibrillary tissue (glial stain), persistence of axis cylinders (silver stain), numerous blood vessels (diffuse stains), no active myelin degeneration (Marchi stain), and an abrupt transition to normal tissue. In acute lesions,

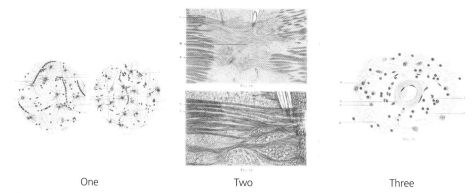

One   Two   Three

Fig. 16.1 [One]: Glia changes in a completely demyelinated area in the cortex. a: Proliferated glia cells with protoplasm and processes differentiated into fibrils; b: capillaries with glia fibrils attached to their outer membrane; c: ganglion cells; d: small glia cells forming nests around the remains of ganglion cells; e: degenerated ganglion cells; f: retained axis cylinders. Note that the normal cytoarchitecture of the tissue is preserved. **[Two]** Persistence of axis cylinders across a demyelinated area in the pons. a: line of transition between myelinated and demyelinated fibres; b: median raphe where axis cylinders intersect. **[Three]** Changes in the blood vessels. a: glia nuclei; b: blood vessel; c: fat granule cell; d: cell containing blood pigment; e: lymphocyte-like cells; f: plasma cells; g: glia tissue; h: connective tissue cell.)

Reproduced from *Transactions of the Royal Society of Edinburgh*, 50, The Royal Society of Edinburgh, p. 517–740, Copyright (1916), with permission from The Royal Society of Edinburgh.

the differences are infiltrated blood vessels, active demyelination with fat granule cells, and transitional zones shading into normal tissue. He illustrates the text with 22 colour and 434 black and white figures (in 78 plates).

Conclusions

Dawson summarizes his ideas on plaque formation around brain inflammation to include a sequence of events that, although not disease-specific, produces recognizable clinical characteristics when directed at glia, leading to degeneration of the myelin sheath with fat granule cell formation, and a reactive change in glia involving cell proliferation with fibril formation culminating in sclerosis.

Critique

Dawson speculated that the inflammatory process is triggered and modified by exogenous factors whose influences fluctuate, causing the characteristic relapses. Remissions depend more on rerouting of synaptic connections—which we would now interpret as plasticity—than remyelination. These comments are prescient.

Perhaps Dawson falls into the trap, which has a distinguished pedigree, of believing that the pathologist can see the cause, effects, and evolution of disease merely by observing snapshots of its end state. Nonetheless, by placing inflammation firmly centre-stage and discarding the 'degenerative hypotheses', Dawson's work set up a theme of research that can be traced through to the modern era of immunological therapies. This is not to say that the argument is fully resolved; still some authors maintain that multiple sclerosis is a degenerative disease with inflammation a secondary phenomenon [15, 16].

16.2 **Evidence for an immune response within the central nervous system in multiple sclerosis**

Main paper: Lowenthal A, Vansande M, Karcher DJ. The differential diagnosis of neurological diseases by fractionating electrophoretically the CSF proteins. *Neurochem* 1960; 6:51–60.

Background

The most consistent laboratory abnormality in multiple sclerosis is the finding of a restricted number of 'oligoclonal' immunoglobulins within the cerebrospinal fluid. These are produced by B cells in the parenchyma of the central nervous system and drift into the cerebrospinal fluid like oil in the sump. The history of their discovery is intimately tied to technological advances, hence our description of the evolution of methods in electrophoresis.

Methods

In 1948, the Nobel Prize for Chemistry was awarded to the Swede, Arne Tiselius, for his application of physical techniques to biological molecules, mainly electrophoresis of proteins. In 1938, he had collaborated with Elvin Kabat who went on, with Harold Landow, to study protein electrophoresis of cerebrospinal fluid from patients with a variety of conditions, including multiple sclerosis, at the Neurological Institute of the College of Physicians and Surgeons at Columbia University in New York. In their 1942 paper, submitted a few days after Landow's death, Kabat and Landlow showed that the ratio of gamma globulin to albumin in cerebrospinal fluid is normally identical to serum, except in patients with neurosyphillis [17]. Rather lyrically, they conclude that 'the data would suggest that some formation of gamma globulin could take place within the tissues of the central nervous system and be poured into cerebrospinal fluid'. This was a new concept; up until then, there was little evidence in humans for an immune response confined to the central nervous system. The researchers commented in passing, within the results section, that of five cases of multiple sclerosis, one had some evidence for intrathecal gamma-globulin synthesis, but they made no more of this.

The Tiselius technique is based on fluid boundaries, requires expensive bulky equipment, and is difficult to perform. From the 1940s onwards, 'zone' electrophoresis was developed, with filter paper used as a substrate. Then, in 1955, Oliver Smithies -an English medical student who failed to complete his degree-developed gel-based electrophoresis [18]. In 2007, he received the Nobel Prize with Mario Capecchi and Martin Evans 'for their discoveries of principles for introducing specific gene modifications in mice by the use of embryonic stem cells'.

Results

The paper we have chosen comes from Lowenthal and colleagues, at the Neurochemical Research Laboratory of the Neurological Department, Antwerp, translated from the

French by Charles Poser, author of another of our top 10 papers. This group pioneered the application of agar electrophoresis to cerebrospinal fluid proteins. They saw, for the first time, multiple sharp gamma-globulin bands (lanes 1, 2 and 3) in the cerebrospinal fluid of patients with multiple sclerosis, which were not present in normal individuals. They distinguished these from the increased lanes 4 and 5 bands seen in subacute sclerosing panencephalitis (Fig. 16.2). They made a point of saying that such bands were rarely seen in cases of African trypanosomiasis (although they confessed that the electrophoresis of these specimens had been delayed by one week because the lumbar punctures were performed in the Belgian Congo). By now, cerebrospinal fluid electrophoresis was being promoted as a diagnostic aid for multiple sclerosis in clinical practice.

Conclusions

Although not commenting on the role of oligoclonal bands in the pathogenesis of multiple sclerosis, this paper made the case that they could be used in the diagnosis of the disease. It is now clear that such bands are found in 90–95% of people with the disease; but also in conditions having an inflammatory basis and, rarely, apparently by chance.

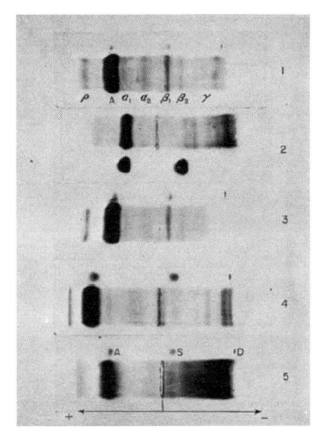

Fig. 16.2 Lowenthal's agar gel micro-electrophoresis pattern of CSF from: 1—multiple sclerosis; 2—subacute sclerosing leucoencephalitis (SSLE); 3—normal; 4—neurosyphilis; 5—African trypanosomiasis.

Reproduced from *J Neurochemistry*, 6, A. Lowenthal, M. Vansande, and D. Karcher, The differential diagnosis of neurological diseases by fractionating electrophoretically the CSF gamma-globulins, p. 51–6, Copyright (1960), with permission from John Wiley and Sons.

Critique

The next technological innovation was isoelectric focusing of agarose-gel electrophoresis, which improved sensitivity yet further. Hans Link and colleagues were early in exploiting this showing, as well as improved definition of the 'oligoclonal bands' (a term that Link coined), that these were largely due to the presence of IgG antibodies [19, 20].

The scientific dividend from the discovery of cerebrospinal fluid oligoclonal bands has been frustratingly small. It seems that there is no consistent antigenic target for the antibodies and they are unaffected by most effective therapies. However, the recent discovery of meningeal B-cell lymphoid follicles and the moderate efficacy of B-cell depleting antibodies has reawakened interest in the role of B cells and antibodies in multiple sclerosis [21].

In clinical practice, the advent of magnetic resonance imaging has reduced the frequency with which it is necessary to test the cerebrospinal fluid in the diagnosis of multiple sclerosis. In the tricky diagnostic case, the finding of cerebrospinal fluid oligoclonal bands can be an indispensable ally, for it remains the only direct clinical test of the pivotal disease process—active inflammation within the central nervous system.

16.3 **Steroid treatment of the acute relapse**

Main paper: Rose AS, Kuzma JW, Kurtzke JF. Cooperative study in the evaluation of therapy in multiple sclerosis: ACTH vs placebo. Final report. *Neurology* 1970; 20:1–19.

Background

> In 1960, at a symposium concerned with the evaluation of drug therapy in neurologic and sensory diseases, the many particular difficulties involved in the clinical trials of therapy in multiple sclerosis were recognized, including those pertaining to the conduct of cooperative studies.

So opens this massive, 59-page report on a trial of adrenocorticotropic hormone (ACTH) as a treatment of multiple sclerosis in relapse. The symposium led to the establishment of an ad hoc committee which reported, in 1965, on the ideal trial for a multiple sclerosis therapy [22]. Five years later, the first application of its principles was published. It represents a landmark in trial rigour and quality, despite a rather unsatisfactory conclusion.

Methods

By 1965, there was agreement that ACTH did not influence multiple sclerosis in the long term, but small-scale reports on its short-term effect on relapses were conflicting. Rose and colleagues suspected that ACTH might have an effect, but of small magnitude, which would require careful trial design to reveal. So, they insisted on a placebo control, and on the use of 10 neurology centres, to maximize recruitment of the required number of patients (eventually197). They described, as a particular strength of the trial:

> a statistical centre office and staff, backed by computer facilities, ensured randomization, diminished bias in data review, and provided opportunity for the multiple analyses that were required for the extensive clinical observations.

Each patient was in hospital for two weeks, receiving twice daily injections of diminishing doses of ACTH or placebo. They were assessed each week, for four weeks, on several scales:

- a rather arbitrary 'estimate of overall condition'
- Kurtzke's Disability Status Scale and Functional Systems Score
- the standard neurological examination
- seven-day symptom score, which attempted to capture what would now be called an 'area under the curve' disability metric
- quantitative examination of neurological function.

Results

Fifty-two pages of charts, tables, and text describe the results of these analyses. Each outcome assessment is compared to another, and across centres, to see which was the most consistent and which scales correlated with each other. In contrast to the detail on outcome measures, there is none on the trial's selection criteria, just a reference to the protocol, published in a previous issue of *Neurology*. Also, there is no discussion at all of statistical technique and power.

The primary outcome measure was comparison of patients' disability at baseline with that at four weeks after starting treatment. There was a significant difference in favour of ACTH, but the authors were not impressed. Firstly, they noted that the size of benefit fell between the third and fourth week, suggesting that it might disappear altogether on extended follow-up. Secondly, they questioned whether the statistically significant difference was clinically significant:

> The treatment results of the study as revealed by extensive analysis of a large mass of data may be considered noteworthy for, although the degree of improvement of the patients treated by ACTH attained statistical significance by each of the several methods of evaluation, at no time was the improvement particularly obvious or outstanding. Indeed, 69% of the patients who were treated by placebo attained improvement, a factor that will not be overlooked by thoughtful investigators.

Conclusions

The authors main conclusion, which has been tested many times ever since and has yet to be bettered, was that:

> the Disability Status Scale, together with the Functional Systems, comprises an adequate system of evaluating change in a therapeutic trial of MS and, of all the measures used in this study, apparently is the most consistent indicator of change.

They also pointed out that:

> It is evident that the 'placebo effect' of a well ordered, seriously applied therapeutic effort, although complex and difficult to define, provides a powerful influence which may qualify treatment results. These observations should serve to temper the enthusiasm of those who would advocate a specific therapy for MS unless the therapeutic trial is adequately and appropriately controlled.

They were doubtful of any real long-term efficacy of steroids in the treatment of relapse.

Critique

Soon, clinicians moved to using synthetic corticosteroids, rather than ACTH, to promote release of endogenous steroids. The lack of extended follow-up in the Rose study was corrected by a study in Wales of 50 people with multiple sclerosis treated with placebo or intravenous methylprednisolone [23], and more still was learned from the effect of steroids on optic neuritis [24–27]. The conclusion of all of these studies is that steroids reduce the duration of a relapse of multiple sclerosis, but have no impact on the extent of residual disability nor of the subsequent disease course.

16.4 **The clinical demonstration of demyelination**

Main paper: Halliday AM, McDonald WI, Mushin J. Delayed visual evoked response in optic neuritis. *Lancet* 1972; i:982–5.

Background

Recording of electrical activity of the brain over the scalp had been pioneered by Hans Berger in the 1920s. The motivation behind his experiments, it seems, was to identify the mechanism underlying telepathic communication with his sister during an accident whilst he was serving with the cavalry. In 1924, he recorded the first human electroen-cephalogram (EEG) [28]. E.D. Adrian, who received the 1932 Nobel Prize in Physiology or Medicine with Sir Charles Sherrington, promoted Berger's work and showed the value of EEG in neurological practice [29]. It was a small step from there to measure scalp potentials over the parietal or occipital lobes following a sensory stimulus or flash of light: somatosensory and visual 'evoked potentials' respectively. George Dawson methodically solved the technical challenges, not the least by introducing a technique to reduce noise by averaging multiple samples of small evoked potentials [30].

Methods

Martin Halliday (Fig. 16.3) set to applying these new methods to the problem of multiple sclerosis, showing, in 1963, that affected individuals have delayed somatosensory evoked potentials [31]. However, the changes were not robust and he soon turned his attention to visual evoked potentials. In the meantime, Ian McDonald working in New Zealand and later, in London, with Tom Sears had demonstrated the electrical consequences of central nervous system demyelination [32, 33]. They showed that direct micro-injection of diphtheria toxin into the spinal cord of the cat produces a highly circumscribed demyelinating lesion which leads to conduction block, or prolongation of the refractory period for transmission and an impaired ability to transmit high-frequency trains of impulses.

Cases were recruited from Ian McDonald's clinic at the Moorfields Eye Hospital. Nineteen patients with unilateral optic neuritis (17 in the acute phase) were studied with flash visual evoked potentials and a new technique, 'pattern' visual evoked potentials (an alternating black and white checkerboard).

Results

In optic neuritis, the mean latency of visual evoked potentials in the affected eye was 155 msec, an increase of 30% over that from healthy people or the unaffected eye; and the peak amplitude was halved at 3.68 microV. In the five patients seen acutely with visual acuities of 6/60 or less, there was no evoked response at all; but, as their vision recovered over weeks, so their visual evoked potential reappeared, although much delayed. Evoked potentials remained delayed, even when visual acuities had recovered to normal, for up to five years. Pattern-evoked potentials elicited more reproducible and sensitive responses than a flash potential.

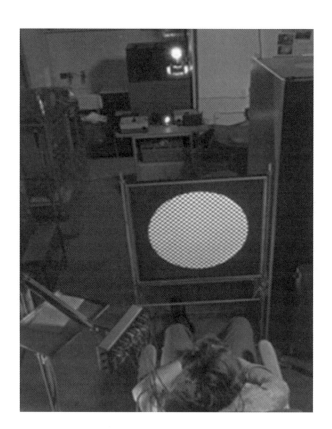

Fig. 16.3a Halliday's equipment for measuring visual evoked potentials.

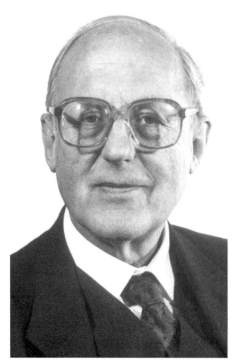

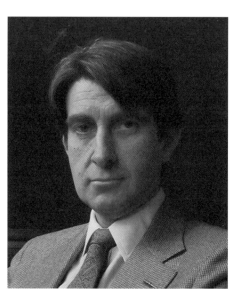

Fig. 16.3b Martin Halliday and Ian McDonald.

Conclusions

The authors concluded:

> Since a persistently increased latency may be present with normal optic discs, fields, and fundi, the technique described here provides a useful objective test for previous damage to the optic nerve. Its potential usefulness in the diagnosis of multiple sclerosis when patients present with clinical evidence of only a single lesion not involving the visual system is obvious.

Critique

Halliday and McDonald went on to test the 'obvious' in a group of unselected multiple sclerosis patients [34]. In 24 individuals with a previous history of optic neuritis, nine had normal discs and all had abnormal visual evoked potentials; therefore abnormal visual evoked potentials are especially reliable indicators of past optic neuritis. Perhaps more usefully, in 27 patients with no history of optic neuritis, 25 had abnormal visual evoked potentials, of whom discs appeared normal in 12. It seems as though abnormal visual evoked potentials provide a sensitive means of identifying previous subclinical optic neuritis. The authors went on to propose diagnostic criteria for multiple sclerosis which incorporated visual evoked potentials [35]. These have evolved, over the years, into the McDonald criteria [36].

To date, it remains true that the only clinical diagnostic test that can demonstrate that a central neurological lesion is *demyelinating* is the cortical evoked potential, of which the pattern-evoked visual potential is by far the most sensitive and robust.

16.5 **The genetics of multiple sclerosis**

Main paper: Naito S, Namerow N, Mickey MR, Terasaki PI. Multiple sclerosis: association with HL-A3. *Tissue Antigens* 1972; 2:1–4.

Background

Discoveries in the genetic basis for susceptibility to multiple sclerosis have followed each increment of technological and statistical innovation in genetics, but the most important association of the disease, with alleles of the human leukocyte antigen system, began to be uncovered in the early 1970s.

Human leukocyte antigens (HLAs) were first identified as serum factors in transplant recipients that reacted against a third party 'tissue', and were associated with transplant rejection. A key figure was Paul Terasaki at UCLA who (having clawed his way into medicine from the low point of being interned as a schoolboy during the war because of his Japanese origins) developed the microcytotoxicity test, a tissue-typing test for organ transplant donors and recipients that required only 1 microlitre each of antisera [37]. (He founded a company to exploit the technology, One Lambda, which grew to generate sufficient income to enable him to make a $50 million donation to UCLA in 2010.)

In 1970, Terasaki organized the Fourth Histocompatibility Workshop in Los Angeles which brought together 15 different laboratories testing 116 highly selected antisera. The conclusion was that there were 11 official HL-A specificities (HL-A1, 2, 3, 5, 7, 8, 9, 10, 11, 12, and 13) and perhaps eight other specificities.

Methods

Shortly after this workshop, Terasaki turned his attention to multiple sclerosis. His group concluded, from 94 patients and 871 controls, that HL-A3 was overrepresented [38]. Furthermore, they demonstrated that the geographical variation in prevalence of multiple sclerosis paralleled the prevalence of HL-A3; for instance, both are high in Scandinavian countries, middle range in America, and low in 'oriental' countries.

Conclusions

They summarized some of the epidemiology suggesting an environmental cause for multiple sclerosis and concluded that 'the evidence to date on MS, however, is still consistent with the idea that a genetic difference in susceptibility underlies some environmental influence.'

Critique

Soon after this paper, Caspar Jersild and colleagues from Copenhagen wrote a brief letter to the *Lancet*, to make some generic points around HLA genetics [39]. They described correction for multiple testing, the need for replication datasets, and the usefulness of meta-analyses. Illustrating their argument, they announced the results of HLA serotyping in 36 Danish patients with multiple sclerosis followed by a replication set in 71 other patients.

From these analyses, HL-A7 emerged as most associated with multiple sclerosis. However, when the Danes merged their data with that from the Terasaki study, and corrected for multiple testing, only HL-A3 retained significance. This set the tone for the years to follow of underpowered studies leading to false positive results and real associations revealed by combining datasets.

Paul Terasaki returned to multiple sclerosis with the discovery of the B-lymphocyte alloantigen serotypes. In 1976, both his group and one of the authors of this chapter discovered the association with what would come to be called the class II allele HLA-DR15 [40, 41]. (This explains, at least in part, the finding by Naito et al. of an association of multiple sclerosis with HL-A3 serotype; in Western Eurasia, A3 is part of the longest known multigene haplotype, A3-B7-DR15-DQ6.) HLA-DR15 remains the best characterized candidate susceptibility gene for multiple sclerosis. After 1976, several decades of increasingly large, expensive, and sophisticated molecular genetic studies followed; all confirmed the association with DR15, but very little else. Only in the last few years has there been sufficient power in the techniques and cohorts, forged through large collaborations (especially studies from the International MS Genetics Consortium), to uncover the much smaller individual genetic contributions of a host of other alleles [42].

The finding that multiple sclerosis is associated with the HLA system implicates the immune system in its pathogenesis; explains some of the geographical variation of the disease; provides a molecular substrate for the interaction of genetics and environment; and suggests treatment directed at the T-lymphocyte, the T-cell receptor, and the class II Major Histocompatibility Complex molecule.

16.6 **Remyelination in multiple sclerosis**

Main paper: Gledhill RF, Harrison BM, McDonald WI. Pattern of remyelination in the CNS. *Nature* 1973; 244(5416):443–4.

Background

A principal hope of people affected by multiple sclerosis is not only control of their disease but reversal of any damage already accrued: repair, possibly facilitated by therapy. Although not yet an everyday reality, trials of potential remyelinating therapies are being conducted. Key steps that made such therapies possible were the demonstrations that remyelination occurs naturally in the central nervous system; that this was mediated by the oligodendrocyte precursor; and that it was accompanied by functional improvement. We could have chosen one of several studies which contribute to this narrative. We have chosen the paper which definitively demonstrated remyelination in the adult mammalian central nervous system, and—perhaps most importantly—showed how to identity demyelinated fibres.

Critical work had already been done by Dick and Mary Bunge [43] who studied myelin repair in cats following demyelination induced by cerebrospinal fluid barbotage. They showed that the remyelinating cell differed from the mature oligodendrocyte and, proposed incorrectly as it turned out, that mature oligodendrocytes de-differentiated into a cell capable of remyelination. Perier and Gregoire [44] showed, from electron microscopic multiple sclerosis plaques, that axons were surrounded by thin myelin lamellae, which they considered to be evidence for remyelination.

Methods

The paper we have chosen comes from Richard Gledhill, Barry Harrison, and Ian McDonald [45]. They compressed the spinal cord of three adult cats, which causes early demyelination with retained axons, and systematically studied subsequent histological changes. Their main technical discovery, under the electron microscope, was that the remyelinated sheath is abnormally thin and has an intermodal distance reduced by 50% compared to control fibres of the same diameter. Under the light microscope, they found no evidence for the presence of Schwann cells, so concluded that oligodendrocytes had been responsible for the remyelination.

Results

Remyelination can occur in the adult mammalian central nervous system approximately three weeks after demyelination.

Conclusions and critique

A key outcome of this work was the definition of the ultrastructural characteristics of remyelination (as opposed to the partially demyelinated axons) used today: reduced internode distance and inappropriately thin myelin. The next important step in the history of remyelination studies was the demonstration that such remyelinated axons could restore function. This work was also supervised by Ian McDonald, working with the electrophysiologist, Ken Smith [46, 47].

16.7 **The epidemiology of multiple sclerosis**

Main paper: Kurtzke JF. Geography in multiple sclerosis. *J Neurology* 1977; 215(1):1–26.

Background

Epidemiology is less dependent upon technological advances than other disciplines represented in this chapter, and more reliant on the steady accumulation of disparate data. So, it is less easy to identify one paper which has made a seminal impression on the field. We could have chosen something from the oeuvre of Geoffrey Dean, who published on multiple sclerosis from 1949 to 2002, focusing especially on the effect of migration on the risk of multiple sclerosis—initially on migration to South Africa; then from Asia, the Caribbean, and Africa to the United Kingdom [48–50]. We chose, instead, one of John Kurtzke's key papers.

John Kurtzke saw action in the Second World War as a pharmacist's mate (2nd class). On discharge, he went to medical school and spent most of his professional life as a neurologist in the Veteran's Administration Service, remaining in the Naval Reserve and achieving the rank of Rear Admiral. He wrote his first paper on multiple sclerosis in 1953 [51] and is still publishing [52]. He is responsible for producing the industry-standard 'Kurtzke Scale' of disability in multiple sclerosis [53–55] and he organized the first placebo-controlled clinical trial (of isoniazid) in multiple sclerosis [56]. However, his principal contribution has been the careful documentation and analysis of the varying prevalence of multiple sclerosis around the world and especially within the cohorts of American military personnel. Characteristic of his papers are distrust of complex statistics and meticulously presented hand-drawn charts.

Methods

In this paper, which is part review and partly based on original data, Kurtzke lays out the big picture of multiple sclerosis epidemiology (Fig. 16.4). He points out that the assertion of the day, that latitude determined multiple sclerosis prevalence, is incorrect. In Asia and the Pacific, latitude seemed not a factor at all and 'at 40° north, for example, MS is high in America, medium in Europe, and low in Asia'. In Europe and North America, there are zones of high frequency of multiple sclerosis between 65° and 45° north latitude. Neighbouring these (in Europe to the north, east, and south; in southern America; and the remainder of Australia) are zones of medium frequency; everywhere else is of low frequency.

Results

Measured serially in the same small region, Kurtzke asserts that the prevalence of multiple sclerosis appears stable over time, although our experience in East Anglia, UK, for example, is different [57]. One area stands out as having a high prevalence of multiple sclerosis (the Fennoscandian focus):

> . . . from the waist and southeastern mountain plains of Norway eastward across the inland lake area of southern Sweden, then across the Bay of Bothnia to southwestern Finland, and then back to Sweden in the region of Umea . . . This clustering, as well as the broader geographic distributions already considered, mean to me that the occurrence of MS is intrinsically related to geography, and therefore that MS is an acquired, exogenous, environmental disease.

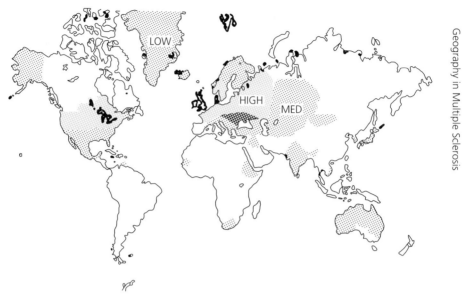

Fig. 16.4 John Kurtzke's map of multiple sclerosis prevalence.
Reproduced from *J Neurology*, 215, JF Kurtzke, Geography in multiple sclerosis, p. 1–26, Copyright (1977), with permission from Springer.

To determine when this disease might be acquired, Kurtzke turned to the migration studies, both his own and those of others. By comparing the age at which migration alters the risk of acquiring multiple sclerosis, he concluded that the key exposure occurs between the ages of 10 and 15 years, and that there is an 'incubation' period of some 20 years before the disease manifests. He then presents new data on the risk of multiple sclerosis in veterans by race and gender, showing that it is greatest in white women. Kurtzke argues that if multiple sclerosis is due to an infectious agent, rather than a toxin, transmissibility should be evident. This is why he is so keen to discuss possible 'epidemics' of multiple sclerosis.

Conclusions

'MS is the white man's burden spread from western Europe.'

Critique

In 1977, Kurtzke had just returned from a second visit to the Faroe Islands, where there seemed to be a cluster of new cases of multiple sclerosis following the stationing of British troops. He was to visit the Faroes many more times, and has just recently advanced the idea that gastrointestinal infections mediated the transmission between British troops and Faroese [58].

Kurtzke's interpretation of the Faroese epidemic of multiple sclerosis has been the most controversial aspect of his work, with other commentators suggesting more prosaic explanations, for instance, increased diagnostic vigilance resulting from improved medical services [59, 60]. However, that should not detract from the enormous service John Kutzke has made in marshalling the huge and complex multiple sclerosis epidemiological dataset into digestible synopses, of which this paper is a prime example.

16.8 **Immunotherapy of multiple sclerosis**

Main paper: Jacobs L, O'Malley J, Freeman A, Ekes R. Intrathecal interferon reduces exacerbations of multiple sclerosis. *Science* 1981; 214:1026–8.

Background

> There is evidence that multiple sclerosis is caused (at least partially) by a viral infection of the central nervous system that acts as a 'trigger' for repeated exacerbations of neurologic symptoms characteristic of the disease. Interferon is a naturally occurring biologic product with potent antiviral activities. It does not cross the blood-brain barrier in significant quantity when administered systemically, but can be safely administered intrathecally.

So opens Larry Jacobs' landmark paper on the use of interferon as a treatment of multiple sclerosis.

This was not the first study of interferons in multiple sclerosis; although not acknowledged in the paper, Verveken had used interferon-beta i.m. in three patients with 'chronic progressive multiple sclerosis' [61] and Fog tested interferon-alpha s.c. in six patients with a similar disease type [62]. No benefit was seen in either of these studies.

The 'interferons' had been identified in 1957 [63] as products that interfere with viruses. Human interferon could be made, with difficulty, in the laboratory, by 'superinduction' of human fibroblasts, and purified by affinity chromatography, to generate a 'natural' interferon, so-called to distinguish it from the subsequent recombinant interferons. One such laboratory was the Roswell Park Memorial Institute (now Roswell Park Cancer Institute) in Buffalo, New York. From this unit came the first evidence, in 1979, that interferons can ameliorate chronic active hepatitis and kill tumour cells *in vitro* [64, 65]. At around that time, Larry Jacobs arrived as a young neurologist in Buffalo, from his residency at Mount Sinai, to work at the Dent Neurologic Institute. With colleagues, he initially contemplated using interferon from the Roswell Park Memorial Institute to treat amyotrophic lateral sclerosis, but their attention soon turned to multiple sclerosis.

Methods

Verveken suggested that interferon failed because it does not cross the blood–brain barrier, and suggested that administration should be intrathecal. Larry Jacobs took up this suggestion, no doubt aware that a group at Roswell Park were using intrathecal interferon to treat meningeal leukaemia [66]. His study group consisted of 20 patients, four with relapsing-remitting disease, four with relapsing-progressive disease, and 12 who were 'stable with residua'. Ten received natural interferon-beta by lumbar puncture, twice a week for four weeks, then monthly for five months; 10 patients were used as unblinded controls. Patients were followed up for over a year.

Results

At the end of the study, two of the interferon-treated patients had experienced four relapses, compared to 10 relapses from six controls—a hint that the relapse rate in multiple sclerosis might be modified.

Conclusions

For the first time, an intervention (intrathecal interferon-beta) was shown to suppress disease activity in multiple sclerosis.

Critique

There are many problems with this paper. Its premise, that viral infections are the remedial cause of multiple sclerosis, is probably incorrect; its analysis is flawed; and, rightly, it met with considerable controversy, for instance from Charles Berry from University of California San Francisco [67]. There are simple arithmetical errors in the tables and the primary outcome is not statistically significant, as was erroneously claimed. Jacobs' reliance on a change in relapse rate before and after treatment is potentially distorted by regression to the mean. Not easily understood by modern readers, there is no explanation for the death of one patient receiving interferon in the first month of the study, other than to say it was unrelated to treatment.

However, the data were encouraging and more studies, led by Jacobs, followed. He went on to produce a much more rigorous trial, including placebo-injection lumbar punctures, in 69 patients with relapsing-remitting disease [68] and did show a definite effect. However, a few years later, a trial of natural interferon-beta had to be stopped early because it exacerbated rather than ameliorated multiple sclerosis disease activity [69]. There was a sense of growing concern over the need for intrathecal injections and the biological variability of human-derived interferon. Thereafter, interferons derived from recombinant technology were given systemically. Still there were problems. Recombinant interferon-alpha was shown to have no efficacy in 1986 [70] and recombinant interferon-gamma (Immuneron, Biogen) provoked relapses [71].

Larry Jacobs was undeterred. He set up the Multiple Sclerosis Collaborative Research Group to test Biogen's recombinant interferon-beta 1a. He designed a large trial, with some innovative features, which eventually led to a product licence for Avonex in 1996 in the USA and in the EU from 1997. However, he was pipped to the post by Ken Johnson, another key figure in the interferon story. With Berlex laboratories, Johnson had managed to get another recombinant, interferon-beta 1b (Betaseron), licensed in 1993 [72, 73].

In 1998, Larry Jacobs became the first holder of the Irvin and Rosemary Smith Chair in Neurology at Buffalo School of Medicine and Biomedical Sciences, which had been established through a $1.5 million endowment by Biogen. He died in 2001, aged 63.

The introduction of the interferons as disease-modifying treatments of multiple sclerosis brought many benefits to people affected by the disease, other than a modest reduction in disease activity and an uncertain effect on its long-term course; not the least the attention of the pharmaceutical companies to the potential marketplace for novel therapies, and the requirement for an infrastructure of neurological and nursing support, improved the generic care of people affected by multiple sclerosis.

16.9 **Diagnostic criteria**

Main paper: Poser CM, Paty DW, Scheinberg L, et al. New diagnostic criteria for multiple sclerosis: guidelines for research protocols. *Ann Neurol* 1983; 13(3):227–31.

Background

The first attempt at systematic criteria for the diagnosis of multiple sclerosis came from Allison and Millar (1954) who classified the disease as *early* (few physical signs but a recent history of remitting symptoms); *probable* (soon changed to early probable or latent: no reasonable doubt about the diagnosis); *possible* (findings suggesting the diagnosis and no other cause found but the history static or progressive and with insufficient evidence for scattered lesions); and *discarded* [74, 75].

However, then as now, neurologists have not felt the need to be constrained by criteria when making the diagnosis of multiple sclerosis. As Charles Poser wrote in 1965:

> . . . many clinicians thus insist that there is, in arriving at any diagnosis, and certainly in diagnosing MS, an intangible, unpredictable, highly personal and almost mystic diagnostic item frequently referred to as the 'feel' or the 'smell' of the patient, and which can best be characterized by the almost classical, pontifical pronouncement: 'Don't ask me why I think that this patient has MS, I just know!' [76]

Poser was not impressed. In his huge multiple sclerosis practice, he frequently encountered misdiagnosis, against which he battled all his life. He died in November 2010, at the age of 86. After escaping Nazi-occupied Belgium with his family, he grew up in New York City and attended George Washington High School and City College. After returning from Army service in World War II, he trained at the New York Neurological Institute under Dr H. Houston Merrit.

Methods

Poser's motivation to introduce diagnostic criteria for multiple sclerosis was to improve research, in particular the quality of epidemiological studies. He set out his stall in a classic paper in 1965 [76]. He asked 190 neurologists in 53 countries to read 30 case records and decide if they had 'probable', 'possible', or 'unlikely' multiple sclerosis. In fact, the cases had all come to post-mortem and included 25 with pathologically proven multiple sclerosis, three cases with other conditions mimicking multiple sclerosis, and in two in whom multiple sclerosis coexisted with another condition.

Results

Of the 108 doctors who replied (including only two from England—Dr Donald Acheson from Oxford and Dr Hugh Garland from Leeds), there was consistent two thirds diagnostic accuracy across the board, regardless of geography and experience (except that Swedes, and those trained in Sweden, were less confident in making a diagnosis of 'probable' multiple sclerosis). Somewhat embarrassingly, people regarded as multiple sclerosis experts performed rather worse than general neurologists. However, between individual diagnosticians, there was a great deal of variety. So, Poser analysed symptoms and signs that neurologists find helpful in making the diagnosis of multiple sclerosis, both in negative and positive terms.

Conclusions

From this exercise, Poser derived a rather complex scoring system to refine the clinician's suspicion of multiple sclerosis. Immediately, he recognized that his algorithm could be fooled by conditions such as brainstem glioma mimicking multiple sclerosis, so he mandated at least two years since the onset of symptoms before the diagnosis of multiple sclerosis could be made.

Critique

Ultimately, Poser's scoring system was too complex and it never took off. In the USA, neurologists continued to use the Schumacher 1965 criteria; however, this focused just on the 'probable' group and did not incorporate the growing literature on paraclinical tests or imaging [22]. In the UK, the McDonald and Halliday (1977) criteria gained favour, as they recognized the value of, for instance, evoked potentials [35].

Poser was not satisfied, so he set out, in 1982, to come up with comprehensive diagnostic criteria for research:

> The main reason for establishing these criteria is to restrict therapeutic trials and other research protocols to patients with definite MS; the category of probable is designed for the purpose of prospectively evaluating new diagnostic methods.

So, Poser gathered, at Washington, the luminaries of multiple sclerosis, including George Ebers, Ian MacDonald, and Donald Paty. They proposed four categories of multiple sclerosis: 'clinically definite, laboratory-supported definite, clinically probable and laboratory-supported probable'. At last, 'paraclinical' evidence of a lesion could be substituted for clinical evidence; for instance, typical abnormalities on computed tomography (CT) or nuclear magnetic resonance (NMR) imaging, evoked potentials, and induced hyperthermia (the 'hot bath test'). Thus, *laboratory-supported definite* multiple sclerosis could be diagnosed after one attack only, with paraclinical evidence of a subsequent new lesion affected (for instance, an evoked potential that becomes abnormal) *and* oligoclonal bands. *Clinically probable* required two attacks with clinical evidence of one lesion, or one attack and clinical or paraclinical evidence of two separate lesions, separated in time. *Laboratory-supported probable* required two attacks and the presence of oligoclonal bands.

Poser's criteria lasted nearly two decades until replaced by the 2001 McDonald criteria, which were themselves modified in 2005 and, most recently, in 2010 [36, 77, 78]. Much of Poser's thinking remains, but he did not agree with the elevation in importance of magnetic resonance imaging (MRI):

> One of the big problems I see now is the numbers of patients who have minimal symptoms, and maybe some abnormal MRI findings, who have been treated for MS for years and who have never had it. I see people like this every week in my office [79].

Of critical importance for the writers of the new McDonald criteria is the ability to make the diagnosis of multiple sclerosis as early as possible, to allow the introduction of therapies. As a result, the absolute requirement for a second clinical (or paraclinical) attack has been dropped; instead, any new MRI disease activity after a clinically isolated syndrome now fulfils the criteria to diagnose multiple sclerosis. This process has reached its apotheosis under the 2010 criteria, where it is proposed that evidence of dissemination *in time* can be derived from a single MRI scan *during* a clinically isolated syndrome—if it shows the simultaneous presence of asymptomatic gadolinium-enhancing lesions and non-enhancing lesions at any time.

16.10 **Magnetic resonance imaging in multiple sclerosis**

Main paper: Miller DH, Rudge P, Johnson G, et al. Serial gadolinium enhanced magnetic resonance imaging in multiple sclerosis. *Brain* 1988; 111:927–39.

Background

In 1973, a paper appeared in *Nature*, having been previously rejected as of insufficient general interest by the editor, entitled 'Image formation by induced local interaction; examples employing magnetic resonance' [80]. The author was Paul Lauterbur, a chemist at the State University of New York at Stony Brook. Peter Mansfield, a physicist from Nottingham University, systematically solved the many problems of transforming this observation to a medical imaging system and produced, in 1976, the first 'nuclear magnetic resonance' image of a human part (a cross-section of the finger) [81]. Thus arrived the definitive method for studying human tissue structure and function in health and disease for which Lauterbur and Mansfield received the Nobel Prize for Physiology or Medicine in 2003.

MRI was first explored in multiple sclerosis through a collaboration between the Hammersmith Hospital in London and the Central Research Laboratories, Thorn-EMI Ltd in Hayes, Middlesex. Their *Lancet* report from 1981 exudes excitement at the vastly improved ability to visualize multiple sclerosis lesions compared to CT. The new technique 'demonstrates abnormalities in MS on a scale not previously seen except at necropsy although the specificity of these abnormalities is uncertain at present' [82]. Other investigators soon picked up on the technique, and early work confirmed and extended its role in supplementing clinical evidence for the diagnosis of multiple sclerosis.

Enthusiasm for the technique soon spread beyond the academic world. The first commercial MR scanner in Europe (from Picker Ltd.) was installed in 1983 at the University of Manchester Medical School. In the same year, the Multiple Sclerosis Society of Great Britain and Northern Ireland funded the first MRI scanner in the world to be solely dedicated to multiple sclerosis research, at the National Hospital for Neurology and Neurosurgery at Queen Square, London. Ian McDonald led the group and their early work emphasized the number of 'silent lesions' visible on MRI scans at presentation in multiple sclerosis and in clinically isolated syndromes [83].

The paper we have chosen comes from Ian McDonald's group. Its importance lies in the insights it gave to the natural history of multiple sclerosis, particularly to the realization that there is continued disease activity even during periods of clinical stability. The problem that David Miller and colleagues sought to solve was how to judge the age of an individual MRI lesion. They argued that distinguishing between new and old lesions would help in two contexts: first, in the assessment of the patient with a clinically isolated syndrome (where lesions of different age would suggest dissemination in time and, hence, the probability of multiple sclerosis); and, secondly, in therapeutic trials. They turned to the paramagnetic agent, gadolinium DTPA, which Donald Silberberg's group at the University of Pennsylvania had shown more frequently to demonstrate abnormalities in patients with clinical disease activity than unenhanced scans [84].

Methods

Ten patients with multiple sclerosis were scanned initially, eight of whom were experiencing a relapse at the time. Fifty-six contrast-enhancing lesions were observed in total, compared to none in the two non-relapsing patients. In six out of eight patients, an enhancing lesion was seen which was anatomically congruent with the relapse phenotype. A second scan was performed between three and five weeks later in nine of these patients. Of the previous 54 enhancing lesions, only 12 persisted, but 12 new lesions had appeared (including four previous lesions where enhancement extended into previously unaffected brain areas). Six months later, eight patients were rescanned and 15 new lesions seen on unenhanced scans, of which eight showed enhancement. In passing, the authors note that some enhancing lesions were seen in the cortex, and one enhancing spinal cord lesion is shown.

Results

For the first time, the dynamics of plaque formation could be studied and some of the controversies arising from static pathological studies resolved. The observation that enhancement was seen as the first abnormality in every new lesion which appeared on interval scans placed breakdown of the blood–brain barrier as an initiating event in the evolution of the plaque. David Miller and colleagues suggested that the elevated T1/T2 ratio of enhancing lesions reflected the increased intracellular water associated with acute inflammation; and the low T1/2 ratio of old non-enhancing lesions might reflect increased extracellular water from leakage of an incompletely repaired blood–brain barrier. Cortical plaques, which were known from pathological studies but had not been seen on unenhanced scans, could now be visualized with the use of gadolinium.

Conclusions and critique

MRI of the brain has become an invaluable technique for the diagnosis and management of people with multiple sclerosis, as well as into research of its pathogenesis and treatment. The paper we have selected is not the first study of multiple sclerosis using MRI but it is, in our view, the first MRI study to bring new understanding of the pathogenesis of multiple sclerosis.

For most contemporary readers, the big news was the revelation on the frequency of new lesions in people apparently with stable multiple sclerosis. This had several implications. For research, MRI provided a sensitive measure of brain inflammation. Don Paty, at the University of British Columbia in Vancouver, was the first to correlate active lesions with changes in peripheral immune function [85]. However, the most obvious conclusion was that gadolinium- enhancing lesions could be used to reduce the duration and cohort sizes of clinical trials.

The findings of this paper were soon ratified. Henry McFarland at the National Institutes of Health (Bethesda) produced a study of six patients with 'early, mild, relapsing-remitting multiple sclerosis', scanned monthly for 8–11 months, and showed that 'numerous enhancing lesions were observed irrespective of clinical activity'; and, again, he suggested that these lesions be used as an outcome measure in clinical trials [86].

Key unanswered questions

1 What causes multiple sclerosis?

Following the most recent study of the genetic susceptibility of multiple sclerosis [42], 110 risk variants have been identified at 103 discrete loci outside of the major histocompatibility complex, and many of relate to T-cell immunology. Yet, the authors estimate that these genes explain only 20% of the genetic risk for the disease. It is likely that more genes will be found, as technology improves and the size of DNA collections increase, but presumably the strength of the associations will be lower also. Beyond this discovery phase lies the task of making functional sense of the implicated pathways. This has only just begun, with some understanding of the role of IL7R [87] and TNFR [88] variants in causing multiple sclerosis.

Approaches to the study of environmental causes of multiple sclerosis currently lack the sophistication and power of genetic studies, and their discovery rate is low. Yet there is hope that such work might identify modifiable factors; for instance, the relationship between early sun exposure, vitamin D, and disease risk [89].

2 Is multiple sclerosis one disease or many?

The finding that a disease such as neuromyelitis optica, once considered a 'variant' of multiple sclerosis, has a distinct pathogenesis unrelated to multiple sclerosis [90], has encouraged some to consider multiple sclerosis as a heterogeneous disorder ripe for 'splitting'. An obvious candidate is primary progressive multiple sclerosis; but all attempts to find a distinct genetic basis of this rare form of multiple sclerosis have proved elusive. A study claiming that the pathology of multiple sclerosis is composed of four types [91] has provoked the debate, which remains unresolved as other investigators find lesion homogeneity [92].

The importance in determining heterogeneity lies in the implications for treatment, and the Mayo Clinic group have consolidated their position by showing that only people whose multiple sclerosis lesions follow the antibody-rich 'Type II' pattern respond to plasma exchange [93]. Initially, there was much excitement around the observation that treatment response to interferon-beta might be predicted by peripheral immunophenotype [94, 95]; but this has not been replicated by further work [96, 97].

3 What is the relationship between inflammation and neurodegeneration in multiple sclerosis?

That inflammation causes demyelination in multiple sclerosis is not seriously disputed, but there is genuine uncertainty about the relationship between these processes and the chronic loss of axons that occurs over time. Direct immune attack of axons is possible, as is axonal death secondary to the loss of trophic support of myelin [98], or the metabolic consequences of demyelination [99]. However, students of the natural history of multiple sclerosis speculate that neurodegeneration may be an autonomous process in the disease, uncoupled from inflammation, to account for the apparent lack of association between relapse frequency and the appearance of secondary progressive multiple sclerosis [15, 100]. These considerations lead to the next unanswered question.

4 What causes the progressive phase of multiple sclerosis?

Until recently, the consensus was clear: progressive multiple sclerosis reflected the slow death of axons, the radiological correlate of which was cerebral atrophy. The disappointing experience of treating progressive disease with powerful immunotherapies suggested that inflammation was irrelevant [101]. However, recently, several investigators have proposed that confinement of inflammation to the central nervous system drives progressive multiple sclerosis. This thinking started with the observation of lymphoid follicles in the meninges of people with progressive multiple sclerosis [102]. Hans Lassman has suggested that inflammation gets 'trapped' behind the blood–brain barrier and so is inaccessible to conventional immunotherapies which act only on the peripheral immune system [103]. All of which leads to the key unanswered question in multiple sclerosis.

5 Does early aggressive immunotherapy of multiple sclerosis prevent the secondary progressive phase of the disease?

The greatest burden of multiple sclerosis, by any measure, occurs among those with secondary progressive disease. Most people with relapsing-remitting multiple sclerosis would be prepared to consider high-risk therapies to prevent this. At present, the only therapies available to people with multiple sclerosis modulate the immune system. It follows that the relationship between inflammation and progressive disability is a clinically important issue. Those treatments for which we have long-term data (interferon-beta and glatirmaer) are only partially effective in suppressing inflammation and do not seem to have a long-term effect on disability [104]. More aggressive therapies are certainly better at slowing the accumulation of disability in the short term, over 2–5 years [105–107], but no formal trial has yet been sufficiently prolonged to examine whether they also reduce the numbers developing progressive disease. Although this is understandable, given the costs and difficulties of following patients over 20 years, it leaves the most critical question in multiple sclerosis unanswered.

References

1 **McDonald WI.** Chance and design. *J Neurol* 1999; **246**(8):654–60.

2 **Dejerine J.** Etude sur la sclérose en plaques cerebro-spinale. A forme de sclérose laterale amyotrophique. *Rev Med (Paris)* 1894; **iv**:193–212.

3 **Williamson RT.** The early pathological changes in disseminated sclerosis. *Med Chron (Manchester)* 1894; **19**:373–9.

4 **Williamson RT.** *Diseases of the Spinal Cord.* Oxford: Oxford University Press and Hodder & Stoughton; 1908.

5 **Marie P.** Sclérose en plaques et maladies infectieuses. *Progrès Med* 1884; **12**:287–9, 305–7, 349–51, 365–6.

6 **Bielschowsky M.** Zür Histologie der multiplen sklerose. *Neurolisches Zentralblatt* 1903; **22**:770–7.

7 **Strumpell A.** Zür pathologie den multiplen sklerose. *Neurolisches Zentralblatt* 1896; **15**:961–4.

8 **Bramwell B.** On the relative frequency of disseminated sclerosis in this country (Scotland and the North of England) and in America. *Rev Neurol Psych Edinb* 1903; **i**:12–7.

9 **Muller E.** Uber sensible Reizerscheinungen bei beginnender multipler sklerose. *Neurolisch Centralblatt* 1910; **29**:17–20.

10 **Charcot JM.** Histologie de la sclérose en plaques. *Gazette Hôpitaux* 1868; **41**:554–8.

11 **Redlich E.** Histologisches detail zur grauen degeneration von gehirn und rückenmark. *Neurolisches Zentralblatt* 1896; **15**:961–4.

12 **Huber O.** Zur patholïschen anatomie der multiplen sklerose der ruckenmarks. *Arch Pathol Anat* 1895; **140**: 396–410.

13 **Rindfleisch E.** Histologisches detail zur grauen degeneration von gehirn und rückenmark. *Arch Pathol Anat Physiol Klin Med (Virchow)* 1863; **26**:474–83.

14 **Marburg, Otto.** Die sogenannte akute multiple Sklerose (Encephalomyelitis periaxialis scleroticans). F. Deuticke, 1906.

15 **Confavreux C, Vukusic S.** Age at disability milestones in multiple sclerosis. *Brain* 2006; **129**(Pt 3):595–605.

16 **Barnett MH, Prineas JW.** Relapsing and remitting multiple sclerosis: pathology of the newly forming lesion. *Ann Neurol* 2004; **55**(4):458–68.

17 **Kabat EA, Moore DH, Landow H.** An electrophoretic study of the protein components in cerebrospinal fluid and their relationship to the serum proteins. *J Clin Invest* 1942; **21**(5):571–7.

18 **Smithies O.** Zone electrophoresis in starch gels: group variations in the serum proteins of normal human adults. *Biochem J* 1955; **61**(4):629–41.

19 **Link H.** Immunoglobulin G and low molecular weight proteins in human cerebrospinal fluid. Chemical and immunological characterisation with special reference to multiple sclerosis. *Acta Neurol Scand* 1967; **43**(Suppl 28):1–136.

20 **Link H.** Oligoclonal immunoglobulin G in multiple sclerosis brains. *J Neurol Sci* 1972; **16**(1):103–14.

21 **Cross AH, Wu GF.** Multiple sclerosis: oligoclonal bands still yield clues about multiple sclerosis. *Nat Rev Neurol* 2010; **6**(11):588–9.

22 **Schumacher GA, et al.** Problems of experimental trials of therapy in multiple sclerosis: report by the Panel on the Evaluation of Experimental Trials of Therapy in Multiple Sclerosis. *Ann NY Acad Sci* 1965; **122**:552–68.

23 **Milligan NM, Newcombe R, Compston DA.** A double-blind controlled trial of high dose methylprednisolone in patients with multiple sclerosis: 1. Clinical effects. *J Neurol Neurosurg Psychiatry* 1987; **50**(5):511–6.

24 **Beck RW, et al.** A randomized, controlled trial of corticosteroids in the treatment of acute optic neuritis. The Optic Neuritis Study Group. *N Engl J Med* 1992; **326**(9):581–8.

25 **Beck RW, et al.** The effect of corticosteroids for acute optic neuritis on the subsequent development of multiple sclerosis. The Optic Neuritis Study Group. *N Engl J Med* 1993; **329**(24): 1764–9.

26 **Optic Neuritis Study Group.** Visual function 15 years after optic neuritis: a final follow-up report from the Optic Neuritis Treatment Trial. *Ophthalmology* 2008; **115**(6):1079–82 e5.

27 **Keltner JL, et al.** Visual field profile of optic neuritis: a final follow-up report from the Optic Neuritis Treatment Trial from baseline through 15 years. *Arch Ophthalmol* 2010; **128**(3):330–7.

28 **Berger H.** Über das elektroenkephalogramm des menschen. *Archiv Psychiatrie Nervenkrankheiten* 1929; **87**:527–70.

29 **Adrian EDM, Matthews BHC.** The Berger rhythm: potential changes from the occipital lobes in man. *Brain* 1934; **57**:355–85.

30 **Dawson GD.** A summation technique for the detection of small evoked potentials. *Electroencephalogr Clin Neurophysiol* 1954; **6**(1):65–84.

31 **Halliday AM, Wakefield GS.** Cerebral evoked potentials in patients with dissociated sensory loss. *J Neurol Neurosurg Psychiatry* 1963; **26**: 211–9.

32 **McDonald WI, Sears TA.** Focal experimental demyelination in the central nervous system. *Brain* 1970; **93**(3):575–82.

33 **McDonald WI, SearsTA.** The effects of experimental demyelination on conduction in the central nervous system. *Brain* 1970; **93**(3):583–98.

34 **Halliday AM, McDonald WI, Mushin J.** Visual evoked response in diagnosis of multiple sclerosis. *BMJ* 1973; **4**(5893):661–4.

35 **McDonald WI, Halliday AM.** *Diagnosis and classification of multiple sclerosis. Br Med Bull* 1977; **33**(1):4–9.

36 **Polman CH, et al.** Diagnostic criteria for multiple sclerosis: 2010 revisions to the McDonald criteria. *Ann Neurol* 2011; **69**(2):292–302.

37 **Terasaki PI, McClelland JD.** Microdroplet assay of human serum cytotoxins. *Nature* 1964; **204**:998–1000.

38 **Naito S, et al.** Multiple sclerosis: association with HL-A3. *Tissue Antigens* 1972; **2**(1):1–4.

39 **Jersild C, Svejgaard A, Fog T.** HL-A antigens and multiple sclerosis. *Lancet* 1972; **1**(7762): 1240–1.

40 **Terasaki PI, et al.** Multiple sclerosis and high incidence of a B lymphocyte antigen. *Science* 1976; **193**(4259):1245–7.

41 **Compston DA, Batchelor JR, McDonald WI.** B-lymphocyte alloantigens associated with multiple sclerosis. *Lancet* 1976; **2**(7998):1261–5.

42 **Sawcer S, et al.** Genetic risk and a primary role for cell-mediated immune mechanisms in multiple sclerosis. *Nature* 2011; **476**(7359):214–9.

43 **Bunge MB, Bunge RP, Ris H.** Ultrastructural study of remyelination in an experimental lesion in adult cat spinal cord. *J Biophys Biochem Cytol* 1961; **10**:67–94.

44 **Perier O, Gregoire A.** Electron microscopic features of multiple sclerosis lesions. *Brain* 1965; **88**(5):937–52.

45 **Gledhill RF, Harrison BM, McDonald WI.** Pattern of remyelination in the CNS. *Nature* 1973; **244**(5416):443–4.

46 **Smith EJ, Blakemore WF, McDonald WI.** Central remyelination restores secure conduction. *Nature* 1979; **280**(5721):395–6.

47 **Smith KJ, McDonald WI.** Spontaneous and mechanically evoked activity due to central demyelinating lesion. *Nature* 1980; **286**(5769):154–5.

48 **Dean G, Elian M.** Age at immigration to England of Asian and Caribbean immigrants and the risk of developing multiple sclerosis. *J Neurol Neurosurg Psychiatry* 1997; **63**(5):565–8.

49 **Dean G, Kurtzke JF.** On the risk of multiple sclerosis according to age at immigration to South Africa. *BMJ* 1971; **3**(5777):725–9.

50 **Elian M, Nightingale S, Dean G.** Multiple sclerosis among United Kingdom-born children of immigrants from the Indian subcontinent, Africa and the West Indies. *J Neurol Neurosurg Psychiatry* 1990; **53**(10):906–11.

51 **Berlin L, Kurtzke JR, Guthrie TC.** Acute respiratory failure in multiple sclerosis and its management. *J Nerv Ment Dis* 1953; **117**(2):160–1.

52 **McLeod JG, Hammond SR, Kurtzke JF.** Migration and multiple sclerosis in immigrants to Australia from United Kingdom and Ireland: a reassessment. I. Risk of MS by age at immigration. *J Neurol* 2011; **258**(6):1140–9.

53 **Kurtzke JF.** A new scale for evaluating disability in multiple sclerosis. *Neurology* 1955; **5**(8):580–3.

54 **Kurtzke JF.** On the evaluation of disability in multiple sclerosis. *Neurology* 1961; **11**: 686–94.

55 **Kurtzke JF.** Rating neurologic impairment in multiple sclerosis: an expanded disability status scale (EDSS). *Neurology* 1983; **33**(11):1444–52.

56 **Berlin L, Kurtzke JF.** Isoniazid in treatment of multiple sclerosis. *JAMA* 1957; **163**(3):172–4.

57 **Robertson N, et al.** Multiple sclerosis in south Cambridgeshire: incidence and prevalence based on a district register. *J Epidemiol Community Health* 1996; **50**(3):274–9.

58 **Wallin MT, Heltberg A, Kurtzke JF.** Multiple sclerosis in the Faroe Islands. 8. Notifiable diseases. *Acta Neurol Scand* 2010; **122**(2):102–9.

59 **Poser CM, Hibberd PL.** Analysis of the 'epidemic' of multiple sclerosis in the Faroe Islands. II. Biostatistical aspects. *Neuroepidemiology* 1988; **7**(4):181–9.

60 **Poser CM, et al.** Analysis of the 'epidemic' of multiple sclerosis in the Faroe Islands. I. Clinical and epidemiological aspects. *Neuroepidemiology* 1988; **7**(4):168–80.

61 **Ververken DCH, Billiau, A.** Intrathecal administration of interferon in MS patients. In: Karcher D, Strosberg AD, (ed). *Humoral Immunology in Neurological Disease*. New York: Plenum; 1979; 625–7.

62 **Fog T.** Interferon treatment of multiple sclerosis patients: a pilot study. In: Boese A, (ed). *Search for the Cause of Multiple Sclerosis and Other Chronic Diseases of the Nervous System*.Weinheim: Verlag Chemie; 1980; 491–3.

63 **Isaacs A, Lindenmann J.** Virus interference. I. The interferon. Proc R Soc Lond B Biol Sci. 1957 Sep 12; **147**(927):258–67.

64 **Dolen JG, et al.** *Fibroblast interferon treatment of a patient with chronic active hepatitis. Increased number of circulating T lymphocytes and elimination of rosette-inhibitory factor. Am J Med* 1979; **67**(1):127–31.

65 **Horoszewicz JS, Leong SS, Carter WA.** Noncycling tumor cells are sensitive targets for the antiproliferative activity of human interferon. *Science* 1979; **206**(4422):1091–3.

66 **Misset JL, Mathe G, Horoszewicz JS.** Intrathecal interferon in meningeal leukemia. *N Engl J Med* 1981; **304**(25):1544.

67 **Berry CC.** Intrathecal interferon for multiple sclerosis. *Science* 1982; **217**(4556):269–70.

68 **Jacobs L, et al.** Multicentre double-blind study of effect of intrathecally administered natural human fibroblast interferon on exacerbations of multiple sclerosis. *Lancet* 1986; **2**(8521–2):1411–3.

69 **Milanese C, et al.** Double blind study of intrathecal beta-interferon in multiple sclerosis: clinical and laboratory results. *J Neurol Neurosurg Psychiatry* 1990; **53**(7):554–7.

70 **Camenga DL, et al.** Systemic recombinant alpha-2 interferon therapy in relapsing multiple sclerosis. *Arch Neurol* 1986; **43**(12):1239–46.

71 **Panitch HS, et al.** Exacerbations of multiple sclerosis in patients treated with gamma interferon. *Lancet* 1987; **1**(8538):893–5.

72 **Paty DW, Li DK.** Interferon beta-1b is effective in relapsing-remitting multiple sclerosis. II. MRI analysis results of a multicenter, randomized, double-blind, placebo-controlled trial. UBC MS/MRI Study Group and the IFNB Multiple Sclerosis Study Group. *Neurology* 1993; **43**(4):662–7.

73 **The IFNB Multiple Sclerosis Study Group.** Interferon beta-1b is effective in relapsing-remitting multiple sclerosis. I. Clinical results of a multicenter, randomized, double-blind, placebo-controlled trial. The IFNB Multiple Sclerosis Study Group. *Neurology* 1993; **43**(4):655–61.

74 **Allison RS, Millar JH.** Prevalence of disseminated sclerosis in Northern Ireland. *Ulster Med J* 1954; **23**(Suppl. 2):1–27.

75 **Millar JH, Allison RS.** Familial incidence of disseminated sclerosis in Northern Ireland. *Ulster Med J* 1954; **23**(Suppl. 2):29–92.

76 **Poser CM.** Clinical diagnostic criteria in epidemiological studies of multiple sclerosis. *Ann NY Acad Sci* 1965; **122**:506–19.

77 **McDonald W, et al.** Recommended diagnostic criteria for multiple sclerosis: guidelines from the international panel on the diagnosis of multiple sclerosis. *Ann Neurol* 2001; **50**(1):121–7.

78 **Polman CH, et al.** Diagnostic criteria for multiple sclerosis: 2005 revisions to the 'McDonald Criteria'. *Ann Neurol* 2005; **58**(6):840–6.

79 **Poser CM.** Revisions to the 2001 McDonald diagnostic criteria. *Ann Neurol* 2006; **59**(4):727–8.

80 **Lauterbur PC.** Image formation by induced local interactions: examples employing nuclear magnetic resonance. *Nature* 1973; **242**:190–1.

81 **Mansfield P, Maudsley AA.** Line scan proton spin imaging in biological structures by NMR. *Phys Med Biol* 1976; **21**(5):847–52.

82 **Young IR, et al.** Nuclear magnetic resonance imaging of the brain in multiple sclerosis. *Lancet* 1981; **2**(8255):1063–6.

83 **Ormerod IE, et al.** The role of NMR imaging in the assessment of multiple sclerosis and isolated neurological lesions. A quantitative study. *Brain* 1987; **110** (Pt 6):1579–616.

84 **Gonzalez-Scarano F, et al.** Multiple sclerosis disease activity correlates with gadolinium-enhanced magnetic resonance imaging. *Ann Neurol* 1987; **21**(3):300–6.

85 **Oger J, et al.** Changes in immune function in relapsing multiple sclerosis correlate with disease activity as assessed by magnetic resonance imaging. *Ann NY Acad Sci* 1988; **540**:597–601.

86 **Harris JO, et al.** Serial gadolinium-enhanced magnetic resonance imaging scans in patients with early, relapsing-remitting multiple sclerosis: implications for clinical trials and natural history. *Ann Neurol* 1991; **29**(5):548–55.

87 **Gregory SG, et al.** Interleukin 7 receptor alpha chain (IL7R) shows allelic and functional association with multiple sclerosis. *Nat Genet* 2007; **39**(9):1083–91.

88 **Gregory AP, et al.** TNF receptor 1 genetic risk mirrors outcome of anti-TNF therapy in multiple sclerosis. *Nature* 2012; **488**(7412):508–11.

89 **McDowell TY, et al.** Sun exposure, vitamin D intake and progression to disability among veterans with progressive multiple sclerosis. *Neuroepidemiology* 2011; **37**(1):52–7.

90 **Lennon VA, et al.** IgG marker of optic-spinal multiple sclerosis binds to the aquaporin-4 water channel. *J Exp Med* 2005; **202**(4):473–7.

91 **Lucchinetti C, et al.** Heterogeneity of multiple sclerosis lesions: implications for the pathogenesis of demyelination. *Ann Neurol* 2000; **47**(6):707–17.

92 **Breij EC, et al.** Homogeneity of active demyelinating lesions in established multiple sclerosis. *Ann Neurol* 2008; **63**(1):16–25.

93 **Keegan M, et al.** Relation between humoral pathological changes in multiple sclerosis and response to therapeutic plasma exchange. *Lancet* 2005; **366**(9485):579–82.

94 **Axtell RC, et al.** T helper type 1 and 17 cells determine efficacy of interferon-beta in multiple sclerosis and experimental encephalomyelitis. *Nat Med* 2010; **16**(4):406–12.

95 **Lee LF, et al.** IL-7 promotes T(H)1 development and serum IL-7 predicts clinical response to interferon-beta in multiple sclerosis. *Sci Transl Med* 2011; **3**(93):93ra68.

96 **Hartung HP, et al.** Interleukin 17F level and interferon beta response in patients with multiple sclerosis. *JAMA Neurol* 2013; **70**(8): 1017–21.

97 **Bushnell SE, et al.** Serum IL-17F does not predict poor response to IM IFNbeta-1a in relapsing-remitting MS. *Neurology* 2012; **79**(6):531–7.

98 **Lappe-Siefke C, et al.** Disruption of Cnp1 uncouples oligodendroglial functions in axonal support and myelination. *Nat Genet* 2003; **33**(3):366–74.

99 **Bechtold DA, Smith KJ.** Sodium-mediated axonal degeneration in inflammatory demyelinating disease. *J Neurol Sci* 2005; **233**(1–2):27–35.

100 **Confavreux C, et al.** Relapses and progression of disability in multiple sclerosis. *N Engl J Med* 2000; **343**(20):1430–8.

101 **Coles AJ, et al.** The window of therapeutic opportunity in multiple sclerosis: evidence from monoclonal antibody therapy. *J Neurol* 2006; **253**(1):98–108.

102 **Magliozzi R, et al.** Meningeal B-cell follicles in secondary progressive multiple sclerosis associate with early onset of disease and severe cortical pathology. *Brain* 2007; **130**(Pt 4):1089–104.

103 **Lassmann H, van Horssen J, Mahad D.** Progressive multiple sclerosis: pathology and pathogenesis. *Nat Rev Neurol* 2012; **8**(11):647–56.

104 **Greenberg BM, et al.** Interferon beta use and disability prevention in relapsing-remitting multiple sclerosis. *JAMA Neurol* 2013; **70**(2):248–51.

105 **Coles AJ, et al.** Alemtuzumab more effective than interferon beta-1a at 5-year follow-up of CAMMS223 clinical trial. *Neurology* 2012; **78**(14):1069–78.

106 **Coles AJ, et al.** Alemtuzumab for patients with relapsing multiple sclerosis after disease-modifying therapy: a randomised controlled phase 3 trial. *Lancet* 2012; **380**(9856):1829–39.

107 **Polman CH, et al.** A randomized, placebo-controlled trial of natalizumab for relapsing multiple sclerosis. *N Engl J Med* 2006; **354**(9):899–910.

Index

Notes:
vs. indicates a differential diagnosis or comparison
The following abbreviations have been used:
    ALS - amyotrophic lateral sclerosis
    MRI - magnetic resonance imaging
    PET - positron emission tomography

Note: The letter 'f' and 't' following locators refers to figure and table.

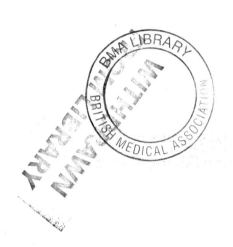